D1207133

A PREEMINENTLY HEALTHY PLACE

A History of Medicine in Travis County, Texas

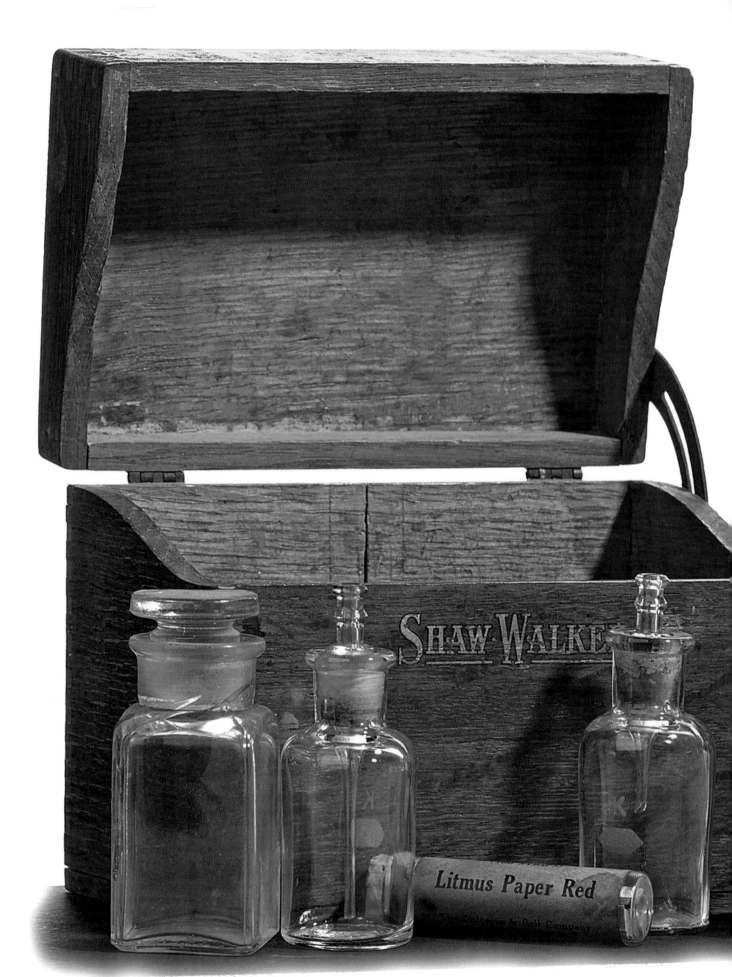

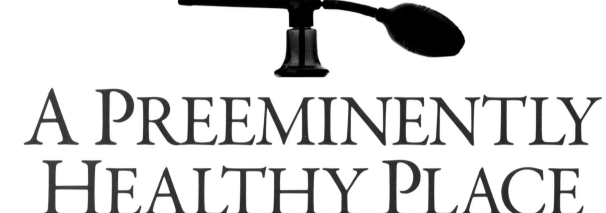

A PREEMINENTLY HEALTHY PLACE

A History of Medicine in Travis County, Texas

MARILYN BAKER

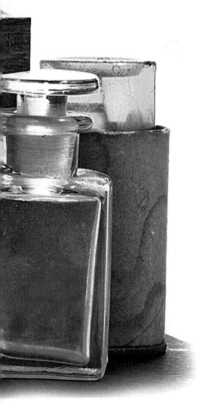

ASSOCIATION PUBLISHING COMPANY
Birmingham, Alabama

A PREEMINENTLY HEALTHY PLACE

Published By
ASSOCIATION PUBLISHING COMPANY
100 Oxmoor Road, Suite 110, Birmingham, Alabama 35209 • (205) 941-4623

JOHN COMPTON, *Publisher*

Published with the cooperation and assistance of
TRAVIS COUNTY MEDICAL SOCIETY
MARSHALL COTHRAN, CEO
BELINDA CLARE, COO

Written By
MARILYN BAKER

Profile Writers
LAURA DOYLE, ADRIENNE SOBOLAK DEWOLFE, ELISA ROBIN MALINOVITZ ELIASOPH,
KAREN STEEDE TERRY, BARBARA WRAY

Design By
ROBIN McDONALD

Editor
ALISON GLASCOCK

Photo Editor
DONNA COATES

Index
JIM SUMMERVILLE

Printed in the United States of America by
TAYLOR PUBLISHING COMPANY, DALLAS, TEXAS

FIRST EDITION

ISBN 978-0-9668380-7-7

Library of Congress Control Number: 2007939923

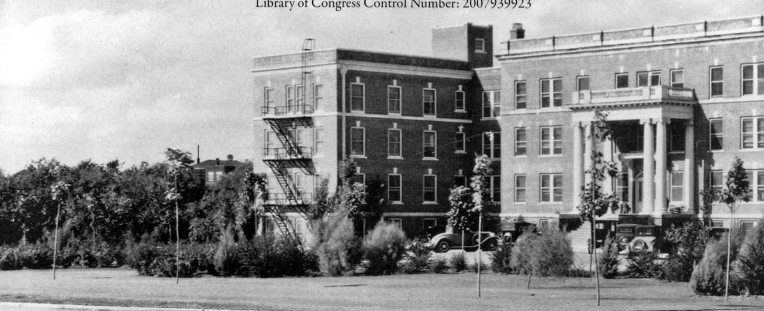

A PREEMINENTLY HEALTHY PLACE

TABLE OF CONTENTS

FOREWORD

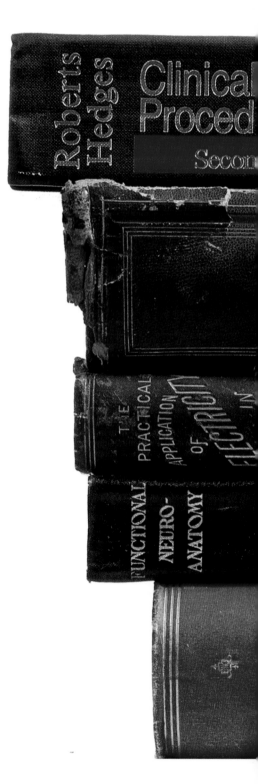

I T IS WITH GREAT PLEASURE THAT WE, as the Travis County Medical Society, present to you this history of the practice of medicine in Travis County. There have been a number of doctors who have written about segments of that history, but this is the first attempt to provide a more comprehensive view over 150 years of the progress of medicine in Austin and the surrounding communities. From the first doctor making rounds on horseback to our current Star Flight helicopter services, we are staggered by the changes. We look at the influence of the War Between The States, the Spanish American War, and World Wars I and II on the practice of medicine. We view the sweeping changes in infectious diseases, public health, and modern technology on Austin and our neighboring towns. And, of course, there are the firsts. The first doctors, the first hospitals, the first ambulances, the first nursing schools, EKGs, internships, residencies, kidney and heart transplants, joint replacements, and laparo-scopic procedures are all included. We hope you will enjoy the stories of the multiple contributions of the individuals and groups of physicians who have dedicated themselves to medicine, politics, teaching, public health, and to just living in Austin.

A written history is an interesting process. It requires the review of many manuscripts in print as well as gleaning from the memories of many people the facts that bring the continuum to life. It is subject to the accuracies of those sources. Our memories are fraught with strange variations. We don't remember even the most dramatic events in the same way. We are indebted to Dr. Kermit Fox, Dr. Maurice Hood, and Dr. Jim Prentice for reviewing this manuscript.

The idea for this project came from John Compton of Association Publishing in Birmingham, Alabama. We are grateful for his initiative. The support of the Travis County Medical Society was crucial to the project and consistent with the mission of the society to promote the health, well-being, and education of the membership.

Most of all we are thankful for the time, energy, and skill of Marilyn Baker in bringing all of this information together. Her background in writing, and specifically her interest in the history of medicine in Texas, has been invaluable in this project. In addition, we greatly appreciate Betsy Tyson's research and contributions.

It is my hope that this information will provide the perspective needed to see the amazing progress that has been made in our field and therefore the contribution that you, collectively and as individuals, have made to your neighbors' health. Thus, I would hope that it would bring you some joy as you view your unique position in history.

—Christopher S. "Kit" Chenault, M.D.

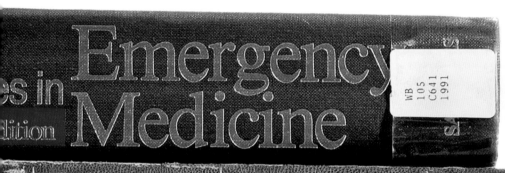
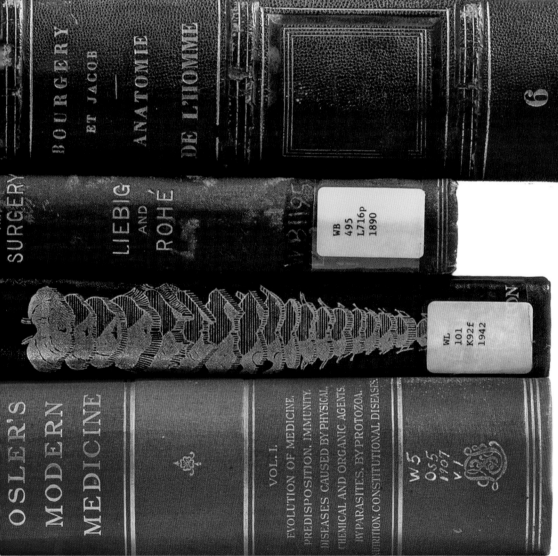

A selection of medical books of various periods from the collection of the Texas Medical Association, photographed by Jim Lincoln.

PREFACE

A YEAR AFTER THE GRID FOR THE CAPITAL of Texas was laid out in 1839, the Republic of Texas established Travis County, carving the territory from the governance of Bastrop County. Webber's Prairie, which would become Webberville, thus became a Travis County town. As the home of Dr. Thomas W. Anderson, the first physician known to practice in Travis County, Webberville developed a lively population and was an early center of medical activity. Physicians in the vicinity, including those arriving in the rustic town of Austin to its west, would become leaders in movements to build a medical infrastructure in the Lone Star State.

Physicians worked to establish Texas government, health and sanitary laws, the regulation of medicine, and tougher standards in medical education. They also set up and managed the earliest hospitals. After the capital area began to see more stability and security, Travis County doctors launched a private effort in 1853 to establish a state medical association. The result was the Texas Medical Association, which formed two district organizations—Travis Medical Society and Bexar Medical Society. Although after two meetings, the association failed to thrive for sixteen years—it was revived by physicians in Washington and Harris counties in 1869—the small group of Travis County doctors had achieved something no earlier group had accomplished.

This panoramic view of downtown Austin was taken around 1910. On the left is Congress Avenue, leading up to the imposing Texas State Capitol.

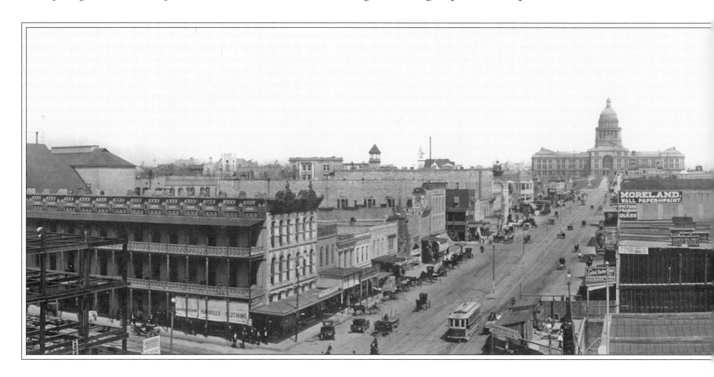

In Travis County today, signs on roads, creeks, buildings, and museums whisper of old tales of medical struggles. The site of Josiah Wilbarger's scalping, once in the westernmost wilderness of Stephen F. Austin's Little or Upper Colony, lies within the city limits of Austin at 51st Street and Manor Road. This man of Texas legend had been cared for by Dr. Anderson. The legacy of settlers in Hornsby Bend, Webberville, and Manor even today includes a distinguished medical cadre in Austin.

Writing or reporting history is a treacherous assignment, for the road to accuracy and truth is fraught with misleading and confusing forks and "facts." As memory grows dimmer, even an individual's own information sometimes contains conflicting data. Further, the language of the participants and the context in which they lived are different from that of the current reader. As historians say, venturing into historical research is like going to a foreign country. Words are spelled differently, used differently, and often have different meanings than modern readers assume. William Strunk, Jr., the writer of the classic book, *The Elements of Style*—known to many authors and editors simply as "Strunk and White"—once observed, "The language is perpetually in flux: it is a living stream, shifting, changing, receiving new strength from a thousand tributaries, losing old forms in the backwaters of time." And so it is that, when one reads the terminology of the earlier decades and centuries, the words may sound quaint and even incorrect. Likewise, medical understanding has changed vastly.

Even "contemporary" history has its own dangers. Students in many fields, including those in beginning journalism, learn that viewers of a single car accident can report widely varying stories. In *A Preeminently Healthy Place: A History of Medicine in Travis County, Texas*, efforts have been made to clarify as much fact as possible, but readers no doubt will have different perspectives or information not uncovered or not possible to include in this short history.

We hope nevertheless that the reader will have as fascinating a journey through the history of medicine in Travis County as we have had during our explorations.

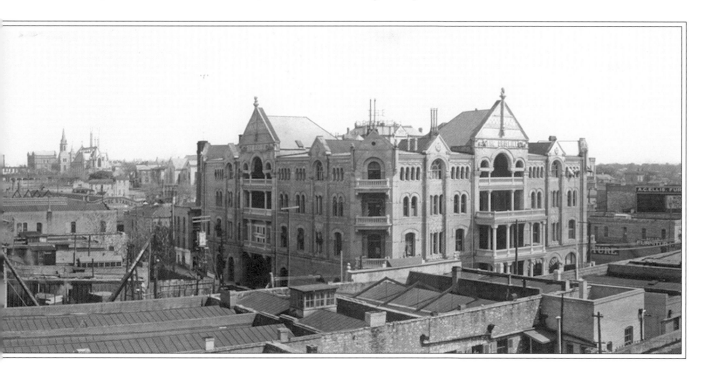

ACKNOWLEDGMENTS

WE ARE PARTICULARLY GRATEFUL to the reviewers of the manuscript, Drs. Christopher "Kit" Chenault, James A. Prentice, Kermit W. Fox, and R. Maurice Hood, and to Belinda Clare and everyone who patiently provided information and interviews. Our thanks go to Austin writer, Betsy Tyson, who contributed to this text through her extensive research and writing. Of inherent value were the historical holdings of the Texas Medical Association, including journals, transactions, and archival files the Travis County Medical Society's journals and historical files. Great appreciation goes to Claire Duncan and her staff of the TMA Knowledge Center, Sarita Oertling of the Truman G. Blocker, Jr., History of Medicine Collection, Moody Medical Library, the University of Texas Medical Branch, Galveston; library specialists at the Pflugerville Community Library, the Austin History Center, and the Austin Public Library. Special thanks also go to physician and historian Dr. Chester R. Burns, professor at the Institute of Medical Humanities, UTMB, whose meticulous published research was invaluable and led to special findings regarding the early history of Travis County Medical Society, and to Shari Henson, Texas Medical Association, for her assistance. Further, significant aid was provided via the Internet and the digital publications of numerous organizations, among which were the John P. McGovern Historical Collections and Research Center, Houston Academy of Medicine-Texas Medical Center Library, Houston, and the Texas Physicians Historical Database, Southwestern Medical Center Library, Dallas. Other materials also placed on the Internet were of significant help, such as the University of North Texas Libraries which digitized Gammel's *The Laws of Texas*, and the online and written publications of the Texas State Historical Association, including the *Handbook of Texas* and the *Southwestern Historical Quarterly*. Finally, of particular value also were the insight and guidance of Marshall Cothran, chief executive officer, and Belinda Clare, chief operating officer, Travis County Medical Society, in developing the project.

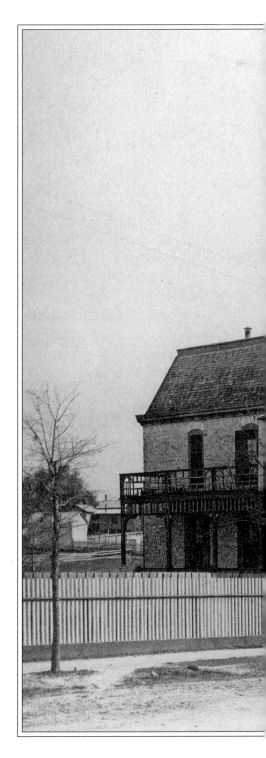

Austin's first public hospital was described as an elegant mansion with red shutters on a street lined with live oak trees and rising "imposingly above its neighbors." The newspaper report noted that it was designed "in the admired Queen Anne style, its gables and turrets" providing a "Victorian flourish worthy" of local leaders' ambitions.

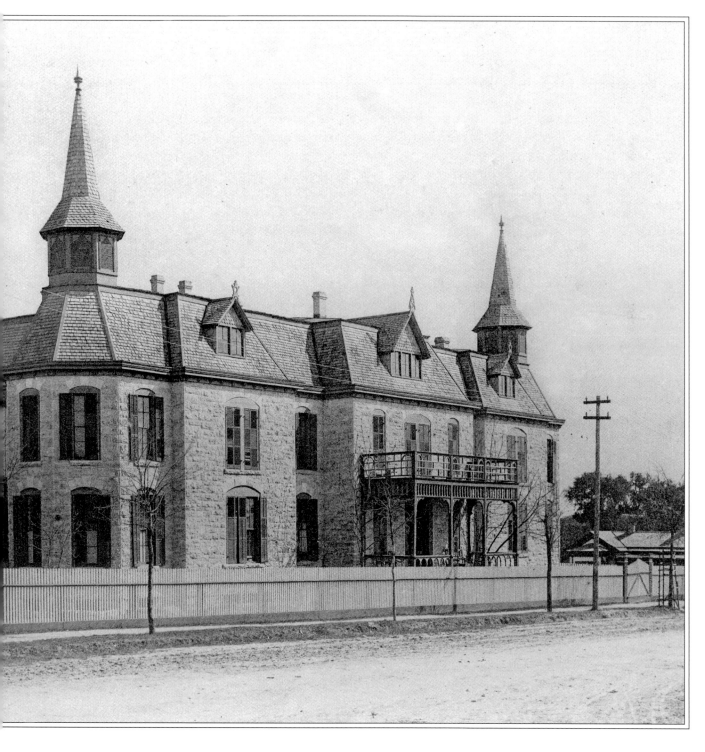

CHAPTER I

TRAVIS COUNTY BY HORSEBACK

D R. THOMAS W. ANDERSON'S arrival in the spring of 1835 was too good to be true. With their only physician absorbed in talks on the Texas Revolution, the plucky settlers around Bastrop sorely needed another doctor. The welcome mat and the rolling hills along the clear Colorado appealed to the Virginia widower with two teenage boys and among those urging him to stay was the hospitable Reuben Hornsby family.

An urgent summons soon drew him to Wilbarger Fort where the owner and former teacher, Josiah Wilbarger, had a poignant tale to tell. Two years earlier, he and four other surveyors had left the Hornsby home to find locations for new land grants, known as headrights, for Stephen F. Austin's upper settlement known as Little Colony. Near the Pecan Springs branch of Walnut Creek, the Comanches ambushed them, killing two of the surveyors. Two escaped, but arrows struck Wilbarger's legs and hip and a musket ball penetrated his neck, exiting the left side of his chin. He was still conscious when the Indians "stripped him naked and tore the scalp from his head," writes Frank Brown in his Travis County annals. After they left him for dead, he dragged his body to a pool, soaking in the water until he was chilled and numb before crawling back to land where he found snails to eat and then slept. Meanwhile, Sarah Hornsby awoke from a startling dream to rouse her husband Reuben whose rescue party found the man of future Texas legend, "a ghastly sight," propped up by a tree. His head wound was covered with a sock he'd pulled from a swollen foot, the only clothing left on him.

Resourcefulness and faith saved Wilbarger, but his pain remained. Molly McDowall writes that he underwent "trepanation," or trephination, in New Orleans but to no avail. The wound never healed completely and the bone under it was infected. Fortunately, Dr. Anderson was able to give relief not previously experienced. Austin pediatrician and historian Dr. James M. Coleman concluded, "It is probable that he curetted out some of the necrotic bone and freshened the edges of the wound."

Dr. Anderson thus brought his modern medical skills to the Wilbargers, Hornsbys, and other settlers above the town of Bastrop (transiently called Mina). Wearing a covering over the small mid-scalp area that never grew back, Josiah Wilbarger lived eleven more years until he struck his head on the low door frame to his gin house. He suffered from exfoliation of the bone, skull exposure, and meningitis. Credited with keeping him alive for so long, Dr. Anderson assessed the cause of death.

Practicing medicine on the western edge of Austin's colonies was foolhardy when Dr. Anderson arrived. Besides sometimes hostile tribes, Mexico's General Antonio López de Santa Anna was on the march from San Antonio. The doctor's sons had signed up to fight for Texas independence and Dr. Anderson also joined the Texas army, remaining to treat the ill and wounded at the Battle of San Jacinto, where son Washington was wounded. For his service, Dr. Anderson received a certificate for land at Webber's Prairie, later Webberville, and continued his medical practice there. Nearby, the Tonkawa, Comanche, and Lipan Apache tribes practiced their own healing arts, adapted from trial

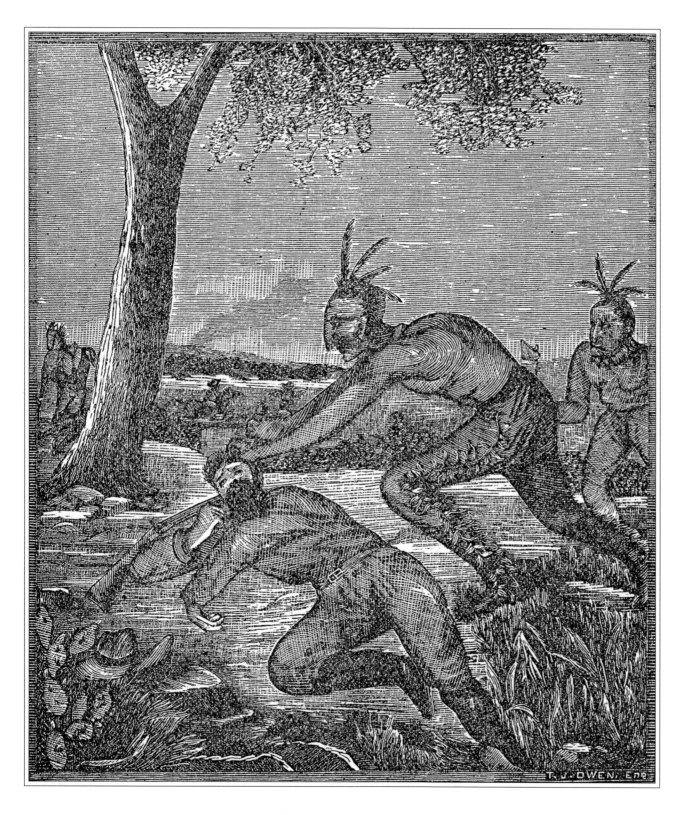

"Scalping of Josiah Wilbarger" from Indian Depredations in Texas *by J. W. Wilbarger, 1890.*

and error. In earlier years, the Spaniards devoted great effort to halting the spread of smallpox by transporting prepared cowpox virus, live and dried, to their colonists for use as a vaccine.

Dr. Anderson had come to Texas with his red morocco medical case and a set of lancets and instruments with tor-toiseshell handles. His "office existed wherever his horse stopped," Dr. Coleman writes. ". . . he would give quinine in horrid bitter powders. If the pulse was fast he would bleed

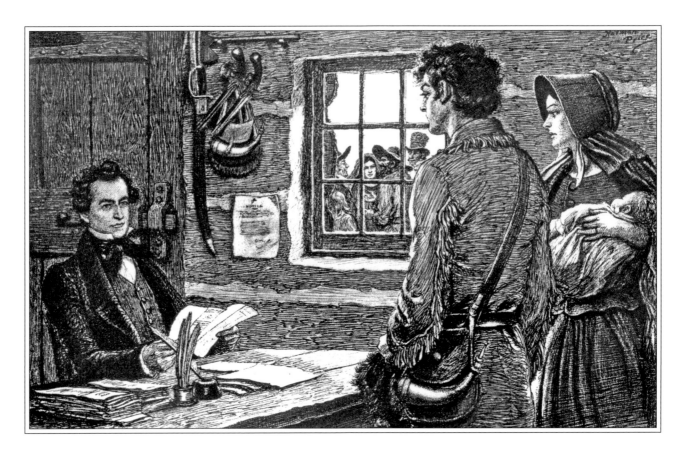

the patient by incising a vein in the arm without benefit of anesthetic." He used a surgical rake to scarify inflamed tonsils, mustard for plasters, and eggs for poultices. He studied the pulse, observed the tongue, sponged and sweated patients, and extracted teeth. ". . . he thumped the chest and listened with his ear against it for the sounds of the heart and the breathing." Working under the Mexican fee system followed in Austin's colonies, he was the only physician practicing west of Bastrop until Dr. J. W. Robertson arrived.

The doctor involved with pre-revolutionary matters when Dr. Anderson first arrived in Bastrop was Dr. Thomas Jefferson Gazley, one of seven physicians signing the Texas Declaration of Independence from Mexico.

Stephen F. Austin had done much to assure good health in his Mexican colonies, having drawn up an 1823 constitution for the Republic of Mexico that included the power to adopt public health measures. His colonists thus wrote regulations for institutions, public places, pond drainage, vital statistics, apothecaries, and physicians. In 1830, vaccination of children became compulsory and a board of medical examiners was set up.

A few months after Texas gained independence, the forty-three-year-old impresario, weakened by overwork, imprisonment in Mexico, and malaria, developed a severe cold. Dr. Branch T. Archer monitored his condition and administered opium. When he worsened, two other physicians, including French physician Dr. Theodore Léger, were consulted. Initially disagreeing on treatment, they concurred on emetics. They administered ipecac, which did not work, and then tartar emetic followed by a blister to his breast. On December 27, 1836, the Father of Texas died.

Doctors' limited armamentaria played into at least one ruse. Noah Smithwick explained how his friend John Ferdinand Webber—for whom Webberville would be named—acquired medical "credentials" during their return from a tobacco-smuggling trip to Mexico. In a Mexican town, they received advice from their host, John Villars, the only Anglo there, that one of the men should become a "doctor" to avert suspicion. Because Smithwick was too "boyish looking," Webber assumed the role. "With an air of importance that would have done credit to a professional, Webber noted the symptoms, shaking his head, knitting his brows, and otherwise impressing the patient with the seriousness of his condition," Smithwick recalled. The "doctor" carried with him, for the most part, calomel, quinine,

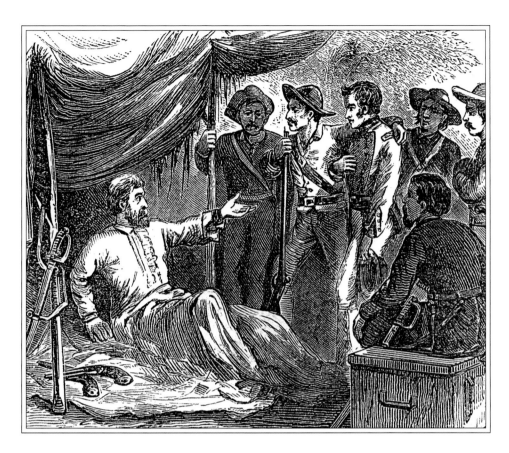

in the lower end of Webber's prairie, whither had preceded me my old time partner, 'Dr.' John F. Webber. He having retired from the practice of medicine, built the first house, a fort in the prairie, which bears his name. Other settlers collected around the pioneer cabin. . . ." Smithwick reported also that "Washington Anderson was there, and with him his father, Dr. Anderson, a noted physician all through the country."

In 1838, physicians striving to establish a scientific approach to medicine in Texas formed the Medical and Surgical Society of Houston opposing quackery and attempting to educate members. They also developed a fee schedule and offered to review disputed fees. Although newspapers remained the primary source of medical information, Dr. Léger published the first medical text in 1838, a pamphlet entitled *"Essay on the Particular Influence of Prejudices in Medicine, Over the treatment of the Disease Most Common in Texas, Intermittent Fever."* He denounced charlatans, hypocrites, and quacks, the "Texian Medicasters, the phrenetic enthusiasm of calomel-givers in Texas," and the hurry to administer purgatives, vomitives, bleeding, and cupping, and to use all the resources of their "pharma-ceutick arsenal." Dr. Léger retired from medicine and became the owner and editor of the *Texas Planter* at Brazoria.

Like Stephen F. Austin, who had longed for a sanctuary in the hill country, Republic of Texas President Mirabeau B. Lamar admired the juncture of the escarpment and the river and asked his site selection commission to consider it for a new capital. In addition to its beauty, natural resources, and economic possibilities, the commission saw the area as a healthful place. The Republic of Texas Congress concurred and the city to be named for Austin was established in 1839. In 1840, it came under a new county dissected from Bastrop and named for Alamo commander William Barret Travis. Dr. Thomas W. Anderson thus became Travis County's first physician.

Top: *Meeting of Sam Houston and Santa Anna after the Battle of San Jacinto.* Above: *Advertisement for "Fresh Drugs and Medicines" from the* Daily Texian *(Austin), December 18, 1841.*

and tartar emetic. "Tartar emetic was the doctor's favorite prescription, and his doses were liberal." Webber soon developed a large practice.

"In the latter part of 1839," Smithwick added, "I took unto myself a helpmeet and established a home on a farm

CHAPTER II

A HEALTHY CAPITAL

PUBLIC HEALTH RECEIVED swift attention in the new capital. Edwin Waller, who began directing surveyors and overseeing construction of public buildings in the spring of 1839, included a hospital block in his grid plan. In December 1839, the Fourth Republic Congress and the first to meet in Austin passed an act of incorporation for the city, giving the mayor and council authority "to erect a hospital for the reception of the sick, and to appoint a physician to attend the same." The city council received authority "to determine the mode of inspection of all comestibles sold publicly in the market or in other places; and to regulate everything relative to bakers, butchers, tavern-keepers or grog-shops." The act is considered the first act of incorporation in a Texas municipality to contain important public health provisions. Still, a public hospital would not be built for more than forty years.

The story of medicine in nineteenth-century Travis County is inextricably tied to the story of Texas. Struggles to conquer the frontier and establish a new government commanded priority and economic realities meant that physicians often had to seek other income. Doctors became soldiers, political leaders, editors and publishers, farmers, preachers, law enforcers, pharmacists, merchants, and even real estate agents. Dr. Coleman described the physician another way, as "pioneer, adventurer, builder, rabble rouser, diplomat, schemer, businessman, organizer, dreamer. He was a Texan."

Historian Dr. Pat Ireland Nixon writes that Texas doctors came from three main sources. Some attended institutions, such as those in Philadelphia, New York, Boston, and Baltimore, with an unusual number from the Transylvania University Medical Department at Lexington, Kentucky, a precursor of the University of Louisville School of Medicine. Others were trained as preceptors with another physician. Some simply labeled themselves physicians. Generally better educated were the European physicians, such as the distinguished Dr. Ferdinand Ludwig von Herff of San Antonio, who arrived a little later.

Having left compatriots on Texas battlefields, most physicians arrived in Austin with responsibilities to the Republic. Others assumed city leadership roles. Dr. John G. Chalmers, a Virginia native who had received his medical education at Scotland's University of Edinburgh, may not have practiced medicine. He became secretary of the treasury under Lamar and later a newspaper publisher. Dr. Moses Johnson, who studied medicine through a preceptorship at Woodstock, New York, was active in community affairs and was elected mayor, serving in 1841. He also was the surgeon for the Austin Artillery Company.

Dr. Joseph W. Robertson was Bastrop's representative to the Fourth Congress in 1839, and, after adjournment, opened a medical practice and a pharmacy on Congress Avenue in Austin. A South Carolina native, he had studied medicine at Kentucky's Transylvania University. The future owners of Boggy Creek Farm found that he had cared for its original owners, James and Elizabeth Smith, who settled on the property in February 1838. Mr. Smith died after being shot and was attended by the doctor during the forty hours before his death. Eight months later, Dr. Robertson also delivered the Smiths' last child, charging twenty-five dollars.

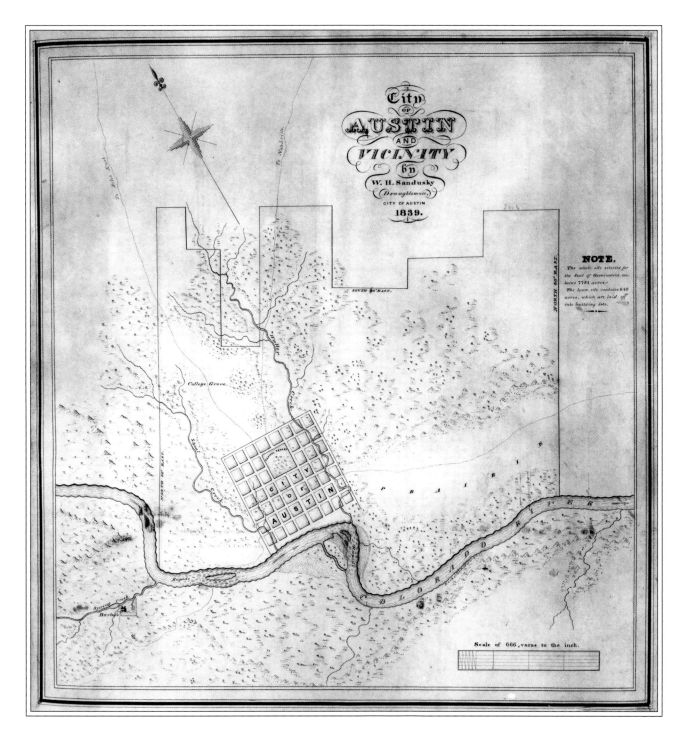

Edwin Waller designed the first plan of Austin in 1839.

Dr. Robertson had been a Texas Ranger and served as Austin's fifth mayor. He also would be remembered for buying the residence of Alphonse de Saligny, the French minister to the Republic of Texas. It became the French Legation Museum on San Marcos Street in the Robertson Hill area. Although death claimed him in 1870, Dr. Robertson's family occupied the home until 1902.

In Austin's first election, Dr. Samuel G. Haynie defeated Dr. Richard Fox Brenham—for whom Brenham, Texas, would be named—to become Travis County's first elected representative in the Republic of Texas Congress. Born in April 1806 in Knoxville, Tennessee, Dr. Haynie came to Austin in 1839 from Independence in Washington County, Texas. He practiced medicine briefly and served as a representative to the Fifth Congress from 1840 to 1842, before returning home.

Physicians like the renowned Drs. Ashbel Smith and Anson Jones had great impact on medicine in Travis County

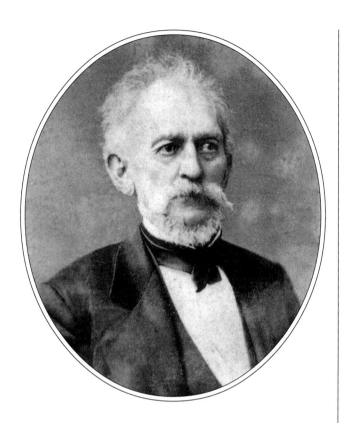

ABOVE: *Dr. Ashbel Smith, pioneer doctor and leader in the development of Texas has been called "the father of Texas medicine."* RIGHT: *Broadside of "Texan Universal Pills," 1838.*

persuaded to stay on the frontier. Practicing in Brazoria, Texas, until the war for Texas independence began, he joined the Texas army as an infantry private and was at the Battle of San Jacinto. He served in various capacities in the army before returning to his medical practice.

He contributed significantly to his profession during the first two sessions of the Republic of Texas Congress. As a petitioner in 1836, he pled for medical licensing, advising representatives that prompt action was required to protect Texans from "individuals assuming to be physicians" who "have neither graduated or been licensed." He urged formation of a medical society or a board of medical censors and a bill regulating fees and "all other matters relating to the Medical Profession." The First Congress failed to regulate medicine but the *Texas Telegraph and Register* spoke out against medical imposters. The editor, Dr. Francis Moore, Jr., an M.D., also offered a prescription: "Establish

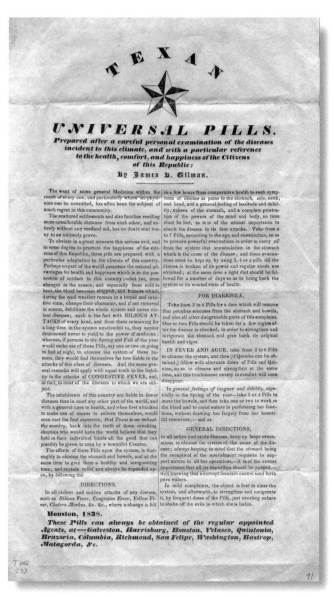

and Texas. Both pressed for institutions of higher learning, standards for practitioners, and professional associations to disseminate information across the isolated settlements.

Born in Hartford, Connecticut, in 1805, Dr. Smith graduated in 1824 from Yale University as a Phi Beta Kappa with a master's degree. Earning his M.D. degree in 1828, he did postgraduate work in England and Paris, the center for medical students of the day. By the time he arrived in Texas in 1837 the revolution was over, but he was appointed surgeon general of the army. He served the government in many capacities including in international diplomacy. In 1839, he wrote an account of yellow fever in Galveston, considered the first book of real scientific merit in Texas. Under Dr. Jones, Dr. Smith became secretary of the Republic.

When Dr. Jones arrived in Austin, he had considerable experience in the Republic. A native of Seekonkville in Great Barrington, Massachusetts, he had chosen medicine as a career because of family wishes. Studying with doctors in Massachusetts and New York, he later earned a degree from Jefferson Medical College, Philadelphia. After practicing in the east, he renounced medicine and moved to New Orleans, but during a trip to the Texas coast, he was

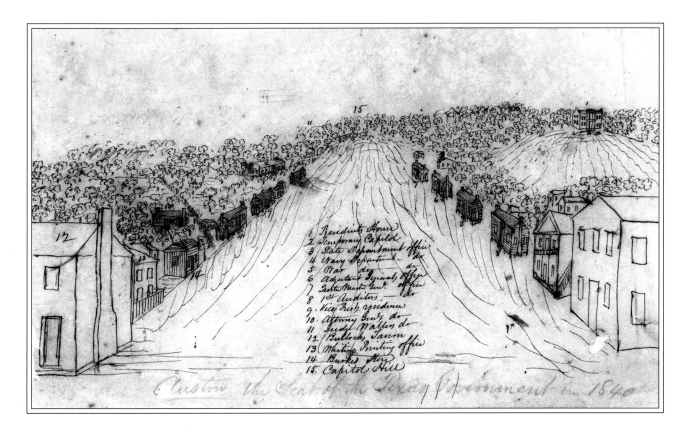

The following labels appear in the drawing:

1. Benedict's House
2. Temporary Capitol
3. State Department office
4. Navy Department
5. War do
6. Adjutant Generals office
7. Justr Master Genl office
8. 1st Auditors do
9. Vice Presd residence
10. Attorney Genls do
11. Judge Wallers do
12. Bullocks Tavrn
13. Whitings Printing office
14. Burkes Store
15. Capitol Hill

Austin the Seat of the Texas Government in 1840

Drawing of Austin attributed to Julia Sinks, 1840.

in each county of Texas a medical society, composed of regular graduates of medical colleges of the United States and Europe, for the purpose of examining and licensing all person(s) duly qualified to practice medicine."

Elected to the Second Congress, Dr. Jones pressed for the law establishing the Board of Medical Censors. On December 14, 1837, the act was signed by Sam Houston, Mirabeau B. Lamar, and Joseph Rowe, a physician and speaker of the House of Representatives. Board members were composed of one physician from each senatorial district, with residence in the latter required. The board set the qualifications and tests to be administered, and the applicant paid a twenty-dollar fee for the license to practice medicine. Among the eleven "medical gentleman" elected by Congress were Drs. Ashbel Smith and Thomas W. Anderson. Dr. Anderson was the representative for the districts of Mina and Gonzales before jurisdictional fate made him a Travis County doctor.

In January 1840, Dr. Jones opened a medical practice on Congress Avenue awaiting completion of his house on Pecan (later Sixth) Street. He soon discovered, however, that Austin residents seemingly needed a doctor less than Houstonians—a reinforcement perhaps of claims that Austin was a healthy place. He became secretary of state in the second administration of Sam Houston and in 1844 was elected president.

Dr. Rowe, who had served in the House of Representatives of the First Congress before being elected speaker, was

born in Caswell County, North Carolina, on June 3, 1802. He apparently came to Travis County in 1845, and would retire as a farmer.

Noah Smithwick declared that "Austin was an exceedingly healthy location, hence poor pickings for medicos, the fraternity being represented by Drs. Cook, Johnson and Chalmers, with old Dr. Anderson of Webber's Prairie to fall back on in critical cases. Nor must 'Old King Cole, the jolly old soul,' be omitted. Being flat broke and afflicted with an ulcer on his leg when he arrived in Austin, a friend set him up in the whisky business with a half barrel for a starter. His kindly disposition soon won him friends and his business thrived apace, enabling him to open the first decent saloon in town." In 1840, there were six doctors in Austin, with seven others "practicing on the side when not fulfilling duties in Congress or appointive office."

In 1842, however, three years after the establishment of the new capital, it was nearly deserted and the only physicians left were Dr. Robertson in Austin and Dr. Anderson in Webberville. The Mexican army had returned, taking San Antonio, Victoria, and Goliad, and President Sam Houston claimed that Austin could not be defended. He whisked the government to Houston and then transferred it to Washington-on-the-Brazos. While most able men in Austin were out hunting the Indians who had been harassing the city, a

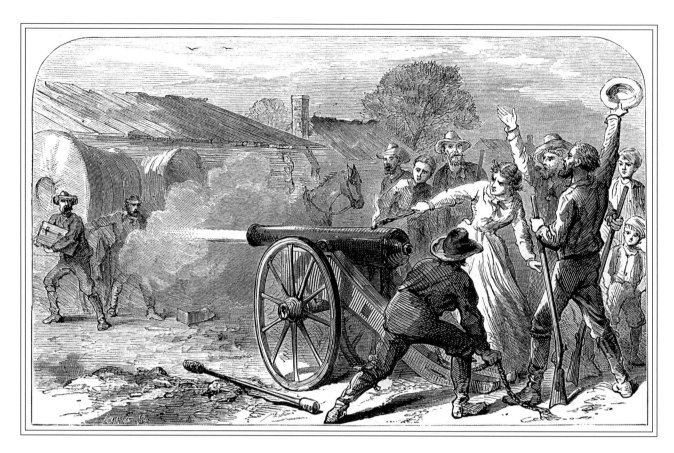

company of rangers arrived on December 29, 1842, to collect the state archives. When Dr. Robertson discovered them loading their wagons, Dr. Coleman writes, he rushed to the hotel to get the cannon. Mrs. Angelina Eberly, however, had heard the rangers and set it off. The able men returned and on New Year's Day the Committee on Safety caught the rangers at Kenney's Fort north of the city and persuaded them to surrender the archives, which were buried in boxes in Austin.

Dr. Robertson became mayor in 1843. Soon after, neighboring tribes isolated the capital. By rationing food and supplies and with help from counties to the east and southeast the city survived. Militias provided protection and Dr. Coleman relays that "On one occasion while the local men were drilling at Barton Springs, a rather large number of Indians appeared in town." Chosen to signal the militia, the doctor stood on the river banks and "called in such stentorian tones that his message was clearly heard two miles away and quickly acted upon."

Meanwhile, the new president, Dr. Anson Jones, called a constitutional convention in Austin on July 4, 1845, to consider annexation to the United States. The presence of the convention attendees and the issue of annexation revived the city. Participants further voted to join the union and chose Austin as the new state capital. Moses Johnson,

treasurer for his friend Dr. Jones, was among the physicians returning to town. He had moved the treasury archives into his home and a week after the convention, fire had destroyed everything. "Dr. Johnson was lonesome for his family," Dr. Coleman reported, "and he found nothing to do in the evenings except to pass from group to group engaged in endless talk and argument.... He was encouraged to resume practice, for there was a call for his service almost every day. One night he spent in the Ogden home where Mrs. Eliza Ogden was very ill. He tried to sleep on a pallet on the floor but the fleas gave him no rest. After the Convention closed he returned to Washington-on-the-Brazos for his family."

There were critical shortages of medicine, with Dr. Johnson complaining that he had been unable to get quinine for his own health. Fortunately, Dr. Samuel G. Haynie came back to Austin with plans to open an apothecary shop. Dr. Chalmers returned with plans to open a newspaper. "Apparently," Dr. Coleman concluded "no doctor was going to be caught with the practice of medicine as his only source of income."

New in town was Dr. John Salmon "Rip" Ford, who faced animosity at first because he had voted against Austin as the capital. Dr. Ford had studied medicine through a preceptorship in Shelbyville, Tennessee, before coming to Texas after the war for independence from Mexico. At age twenty-one, he began practicing in St. Augustine, Texas, using a prepaid medical care system, including at least one situation in which he received a hundred dollars to care for a family and its slaves for a year. Dr. R. Maurice Hood, a future Austin physician and a Ford biographer, observed that the medication in Dr. Ford's journal was typical, reflecting the lack of specific medications and showing reliance on symptomatic treatment. "The exception was quinine which was effective in treating malaria and was the first, disease-specific drug in medical history."

Dr. Ford was elected to the House of Representatives, serving in the Ninth Congress in 1844-1845. He also be-

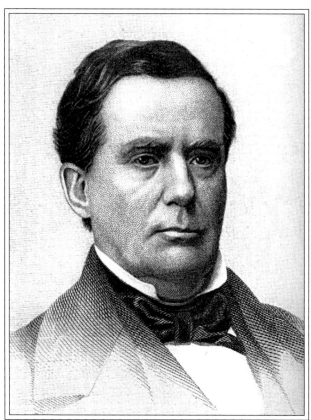

RIGHT: *Anson Jones, doctor, congressman, and the last president of the Republic of Texas.* BELOW: *Painting of Texas pioneer John S. "Rip" Ford. Dr. Ford practiced medicine in St. Augustine until 1844.*

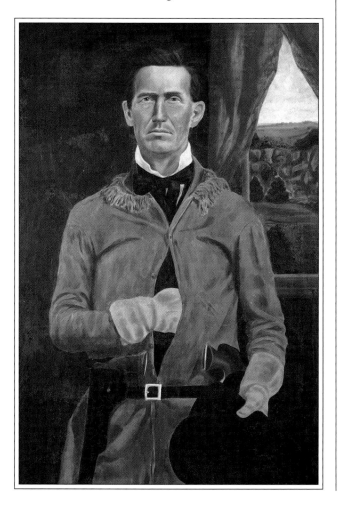

came editor of the *Texas Democrat.* In 1854, he was elected mayor of Austin and from 1876 to 1879 he was superintendent of the School for the Deaf. His other picturesque activities on behalf of Texas, especially as a Texas Ranger, coincided with highlights of Texas history and, in his final years, he wrote extensive memoirs.

Medicine had changed little. Vaccination for smallpox was transferred from arm to arm or by using dry lymph or a scab from a cowpox inoculation. Epidemics, including tuberculosis, often were associated with the migration of settlers. Yellow fever, considered an infectious rather than a carrier-borne disease, rampaged from 1839 until 1907. Dengue fever remained a threat and cholera had a thirty-to eighty-percent mortality rate.

Texas and Travis County were changing rapidly, however. In 1846, Dr. Jones told a tearful crowd on a hillside of the old Capitol, "The Republic of Texas is no more." Lowering the Lone Star flag, he raised that of the United States. Texas was its twenty-eighth state. Judge Alex Terrell reminisced. "The country will never again look as beautiful.... The prairies were clothed with waving grass hip high, and abounded with deer and antelope...."

For the "medicos" who came to Austin—despite the admonition that pickings were slim—there remained much work to be done.

CHAPTER III

A MEDICAL
SOCIETY ON THE
FRONTIER

WITH THE FORMATION OF THE American Medical Association in 1847, medicine and medical education gained new impetus. Travis County physicians, however, probably were more concerned about Indian attacks after massacres at Barton Creek, along Shoal Creek, and at the future state hospital site. To the south, the Mexican-American war was being fought.

More medical texts appeared, but the profession lacked organization, libraries, standards, and journals. During the Second Texas Legislature in 1848, Dr. Ashbel Smith led physicians from Galveston, the state's leading city, hoping to incorporate the Medical and Surgical Society of Galveston. Their request included the power to examine and regulate physicians and to have authority to regulate other areas affecting medical advancement and the good of the community. The

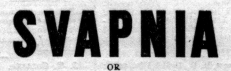

SVAPNIA

OR

PURIFIED OPIUM

☞ **FOR PHYSICIANS USE ONLY.** ☜

Contains the Anodyne and Soporific Alkaloids, Codeia, Narceia and Morphia. Excludes the Poisonous and Convulsive Alkaloids, Thebaine, Narcotine and Papaverine.

SVAPNIA has been in steadily increasing use for over twenty years, and whenever used has given great satisfaction.

To PHYSICIANS of REPUTE, not already acquainted with its merits, samples will be mailed on application.

SVAPNIA is made to conform to a uniform standard of Opium of Ten per cent. Morphia strength.

JOHN FARR, Manufacturing Chemist, New York.

C. N. CRITTENTON, Gen'l Agent, 115 Fulton St., N.Y

To whom all orders for samples must be addressed.

SVAPNIA IS FOR SALE BY DRUGGISTS GENERALLY.

effort evolved into a proposal for a state society but became mired in debate and maneuvering and never gained approval. In 1851, the renowned Dr. Smith was ready to throw up his hands. "We have, so far as I am aware, no medical organization in our State; nor is there much prospect of any change. Each member of the faculty is a separate independency, and sometimes adopts a sort of armed neutrality system."

Scientific progress was far behind that of Europe, where Rudolf Virchow was challenging the existing tenets of the medical world, and before long would produce his elemental work on cellular pathology. No Texas doctor was known to have a microscope. As elsewhere, Travis County healers would practice under various theories or schools of medicine: "regular" or allopathic; homeopathic; eclectic; botanical; mesmeric; and sundry other approaches. Blood-letting was common. Of

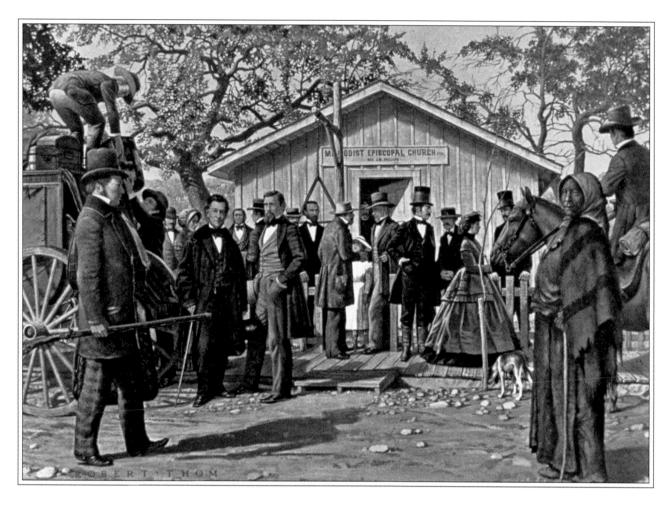

ABOVE: *Painting by Robert Thom of the first meeting of the Texas Medical Association in Austin, January 1853.* OPPOSITE PAGE: *Advertisment for opium. Opium was commonly used for pain relief in the 19th century.*

this mid-nineteenth-century era, Dr. Coleman laments, "Aesculapius looking down through the ages at the practice of this day may have wept, for in the Asklepiaia [sic] of early Greece, rest, food, fresh air and baths were the foundation stone of treatment. Now there was no rest for the patient, no time for food, fresh air was interdicted and baths, if used, were usually sulphurous and nauseating.... That medicine survived this era is surprising, for in the contest between medicine and the patient, the patient lost."

Dr. Richard S. Morgan's casebook for 1851 illustrates this point. Although "bleeding had fallen into disrepute, other revolting practices remained," Dr. Coleman declared. The fees, however, seem modest: scarifying and cupping, $4.00; Oil Ricini (castor oil) and pills, $2.50; Febrifuge (an antipyretic) and blister, $2.50; Quinine, 30 gr. Prescription, $1.00; Quinine, 15 gr. Prescription, $0.50; Febrifuge and cathartic, $3.00; emetic and cathartic $2.50; pain extractor,

$0.50; c(h)amomile flowers, $1.00; night visit with quinine and nitre pills, $9.00; night visit with expectorant mixture, camphor, capsicum, opium and services, $9.00, and office visit without prescription, $1.00.

Scarifying and cupping, a mild form of bloodletting, involved multiple small incisions with a "scarificator" to draw blood from a small vein rather than a large one. A heated glass was placed on the skin to create a vacuum within the vessel to draw out blood. Oil Ricini was a cathartic. Blister therapy was intended to cleanse the system, typically by applying a hot mustard plaster to cause a blister, which was then drained. Quinine from the bark of various species of the cinchona tree had several uses, including fever reduction. Opium was also used commonly in the nineteenth and early twentieth centuries for pain relief, often in the form of laudanum or tincture of opium, a combination of opium and alcohol. Camphor might have been used as a stimulant or sedative. Among emetics for vomiting and purging were ipecac, calomel, jalap, tartar emetic (antimony potassium tartrate), and lobelia. Nitre pills caused patients to perspire and thus were intended to flush the system.

Laboratory aids were crude. Flies around urine might indicate diabetes, or it might be detected by taste or fermentation. "Consequently," Dr. Nixon states, "much store was laid by observation, palpation, and common sense. The pulse was studied very closely. Twenty-one different types of pulse are described by [J. C.] Massie and the diagnostic significance of each is explained. The facial expression, the type of breathing, the shape of the abdomen, the position in bed, the appearance of the sputum and the stools, and many other observations are emphasized."

Arriving in Travis County from diverse locations and backgrounds, more physicians would devote time to the practice of medicine, although that is not to say they didn't have supplementary means of income. In 1850, Austin had at least ten physicians and one druggist, G. W. Gray. Dr. Francis T. Duffau returned to Austin in 1851, went into business with Gray, and became the sole owner of the drug store. Later, he took on another partner.

Doctors and dentists were advertising partnerships, arrivals, and specialties in newspapers or card announcements. Some were simple—as would be insisted upon by medical societies in the future—and others were more effusive, as illustrated by these examples, reported by Dr. Coleman:

S. D. MULLOWMY formerly of Missouri offers his services in the practice of medicine, surgery and obstetrics. Chronic diseases of females and those of infancy and childhood have been much studied.

W. W. PAYNE treats according to the eclectic system. His knowledge is sought from all systems of medical practice freely. Truth is received where found. Medicine used is of a safe salutory [sic] character rather than dangerous and debilitating. Cases will be treated without the use of antimony and mercury in any form.

The 1850 Travis County census described the status of public health for the previous year. Travis County had seen forty deaths during the year ending January 1; ten were of children under age one and eight were of slaves. The causes of death included one each for thrush, a cold, teething,

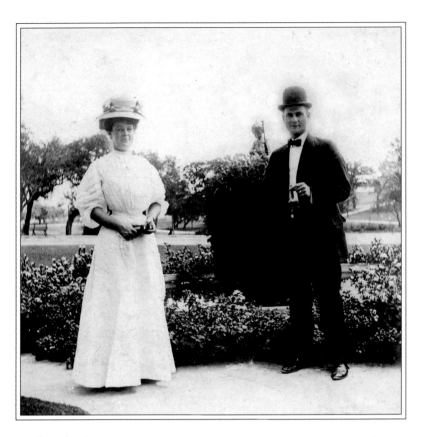

ABOVE: *M. A. (Matthew Addison) and Daisy Bouldin Taylor. Dr. Taylor served as an Austin city alderman.*
OPPOSITE PAGE: *Plan of the city of Austin, 1853.*

croup, congestive fever, inflammation of the brain, inflammation of the bowel, flux, and hives. One explanation was "chronich" and another was "dunat," which could be interpreted in a variety of ways. Four deaths were attributed to fever, three to accidents, two to smallpox, seven to "numonia," two to "worps cough," and four were unknown.

Dr. Thomas Anderson, now in Austin, formed the city's earliest known partnership in 1849 with Drs. William T. Horne and James R. Horne. It was dissolved before long, however, after Dr. James Horne's death. Then, in 1851, Drs. William Horne and R. S. Morgan formed a partnership. Dr. Coleman concluded that the short duration of partnerships showed that doctors had much to learn about working together.

Physicians maintained strong civic roles. Dr. Haynie was elected mayor of Austin, serving two terms from 1850 to 1852. Drs. Duffau, John E. Elgin, James Holiday, R. N. Lane, and M. A. Taylor served as city aldermen. "Dead heats in elections were not unusual," Dr. Coleman observes. "Dr. R. S. Morgan lost a race for alderman in a runoff. ... A tax on hogs within the city limits was defeated and a proposed annual tax of five dollars on attorneys, physicians, dentists and other professional men resulted in a furor. Concern for sanitation manifested itself in ordinances governing the cleanliness of sidewalks and the removal of dead animals." Doctors also became involved in political parties appearing on the frontier, from the Democratic Party to the Know Nothing Party.

By 1852, Austin was more stable, although homes remained log cabins and the Capitol was "an old wooden shack." William M. "Buck" Walton writes, "At that time, we had one policeman and he was seldom on duty. The latch string of every home hung on the outside.... There was no such thing as stealing, robbery or violence toward women.... The Indians visited us frequently, not as hostiles but as friends, bringing hides and furs for trading purposes. They would camp near the city and stay for several days."

Perhaps now physicians could devote more time to their profession. Dr. Samuel K. Jennings, who lived just south of the Colorado River on the site of the future Texas School

for the Deaf, is thought to have called the first of a series of meetings. On May 26, 1852, the participants produced a memorial resolution, with Drs. S. G. Haynie, A. J. Lott, and Wade A. Morris drafting the words to honor Dr. Henry T. Briggs. Then, following the August drowning in San Antonio of Dr. R. C. Moffett, a Texas Rangers' surgeon, Dr. J. R. Simms wrote a resolution honoring him.

As the doctors met, their goals became evident in typical nineteenth-century fashion—through a newspaper. On December 8, 1852, the *Southwestern American* carried the following announcement, "The physicians of this city and county had a meeting yesterday evening with the object of calling a convention for the organization of a State Medical Society."

This "group of farseeing physicians of Austin set on foot a movement," Dr. Nixon noted, that led to the formation of the Texas Medical Association. Instead of taking their petition to the Legislature, however, the Travis County doctors published the following notice in the December 11, 1852, *Texas State Gazette* and four days later in the *Texas Monument*:

The members of the medical profession resident in the city of Austin and county of Travis, had a meeting on the 9th instant [meaning the current month, which was December], to consider of the propriety of assembling a convention of the profession throughout the State at an early day. After due consultation, it was unanimously resolved to issue the following call. The objects to be attained are of an important character, and we commend the subject to the serious consideration, and prompt action of physicians in all parts of the State.

To all regular authorized Physicians of the State of Texas:
We the undersigned, Physicians of the City of Austin and vicinity, being desirous of promoting the advancement and improvement, as well as elevating the standard of our profession within this State, propose an object conducive to that end a State Medical Convention, to meet at the City of Austin on the Seventeenth day of January next; for the purpose of organizing a state medical society, and generally to do and take such action as will be most conducive to these objects.

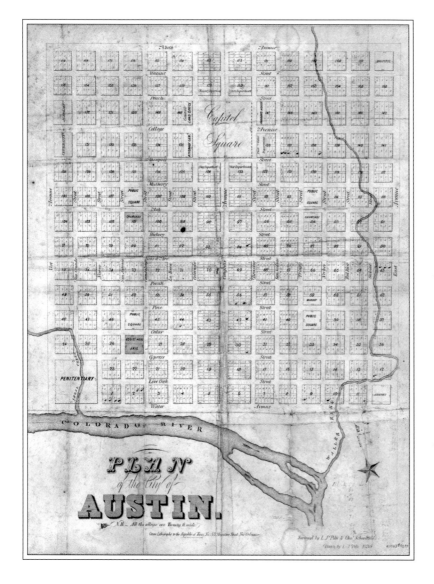

And we furthermore express the wish and hope that all the members of our profession throughout the State who can, will meet with us at the time and place specified, and aid us in the proposed organization.

The notice had been signed on December 8 by ten Travis County doctors: Arthur J. Lott, J. T. Alexander, S. W. Baker, J. P. Duval, S. K. Jennings, Jr., Edward McDonnell, J. M. Litten, R. N. Lane, W. K. Brown, and W. A. Morris. [Although the *Texas State Gazette* of December 11, 1852, cites "S. W. Baker," the noted historian of early Texas medical history, Dr. Pat Ireland Nixon, consistently refers to "S. W. Barker" in his books and writing. It is possible that Dr. Nixon found verification for this name, but citations from other historians and in local records suggest that "Baker" is correct.]

On January 17, 1853, thirty-five doctors answered the Travis County invitation, arriving at the Methodist Church, a board and batten structure on what became the northeast corner of Congress Avenue and Fourth Street (then Cedar Street). Most physicians arrived from nearby counties, but one physician, Dr. Joseph Taylor, traveled more than 300 miles from Harrison County on the Louisiana border to attend the meeting. Although some stagecoach lines were functioning, his trip likely was an arduous one by horseback.

The Texas Medical Association thus was established a little more than a month after Travis County doctors sent out their call. Considering the frontier conditions, the number of physicians arriving so quickly was remarkable. Dr. Jennings chaired the first meeting, with Dr. Lott as secretary. Twelve Travis County physicians were registered, including nine who had signed the invitation plus Drs. S. W. Davis, W. H. Johnson, and R. B. Pumphrey. Four Travis County physicians were elected to officer positions in the new association—Drs. W. A. Morris, first vice president; A. J. Lott, corresponding secretary; R. N. Lane, recording secretary; and J. M. Litten, treasurer. The physician who had ridden the farthest—Dr. Taylor—was elected president.

Dr. Litten served on the committee to draft the constitution, which provided for a single state organization with collateral district societies. Five other members were ap-

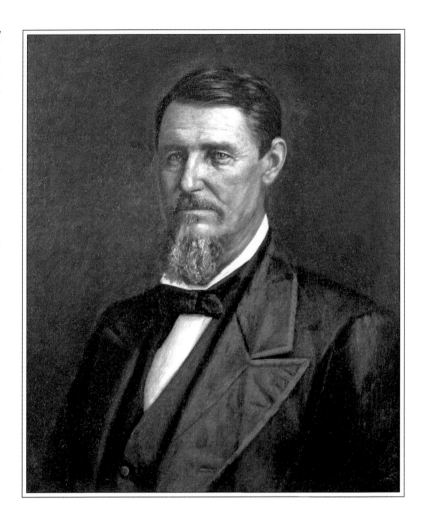

ABOVE: *James Webb Throckmorton was a doctor, a lawyer, and politician. He served as governor of Texas from 1866 to 1867.* OPPOSITE PAGE: Manual of Practice for the Diseases of Texas, *an early medical book published in 1866.*

pointed to petition the state legislature for a simple charter for the private organization.

Convention proceedings were printed in Austin by J. W. Hampton at the *Gazette* office.

Two attendees would become especially prominent in Texas politics: Dr. Ashbel Smith would lead the University of Texas Board of Regents and Dr. J. W. Throckmorton would become governor of Texas.

Two district societies were formed in the fall. On September 22, 1853, the Bexar Medical Society was established with Dr. George Cupples of San Antonio as president, and on October 22, 1853, the Travis Medical Society was formed with Dr. John T. Alexander of Austin as president.

The state association met again in November 1853 at the Methodist Church. In the president's absence, Dr. W. A. Morris of Austin, the vice president, presided. The organization would change its name several times beginning with the second meeting. In 1951, it would return to its original name, the Texas Medical Association (TMA), the citation used throughout this book. The Travis County Medical Society also would have several names. No consistent pattern for county society names would develop until the federation of medicine reorganized in 1903.

A Scotsman, Dr. George Cupples of San Antonio, president of the Bexar Medical Society, was elected the second president of the TMA, and his stirring speech is remembered as a masterpiece, representing the "flowering of medicine" in Texas. Other officers were from Travis County: Drs. S. K. Jennings, Jr., first vice president; John T. Alexander, second vice president; R. N. Lane, recording secretary; M. A. Taylor, assistant recording secretary; A. J. Lott, corresponding secretary; and J. M. Litten, treasurer. On November 28, 1853, the Fifth Legislature granted a state charter. Unlike the previous Galveston request, the new association had not sought power to license physicians or to regulate external medical matters.

Unfortunately, after the two 1853 meetings, the association lapsed until after the Civil War. Speculation as to why this was so has been far ranging from travel distance and poor transportation to economics and the war itself—

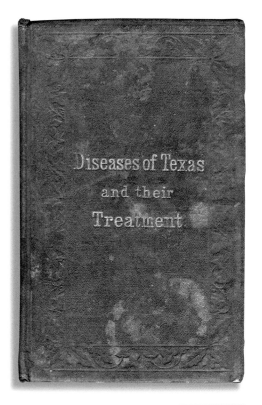

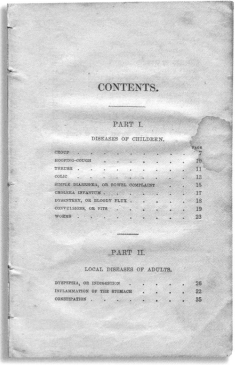

CONTENTS.

committee with Dr. Ferdinand Ludwig von Herff of San Antonio were Travis County members Drs. J. R. Simms of Webberville, and J. T. Alexander, J. W. Robertson, R. N. Lane, W. A. Morris, J. M. Litten, and A. J. Lott, all of Austin. As far as is known, the Travis Medical Society also lapsed until 1870.

Newspapers continued as the outlet for medical news, and the *Tri-Weekly State Times* of December 3, 1853, published a verbatim copy of a Webberville physician's paper. "Dissertation on Post Mortem," delivered by Dr. Simms at the November meeting of the Texas Medical Association, apparently became the first published scientific paper of a Travis County doctor.

Austin physicians were agitators for change. Dr. William T. Horne had been a founder of the Austin Sons of Temperance in 1848. Dr. Haynie joined in 1849 and became a director; and Dr. John Ford also was active. Their work and that of others may have had some effect. In 1853-1854, Texas adopted legislation aimed at reducing alcohol consumption, and Austin's grog shop landscape changed quickly. From fourteen shops in 1853, there were only four by October 1854.

Although there was little thievery, drugs tempted someone. Dr. Ford's *Tri-Weekly State Times* of December 13, 1853, stated that "Some person took the medical saddle bags of Dr. Lott from the door of his office. The individual performing this jocund trick will please return the portable apothecary shop to the owner. The doctor says his drugs are powerful and might do harm in the hands of an injudicious administrator. Carry them home and let such things alone hereafter." Dr. Ford also alerted the citizenry in 1854 about a man

and perhaps a controversy surrounding two Travis County doctors. After two signers of the original invitation developed hard feelings, a TMA resolution declared that they had set out to destroy the association by circulating injurious reports to prevent the accession of members. A committee then was appointed to prepare a positive circular to assure Texas doctors about the new organization. On the

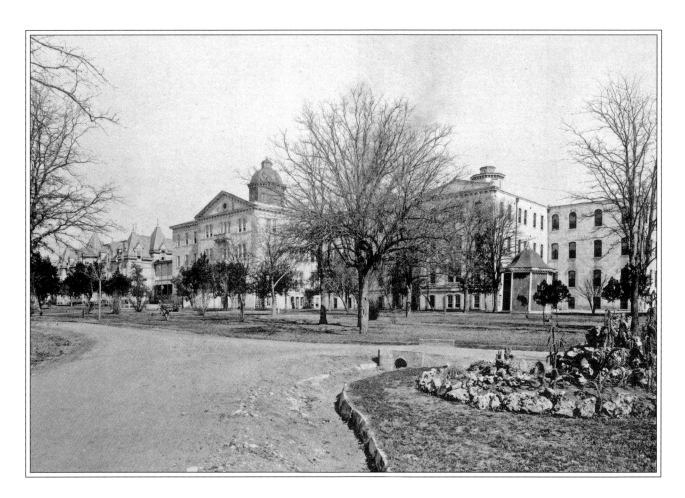

who called himself Dr. Armstrong and allegedly was stealing medical diplomas.

Besides smallpox, cholera, and yellow fever, other epidemics left misery in Texas: scarlet fever in 1849 (it was not known then that it was a result of a *Streptococcus*); measles in 1850; typhoid fever and dengue fever in 1852; and diphtheria in 1860. In 1853, smallpox almost dissolved the Texas Legislature. The *Colorado Tribune* of Matagorda reported the disease "threatened for some time to stop all legislative proceedings, and knock rail roads, rivers, apportionments, and all other bills and schemes into a cocked-hat, for the present. For some time it was seriously urged that there should be an immediate break up and stampede for the legislature, but after grave deliberation, of several hours, with closed doors, it was finally decided better to remain and die the death of martyrs to the shrine of patriotism than to return home and run the risk of contaminating a devoted constituency."

By 1855, Austin had 25 physicians and a population of 2,500. Although many had less than desirable training, the 1 to 100 ratio can be considered favorable. Numerous new homes were being built. Having had much experience in constructing prominent edifices, including the post office,

a mercantile building, and his own home, Dr. S. G. Haynie became one of the two commissioners in charge of building the new Capitol. Dr. Coleman reports that Drs. S. W. Baker and M. A. Taylor were "the moving spirits" behind the Presbyterian Church building.

Like other states, Texas was more active in medical care, and in 1856, the Sixth Texas Legislature approved asylums for deaf, blind, and mentally ill persons.

Two occurrences marked the end of an era. Travis County's first physician, Dr. Anderson, died in Round Rock, probably at his son Washington's home, on April 26, 1857. On January 9, 1858, Dr. Jones told a friend at dinner in the old Capitol Hotel in Houston that his public career had begun there and might close there. Suffering from mental depression, he shot himself to death that night.

In Travis County, mortality figures during 1859 showed that out of 100 cases, 35 were infants under age one and slaves accounted for 50 deaths. The most frequent causes cited were pneumonia, 9; croup, 6; cholera infantum, 6; teething, 5, and pulmonary consumption, 5.

War was on the horizon and physicians were divided about whether Texas should secede from the Union. In Austin, Alex Terrell writes that Union men called "home guards" drilled in 1861 at the first brick house on Congress Avenue, built in 1854 by George Hancock, until "a short time after Fort Sumter was assaulted. Then many of them crossed the Rio Grande." Among those drilling were several judges, a congressman, former Governor E. M. Pease, and several doctors, including Drs. Lane and Litten. "Dr. Litten and a few other Union men remained in Austin until the close of the Civil War," Terrell reported, "but their opposition to secession was not concealed, and that fact made their condition one of great disquiet during the war."

The Union blockade resulted in critical shortages, and Drs. Haynie and Rentfro helped organize a Mutual Supply Association to distribute supplies. A committee to help soldiers' families was established with Dr. M. A. Taylor in charge. Dr. Beriah Graham announced free services for wives and children of soldiers serving the Confederacy. An 1804 North Carolina native, Dr. Graham had studied medicine at Transylvania University in Lexington, Kentucky, and St. Louis Medical College (later Washington University School of Medicine). He had come to Austin in 1859 from Palestine, Texas.

With medicines scarce, the *Austin State Gazette* reported on June 1, 1864, that J. J. Beech on Pecan Street had received a selected stock of staple goods and medicines directly from Monterrey, Mexico. Dr. F. T. Duffau announced on January 11, 1865, that he had received drugs and medicines for sale at reasonable prices, including quinine, morphine, castor oil, opium, and other typical medications. A column on July 13, 1864, extolled the merits of a doctor-owned New Braunfels firm with an agent in Mexico. On April 5, 1865, the headline, "Drugs! Drugs!! Drugs!!!" proclaimed its freshly imported supply.

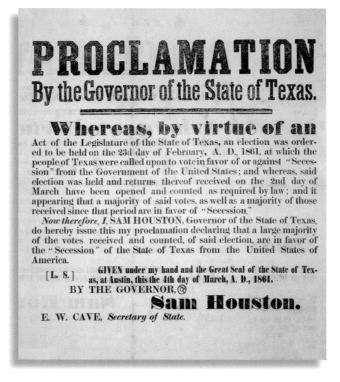

On March 4, 1861, Governor Sam Houston issued this proclamation announcing that the citizens of Texas had voted for secession.

Medical journals also were caught in the blockade and Dr. J. C. Massie's 1854 *Treatise on Eclectic Southern Practice of Medicine* probably served as the primary source of medical information beyond newspapers. Texas doctors had asked the Houston physician to write the book with the belief that diseases behaved differently in Texas.

County commissioners exempted physicians from militia duty, "believing the same are absolutely necessary to the wants of this county." Doctors became surgeons to various military units and groups, however. Strapped for income, some doctors left their profession for mercantile ventures.

By the end of the Civil War, there was a complex system of taxes—poll, property, salary, and occupation—and doctors were among those singled out. "As to the tax on professions, which is the tax nearest to income taxation in the financial history of Texas," E. T. Miller wrote, "Governor Throckmorton later said that its yield was small and that it operated oppressively and unequally. He recommended a minimum exemption with a graduated but moderate rate on the remainder."

Although medical research was nearly halted, progress resulted from battlefield experiences in surgery and anesthesia; on diet and cleanliness; in certain technical areas like photomicrography, from refresher courses required for Confederate doctors; and in the development of scholarly medical works. Dr. J. W. Stalnaker, who later moved to Austin, participated in the preparation of the manual of practice developed by the Confederacy during the war. Also, the scholarly collections from the Army Surgeon General's office, which eventually evolved into the National Library of Medicine, may have been one of the most important advancements. Dr. R. Maurice Hood also writes that the mobile battlefield hospital saw its genesis in this war although refinement was many years away.

CHAPTER IV

PROGRESS AFTER WAR

IN 1867, THE U.S. CONGRESS PASSED THE First Reconstruction Act, citing Texas as "an impediment to progress," and Dr. Throckmorton, who had been inaugurated governor in 1866, was removed from office by General Philip H. Sheridan on July 30, 1867.

Austin, however, had its first hospital, the Military Post Hospital, which had begun operating in 1867 under a Dr. Kirk. The frame structure had twelve beds and an average occupancy of six. The sink was kept "clean and disinfected" and the house had water from public and private cisterns. Patients suffered from chronic rheumatism, contusions, convalescent typhoid, fractured femur, fractured rib, primary syphilis, and insanity.

More Texas medical societies were being established and a private medical school was functioning. In 1856, Soule University at Chappell Hill had been launched by the Methodist Episcopal Church and had planned to include medical education in 1860. Disrupted by the war, the institution later was decimated by a yellow fever epidemic. After the war, Soule University's Medical Department moved to

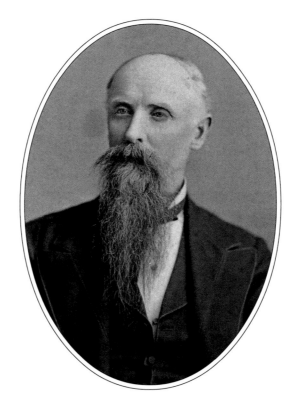

Galveston, becoming Galveston Medical College. In 1866, Dr. Greensville Dowell held the school in his home and leased the old 1845 Island City Hospital for clinical training. In late 1865, he had also begun the state's first medical journal, the *Galveston Medical Journal*, which was published until 1871, with a brief revival in 1880. Dr. Dowell published two books, including one on yellow fever, theorizing that it was spread by mosquitoes. His view preceded by five years Carlos Finlay's findings that mosquitoes were the vectors.

Professional nursing emerged when Catholic nurse volunteers from France arrived in 1866 to open Charity Hospital, later St. Mary's Infirmary, caring for more than a thousand patients with yellow fever in 1867. Their order, the Sisters of Charity of the Incarnate Word, later opened other hospitals in Texas and elsewhere.

Texas doctors again sought to unite their profession. In 1869, Washington County called delegates from local and regional associations to Houston, and the convention resulted in the reorganized Texas Medical Association. The

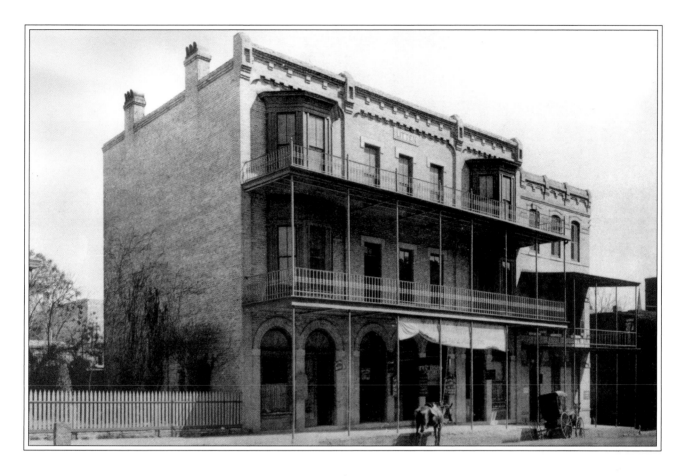

ABOVE: *Litten Block, West 7th, office of Dr. J. M. Litten, Austin's first city physician.* OPPOSITE PAGE: *Dr. J. W. Stalnaker was Austin's second city physician, serving from 1872 to 1876.*

only attendee from the 1853 Travis County meetings was Dr. Ashbel Smith. Although apparently no physicians from Travis County were present, one key participant—Dr. Richard Montgomery Swearingen—later moved to Austin. In 1870, Travis County Medical Society resumed regular meetings and was one of the first societies to affiliate with the reorganized state association.

As construction boomed in the capital, the *Austin Daily Journal* in 1870 declared, "No more visitors are wanted. The City is full and overrun." Keeping visitors out was not likely, however, because the long-anticipated Houston and Texas Central Railroad reached Austin in late 1871, supplementing its existing stagecoach lines. The newspaper's attitude was understandable, however. "Our city was never more besmirched and foul than now," wrote one editor. "Its dirt and filth give forth unwholesome smells wherever we turn and if Austin escapes a large amount of sickness this fall we must thank our lucky stars rather than ourselves." Cows grazed on the Capitol grounds, dogs and hogs ran

the streets, and there was nude bathing at the foot of Congress Avenue, which had no bridge across to the south.

A board of health was appointed in 1871, with Dr. J. M. Litten becoming chairman and Austin's first city physician, followed by Dr. J. W. Stalnaker in 1874.

The state's eleemosynary institutions suffered during the Reconstruction era, with patients at the Texas State Lunatic Asylum enduring crowded and shabby conditions. On the positive side, plans were under way to establish the American Dental College in Austin, with professors of dentistry and two physicians scheduled to teach physiology, anatomy, and surgery. The college, however, was apparently never launched.

In the late 1860s and early 1870s, older doctors were being succeeded by a new group moving to town. "Heretofore we have known our physicians principally through their political activities," Dr. Coleman wrote, "now with the advent of medical journals we are able to evaluate doctors as practitioners of healing." Travis County medicine, he added, had lagged twenty years behind the more enlightened parts of the United States, but after the arrival of journals, "the upgrading of practice was rapid." He credited Drs. B. E. Hadra, J. W. McLaughlin, R. M. Swearingen, David Wallace, and T. D. Wooten, working with Drs.

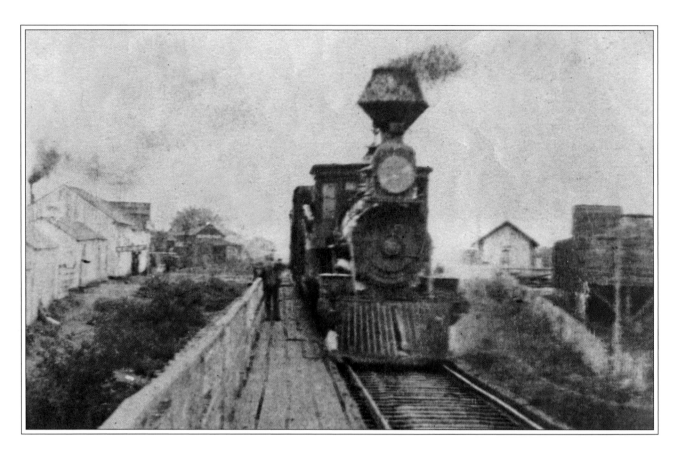

The Houston and Texas Central Railroad began service between Houston and Austin in 1871. Here, passengers are disembarking at the Depot House on Waller Creek.

Haynie, J. M. Litten, W. A. Morris, and M. A. Taylor, with lifting "the quality of medical care to its highest levels in the history of the community."

After practicing for thirty-four years, Dr. Samuel G. Haynie, a former mayor who had come to Austin in 1839, returned to school. His original education was through a preceptorship, but after talking with his colleagues about their war experiences, he enrolled in Soule University's Galveston Medical College. In 1871, at age sixty-five, he graduated with valedictory honors and returned to Austin to practice.

In 1873, Manor, a Travis County town east of Austin, received a new physician, Dr. Richard S. Gregg, a graduate of the University of Louisiana (eventually Tulane University School of Medicine). In 1870, a botanical physician and druggist, Dr. John R. Hammel, was in Austin. He had been preceded in Texas in the 1830s by another botanical physician, Dr. Gideon Lincecum, who had identified 500 plants with medicinal properties in Texas.

Austin was a destination for families escaping the coastal summers and yellow fever. In 1873, however, it had its own yellow fever scare, with threats of quarantine and rumors that trains would be cut off, as had happened already in Navasota. An Austin editor published reassuring words. "An old and experienced physician, J. M. Litten, of our city says that after exhaustive investigation he is able to assert that yellow fever has never generated at an altitude above 400 feet above the level of the sea. Let the panic stricken from the wasted areas come here." Drs. McLaughlin, J. B. Shepherd, Stalnaker, and Taylor also declared the rumor not true.

Although investigators in the long-developing field of microbiology had found significant evidence of microorganisms, most Texas physicians did not yet accept germ theory. Nor was the rest of the United States much different, many scoffing at the effect of bacteria in disease. The first doctor known to bring a microscope to Texas was Dr. Lycurgus Van Zandt, a Civil War veteran, who took it from Bellville to Fort Worth in 1868. In other medical realms, there was apparently no one in Texas who could perform abdominal surgery or remove an appendix.

In 1873, Texas required physicians to have an M.D. degree or be certified by the board of medical examiners in their district. Registration also was required at a fee of one dollar, and county courts were directed to set up boards of examiners of not less than three practicing physicians. A grandfather clause allowed those who had been in practice for five consecutive years to continue without complying with the new educational requirements. Midwives, however, were prohibited from obtaining a license. In response to the new law, the Travis County Board of Medical Examiners was organized on February 4, 1874. Members were Drs. Wade Morris, president; W. A. East, secretary; and Lafayette D. Hill. The licensure law would be amended in 1876 and repealed in 1879, after which county clerks were required only to record all diplomas from recognized medical colleges.

Dr. Berthold Ernest Hadra was among Austin physicians presenting papers at the 1874 Texas Medical Association (TMA) meeting in Dallas. Born in 1842 near Brieg, Silesia, he had studied at the Universities of Breslau and Berlin. After serving as an assistant surgeon in the Prussian Army, he came to America, moving to Austin in 1872. He and other physicians provided the primary impetus for establishing infirmaries for the full-time care of the sick in the capital. In 1873, he opened the city's first private hospital, the Austin Infirmary, in the Wahrmann home near Lavaca and Walnut (later Fourteenth Street). He closed it in 1876, but the following year he opened Austin Hospital at Walnut and Nueces, where he charged one dollar a day. The hospital equipment included inhaling apparatus and a "liberal" number of surgical instruments. It also had a waiting room, a large bathroom with two tubs, seven private rooms, and a twelve-bed ward.

Dr. Hadra brought a more scientific approach to medicine in Travis County and was likely the first to use the microscope as a diagnostic tool, as deduced from a public health notice signed by Drs. James M. Litten, county society president, and Josephus Cummings, secretary, in the early 1870s: "At the regular meeting of the Travis County Medical Society held on the 9th inst. [an abbreviation for "instant," meaning the current month] several cases of trichinosis were brought before the society by Dr. B. Hadra." In language typically used at the time, the notice continued, "The disease is carried by eating pork similarly affected and is one involving

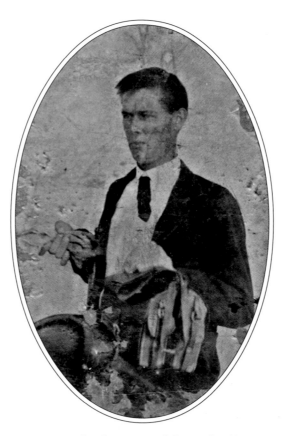

Tintype of a physician with his medical bag.

the welfare of the community. It is due to a small animalicule that is destroyed by high temperature. Consequently as much suffering and death may be avoided we recommend that all pork for table use be thoroughly cooked." Word usage and spelling would evolve and in future language, the notice might have been stated more directly, such as: "The disease can be acquired by eating undercooked pork infected by the larvae of a worm called *Trichinella spiralis*. The parasite can be found coiled in a cyst in the muscles of certain animals, such as pigs."

In a case report to the Texas Medical Association, he observed that the first view of the microscopic field "gave us a most lively picture, it being crowded by the living and true *trichinoe* [sic] *spiralis*. Thus, it will be seen, that this little epidemic had five victims, two of whom died...." Already, American hams sent to Germany had a bad reputation and German butchers were required to have pork examined before selling it. "It would be a praiseworthy act if this Association," Dr. Hadra suggested, "would place matters of this kind under the control of the much hoped for State Board of Health." His was one of many TMA calls for the establishment of the state board.

In 1875, six years after TMA reorganized, Austin was the meeting site for the first time since 1853. Physicians gathered in the House of Representatives Chamber at the old Capitol, after the Texas Legislature passed an act allowing them to do so. Governor Richard Coke hosted a reception at the Governor's Mansion and the Travis County Medical Society held a banquet at the Raymond House.

Dr. Thomas Dudley Wooten of Austin presented a paper that Dr. Nixon described as clear and forward looking: "In great detail he outlined the known facts about the histological changes that take place in inflammation, quoting Cohnheim, Billroth, and Burton Sanderson." Dr. Wooten, Nixon said, showed that he was familiar with wound cleansing and the use of carbolic acid dressings advocated by Joseph Lister. Dr. Wooten also had used chloroform as anes-

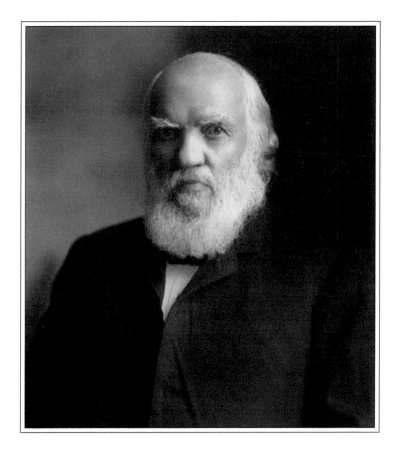

Dr. Thomas Dudley Wooten was a surgeon in the Confederate Army. After the war, he practiced medicine in Paris, Texas, and in Austin in the 1870s. He became one of the original regents of the University of Texas in 1881.

thesia "for twenty odd years" without a death, and discussed the importance of monitoring a patient during surgery. He was certain that the many deaths attributed to chloroform could be traced to carelessness and ignorance.

A frequent presenter, Dr. Wooten had practiced in Kentucky and Missouri before serving the Confederacy as a private soldier, as a surgeon in Missouri, and as medical director of the District of Arkansas. In 1865, he moved to Paris, Texas, and then to Austin in 1876. In 1885, he was named one of the original University of Texas regents and, following the death of Dr. Ashbel Smith, became president of the Board of Regents. He served until his death in 1906 and was considered "one of the most honored, respected, and beloved" of his profession. He was an 1853 graduate of the Medical Department of the University of Louisville, a school founded in part by faculty of the old Transylvania University Medical Department.

Dr. R. M. Swearingen, who arrived in Austin in 1875 from Chappell Hill, Texas, became an outstanding figure in Travis County and also nationally. At the TMA reor-

ganizational meeting in 1869, he became chairman of the Committee on Climatology and Epidemics. Born in Noxubee County, Mississippi, in September 1838, he had moved with his family to Chappell Hill in 1848. He attended the Chappell Hill Male and Female Institute and Centenary College, then at Jackson, Louisiana. A medical student at the New Orleans Medical College (likely the Medical College of Louisiana which became Tulane University School of Medicine), he joined the Confederacy in 1860 and served in several campaigns including the retreat through Georgia. After graduating from medical school in 1867, he had returned to Chappell Hill to practice medicine when yellow fever reached the area. Suffering from glomerulonephritis, he nevertheless worked tirelessly during the epidemic, watching many friends perish.

The 1876 Texas constitution stated that the Legislature could give no preference to any schools [theories] of medicine, which opened a can of worms in Travis County. Allopathic physicians typically referred to themselves as "regular" doctors and opposed "irregular" theories, particularly homeopathic medicine. A district judge, E. B. Turner, however, was planning to appoint a homeopathic physician to the Sixteenth Judicial District Board of Examiners. Representing allopathic doctors, Travis County Medical Society refused to cooperate with "irregular practitioners in establishing a mixed board of medical examiners to regulate the practice of medicine and surgery in the state." An 1877 society resolution asked the Texas Medical Association for support.

After a volatile debate, which also impugned a regular TMA member on the district board, Dr. Ashbel Smith proposed postponing action. The subject was brought up again, however, and Travis County's resolution was unanimously "carried amid applause." Judge Turner, nevertheless, appointed Dr. G. E. Routh, "the homeopath in question," writes Dr. Coleman, "as well as Dr. E. G. Doerr of the despised local branch of the Indianapolis Surgical Institute."

Disagreements on theories would occur more than once, and the editor of the *Statesman*, writes Dr. Coleman, commented that "allopaths believed that a rattling dose of podophyllin is good for a man's soul, while homeopaths hold that a pound of drug poured into the Colorado River at Austin would after a flow of many days fill Matagorda Bay with liver tonic." Despite differences, Travis County physicians worked together. Drs. Bibb and Routh cared for four patients with diphtheria at the governor's mansion, and Dr. Thomas D. Wooten performed an autopsy on a patient of Drs. Bragg and C. E. Fisher, confirming the appropriateness of their diagnosis and treatment. For health reasons, allopathic and homeopathic physicians, together with a botanical doctor, signed a petition opposing expansion of the cemetery.

Evidence of specialization in Travis County is apparent from Dr. T. D. Manning's report on ophthalmology and otology at the 1877 TMA meeting. Dr. W. J. Burt reported reduction of a large fibroid tumor by administering ergotine, and Dr. R. H. L. Bibb observed that infectious diseases were due to "living germs." He warned there was "always danger lurking in water liable to contamination" from animal matter and from evacuations of patients suffering from diseases like cholera or enteric fever.

Dr. Bibb had arrived in Austin in 1873 to become assistant superintendent of the State Lunatic Asylum. An 1872 graduate of Texas Medical College, Galveston, he had also undertaken postgraduate work. He became Austin's city

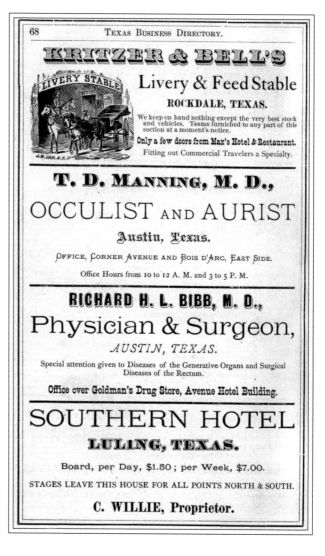

Left: Advertisement for Rucker's Southern Tonic, in Texas Business Directory, 1878-1879. Above: Advertisements for Austin physicians in Texas Business Directory, 1878-1879.

health officer, serving in the late 1870s to the early 1880s, and the state health officer from 1881 to 1885 and in 1899.

In 1878, Austin physician partners, Drs. Swearingen and Manning, responded when yellow fever struck along the lower Mississippi Valley, killing 13,000 people. While assisting in Holly Springs, Mississippi, Dr. Manning died. Memorials revealed that the loss struck his colleagues particularly hard. The next year, Dr. Swearingen participated in a federal board of experts on prevention of epidemic diseases, which increased his stature nationally.

Texas law now allowed the governor to appoint a state medical officer with authority to quarantine an area and the state appropriated $12,000 for quarantine stations along the coast and at main points of entry from other states. In 1879, Dr. Robert Rutherford became the first state health officer.

CHAPTER V

A PREEMINENTLY HEALTHY PLACE

Texas HAD BEGUN TO SET UP an infrastructure for the scientific practice of medicine, but one component, higher education, had been elusive. Economic and other reasons, including yellow fever and transportation, had been problems but, at times, there was almost a pride in ignorance. Ironically, education had been among the ideals of Stephen F. Austin and his colonists. The Texas Declaration of Independence had charged the Mexican government with failure to establish a public system of education and in 1839 the Republic of Texas Congress passed a law directing a foundation for a state university, but there had been no progress and the state constitution did not even mention universities.

In 1858, however, the Legislature called for a state university, including instruction in surgery and medicine. Finally, more than two decades later, by a statewide vote of Texas citizens in 1881, Austin was chosen as the site for the Main University of Texas. Texans, however, wanted their medical department placed elsewhere and Galveston, the largest city in the state, was se-

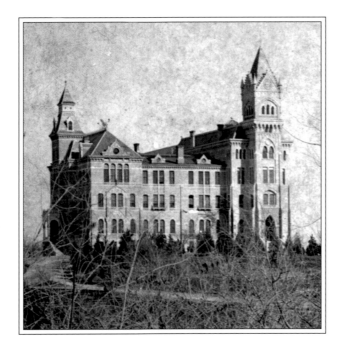

lected. The Main University opened in 1883 and the governor appointed eight regents, three of whom were physicians. All had ties to Austin. Dr. T. D. Wooten was an Austin physician; Dr. Ashbel Smith was quite familiar in Austin; and Dr. B. E. Hadra had practiced in the city.

Dr. Smith, the first president of the University of Texas Board of Regents, strove fiercely to build a high quality faculty and to obtain funding for the medical school. He had favored locating the university in Austin because he considered the city to be "preeminently healthy." However, he also fiercely supported locating the medical department in Galveston because of that thriving city's assets, including its general healthiness. He also based his argument on the existing private medical college in Galveston and its clinical opportunities, including the treatment of ill patients arriving on ships.

About this time, Travis County physicians became embroiled in an internecine matter involving several highly respected colleagues. Texas Ranger Adjutant-General John B. Jones, who had been the commander of the Frontier Battalion, became severely ill from what Nixon says may have been an "amebic abscess of the liver which subsequently ruptured into the right pleural cavity." Drs. J. E. Morris, R. M. Swearingen, E. G. Nicholson, and J. W. McLaughlin treated him but his situation deteriorated. Then, San Antonio's Dr. Ferdinand Herff observed him but found no pus by aspiration. With the patient *in extremis*, Dr. T. D. Wooten was called in, and he found evidence of fluid in the right pleural cavity. He advised aspiration, and forty ounces of pus were withdrawn. Unfortunately, Ranger Jones died the next day, July 19, 1881. The disagreement over his treatment and over who first detected the presence of pus in the pleural cavity was brought before the Travis County Medical Society, where there were heated debates. The prominent Dr. R. H. L. Bibb, as secretary, reported the controversy on forty-five pages of the *Texas Medical and Surgical Record*. Dr. Wooten followed with fifty-two more pages. The matter led the editor of the *Record* to write that "Hereafter articles containing anything of a personal nature, or consuming more than half the available space of the *Record*, must seek some other journal for publication." He later also wrote, "Let us frown down on everything that tends to belittle the individual members of the profession, in the hope that we may thereby add dignity and strength to the body of physicians at large, and to ourselves in particular."

Austin faced a hospital crisis in 1882. Physicians had worked hard to provide care for indigent individuals and the city was contracting with small physician-owned infirmaries to admit charity patients needing constant care. Smaller in-

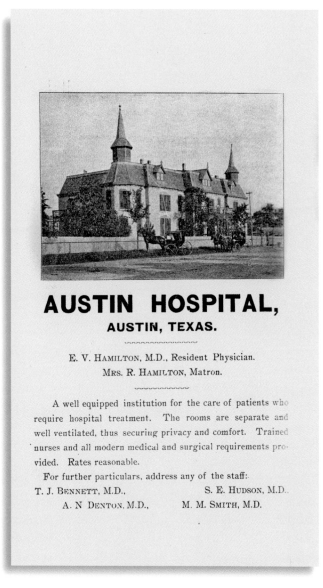

AUSTIN HOSPITAL,
AUSTIN, TEXAS.

E. V. HAMILTON, M.D., Resident Physician.
MRS. R. HAMILTON, Matron.

A well equipped institution for the care of patients who require hospital treatment. The rooms are separate and well ventilated, thus securing privacy and comfort. Trained nurses and all modern medical and surgical requirements provided. Rates reasonable.

For further particulars, address any of the staff:

| T. J. BENNETT, M.D., | S. E. HUDSON, M.D. |
| A. N DENTON, M.D., | M. M. SMITH, M.D. |

ABOVE: *Advertisement for Austin Hospital in* Texas Medical News, *1899.* OPPOSITE PAGE: *Main Building, University of Texas, Austin, ca. 1880s.*

stitutions like the Manning and other infirmaries never had sustained a profit. Dr. Hadra had closed his hospital and moved to Galveston to teach at the Texas Medical College. Further, smallpox had struck, and patients typically were taken south across the river to a pest house. One improvement was the telephone, considered "a great step in quarantine since entry and exit was reduced." The city physician, Dr. Cummings, suggested the construction of a new pest house, which evolved into the idea of a general hospital with a pest cottage attached. The city council, however, had little interest. Drs. J. W. and Frank P. McLaughlin, R. M. Swearingen, and J. J. Tobin offered to build a hospital if the city guaranteed $125 a month for five beds. Although the plan was tabled, finally, in October 1883, a city council committee was authorized to consider plans for a hospital, with the cost not to exceed $10,000.

The intent was to build on the block designated in 1839 by Edwin Waller, but a petition called for the hospital to be built outside the city, based on the belief that the prevailing winds would make it a hazard in the city. After a full review, however, the Waller plan was adopted. A committee of Austin physicians with city and county officials agreed to fund a building project, each contributing $5,000. Thus, in 1884, Austin at last fulfilled Waller's vision, completing its first public hospital on his planned site in the northeast corner of his original Austin grid. It would be the fifth known public hospital established since the founding of the Republic of Texas. The city of Galveston had the first such institution, the Island City Hospital, in 1845.

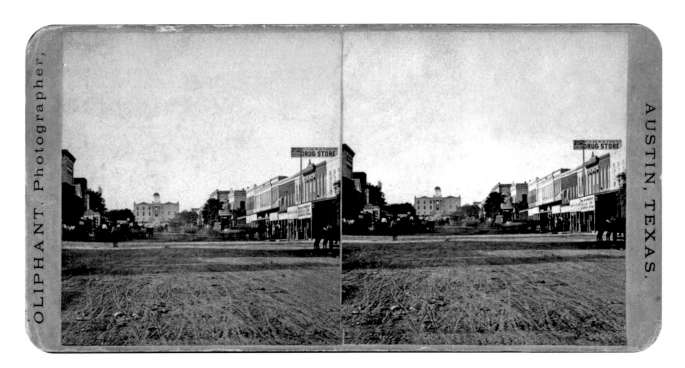

At 1405 Sabine Street, the new City-County Hospital was described as an elegant mansion with red shutters on a street lined with live oak trees, and rising "imposingly above its neighbors." The newspaper report noted that it was designed "in the admired Queen Anne style, its gables and turrets" providing a "Victorian flourish worthy" of local leaders' ambitions. Dr. W. J. Burt accepted responsibility for managing the hospital and by August moved in ten city patients from the building owned by Dr. Cummings. Dr. Burt also suggested appointment of a board of trustees and, after a druggist was accused of knocking down and beating an aged patient, the doctor suggested employing a resident physician. Dr. Frank McLaughlin assumed the position with Matron Alla Wright also living on site. The two-story building had forty beds; sleeping quarters for staff; four private patient rooms on each floor; and wards for public patients. Fifty percent of the first-year patients admitted had consumption, typhoid, dysentery, malaria fever, rheumatism, insanity, or *delirium tremens*. Dr. Burt reported further that the hospital was filled with old patients with chronic incurable diseases and no place to go.

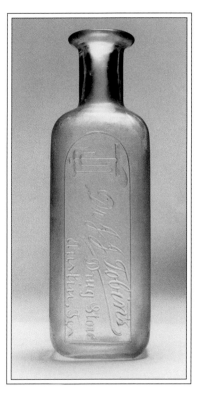

ABOVE: *Congress Avenue, Tobin Drug Store. Stereograph by W. J. Oliphant.*
LEFT: *Prescription bottle from Dr. Tobin's Drug Store.*

In 1886, the Texas Confederate Home for disabled and indigent veterans opened on West Sixth Street. Run by military veterans, it was funded with public contributions until the state assumed responsibility in 1891. A veteran, Dr. Lafayette D. Hill, was one of the first physicians to provide medical service.

Patent medicines with imaginative names and promises of elaborate cures were touted. Dr. J. J. Dulaney had one reminiscent of a future perfume. His "Joy" was supposed to be a medicine "that never fails, throat and lung diseases defied and all the other discoveries thrown in the shade." Supposedly, it was made of Texas plants and was to be a cure for consumption and many other diseases. Such patent medicines were of growing concern and doctors sought regulation of druggists and drug stores through the Texas Medical Association. They also wanted proper labeling on both patent medicines and poisons, with a registry for the sales of poisons.

Specialty hospitals were being built, and in 1883, Dr. J. D. Stansbury opened the "Austin, Texas Sanitarium," a private hospital, at Magnolia and San Jacinto with a focus on chronic and nervous diseases. Dr. Hadra returned to Austin in December 1885 and opened a private hospital for diseases of women, to be called the Ladies Infirmary, at 208 West Fourteenth Street. In 1887, the Austin Sanitarium took over the facilities where Dr. Hadra had his Ladies Infirmary. It was open to everyone except those with contagious diseases. Dr. Hadra continued to manage it with a board of directors that included Walter Tips, proprietor of a hardware business on Congress Avenue, and Drs. Frank P. McLaughlin, Ralph Steiner, and T. J. Tyner. A number of other Austinites also became stockholders, including Dr. J. J. Tobin.

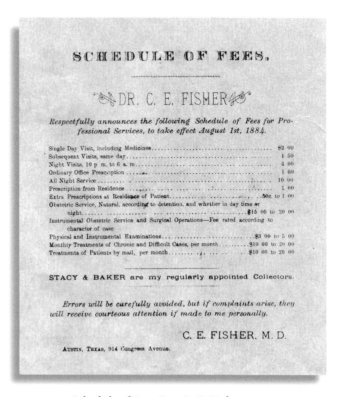

Schedule of Fees, Dr. C. E. Fisher, 1884.

Austin doctors enjoyed outside interests, from raising fine racehorses to having a model stock ranch with imported sheep. Dr. George P. Hachenberg achieved fame across the country for his medical and other scientific publications. He also wrote articles on spontaneous combustion, hygrometers, murders, criminal lawyers, and "the proper handling" of quacks.

City leaders continued to promote Austin as a healthy place, and the city directory for 1883 to 1884 used records left by an Austin physician to support the claim. Residents also enjoyed urban improvements, including water pumped through pipes to households, electric lights, and two ice companies. Gas light glowed on every street corner at night. Dr. J. J. Tobin especially loved the new electric lights and, in 1883, was the first to use colored lights, installing them in his drug store. He also held elaborate garden parties on East Pecan using twinkling lights. Besides having telegraph facilities, Austin also extended its telephone lines to Round Rock. In 1886, physicians were named to a committee to advertise the city as a health and winter resort. Included were Drs. Litten, J. W. McLaughlin, R. M. Swearingen, and T. D. Wooten along with retired physician, Dr. W. H. Tobin, and homeopathic physicians, Drs. T. Howard Bragg

and Charles E. Fisher. The *Statesman* featured the city as a resort in its Christmas edition, distributing copies throughout the country.

Dr. Fisher, who had come to Austin after graduating from a Detroit homeopathic college in 1883, established a homeopathic pharmacy; founded a journal, *The Homeopathic Pellet*; and was president of the state and national homeopathic medical associations. Samuel Hahnemann's homeopathic theory, developed in the late eighteenth century, was based on his "fight like with like theory," or the "law of similars" used in ancient cultures.

Austin became home to at least three pre-1900 journals. Dr. Fisher edited his *Pellet* at 105 East Hickory Street, changing its name to the *Southern Journal of Homeopathy*, and in 1884 selling it to a San Antonio physician. In 1885, Dr. Ferdinand Eugene Daniel launched his popular "Red Back," *Daniel's Texas Medical Journal*, dropping his name from the title in 1893. In 1896, Dr. Daniel and Dr. S. E. Hudson of Austin were listed as "editors and proprietors." The *Texas Medical Journal* served unofficially as the TMA publication until the association launched the *Texas State Journal of Medicine* in 1905 over the colorful Dr. Daniel's protests. His journal, whose theme was "down with quacks of all kinds," would have the longest life of the early entrepreneurial journals, continuing until 1920. It then acquired a new name, *Practical Medicine and Surgery*, with Dr. Daniel's spouse Josephine as the managing editor and publisher through 1924. Subsequently, it combined with *Medical Insurance and Health Conservation*, becoming *Medical Insurance* in 1925.

Born in 1839 in Hicks Ford, Virginia (which became Emporia, Virginia), Dr. Daniel attended common school in Mississippi and graduated in 1862 from the New Orleans School of Medicine. He was appointed surgeon, with the rank of major, and served in the Confederate Army until the end of the Civil War. Having previously studied law, he also became Judge Advocate General of the Army of Tennessee. He was Secretary of the Army Board of Medical Examiners in General Braxton Bragg's Army, and was attached to the staff of General William J. Hardee in the Kentucky campaign. From 1867 to 1868, he was a founder and also professor of surgery at the Texas Medical College in Galveston. He left Texas for almost twenty years to practice medicine, serve as a sanitary inspector for the National Board of Health, and manage the national quarantine station south of Vicksburg, Mississippi. In addition to his publishing and editorial ventures, Dr. Daniel authored numerous articles on a wide range of topics, including "Recollections of a Rebel Surgeon"; "A Plea for Reform in Criminal Jurisprudence"; and "Cause and Prevention of Rape." The editor of the *Texas State Journal of Medicine* extolled him: "A man of strong convictions and the courage to express them, he early gained the reputation of being a fighter...."

In 1891, the *Texas Sanitarian*, a journal of preventive medicine and hygiene, was launched by Austin physicians Drs. Thomas Joshua Bennett, J. W. McLaughlin, R. M. Swearingen (the state health officer), and T. D. Wooten. Dr. Bennett, as editor, wrote in the first issue, "Preventive Medicine has become now a recognized branch of the great science, and its beneficence is felt in lessened mortality, and the disappearance of epidemics." The first issue also contained a comparative study of the users and non-users of tobacco, and examined the physical benefit of not smoking. In 1895, the publication was renamed *Texas Medical News*, with editors Drs. Bennett and McLaughlin. Drs. Matthew M. Smith, A. N. Denton, and T. J. Bennett later were listed as editors. Associate editors included Dr. McLaughlin, then teaching in Galveston, and other physicians from Dallas, Houston, Fort Worth, Waco, and San Antonio.

Born in 1854, Dr. Bennett had graduated from the University of Louisiana's Medical Department (later Tulane University School of Medicine) in 1883 and had begun practicing medicine with Dr. L. D. Hill in Webberville. In 1884, he moved to Austin.

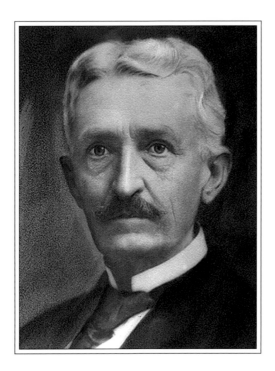

Dr. F. E. Daniel (above) launched Daniel's Medical Journal *(opposite page) in 1885.*

The Texas Medical News Publishing Company, with offices at 101 West Sixth Street in Austin, announced consolidation of several journals in 1900. Citing branch offices in Dallas and Fort Worth, the *News* claimed it had "the largest and best distributed circulation of any Texas medical journal....The *News* furnishes the subscriber more medical reading monthly than any journal in the State, and the returns it can give the advertiser are exceptionally good." Absorbed by the *News* were the *Southwestern Medical and Surgical Reporter*, Fort Worth; the *Texas Medical Practitioner*, Dallas; and the *Southwestern Medical Record*, Houston. Subscription for the *News* was one dollar per year in advance. It was published until 1916.

Dr. R. H. L. Bibb and prominent physicians from San Antonio, Galveston, Fort Worth, Marshall, and Sherman had formed a company to issue the *Texas Medical and Surgical Record*. Its first issue was January 1881 and it served briefly as the official publication for the Texas Medical Association. It apparently had considerable influence in shaping professional opinion about where the University of Texas medical school was to be located. Dr. Bibb announced in 1882 that he was moving to Saltillo in Mexico's state of Coahuila, and received high praise for his achievements in Texas. Besides his city and state duties and devotion to TMA, Dr. Bibb had been president of the Travis County Medical Society and was a member of the Board of Medical Examiners for the Sixteenth Judicial District.

Dr. Joe Rude writes that as the microscope came into general use, it would allow "physicians to take advantage of scientific advances such as the discovery of streptococcus, staphylococcus, and pneumococcus by Pasteur in 1880; Koch's discovery of the tubercle bacillus in 1882; and discovery of typhoid bacillus by Eberth in 1880. The routine use of the microscope in the study of blood and urine elements enabled both surgeons and medical men to proceed with better comprehension." Surgery also had made great strides because of the principles of asepsis and antisepsis shown by Lister in 1867. Advancements in anesthesia through ether, chloroform, nitrous oxide, and cocaine and its derivatives had further helped. At meetings of the Texas Medical Association, surgeons were presenting more than twice the numbers of papers as other doctors.

Physicians often practiced in small Travis County towns. The *History of Texas* in 1893 reported that Dr. W. A. Ellison practiced south of Austin in Manchaca and also was a merchant there. He was born in Caldwell County, studied under an uncle, and in 1876 and 1877, attended lectures at Missouri Medical College in St. Louis. "He then practiced medicine under a certificate in Manchaca until 1883, and in that year entered the Louisville Medical College, graduating...in February, 1884, receiving two gold medals. Since that time Mr. Ellison has practiced medicine in this city. In 1889, in company with P. Von Rosenberg, he embarked in the mercantile and drug business, but in January, 1893, purchased his partner's interest, since which time he has continued the business alone." Louisville Medical College merged into the University of Louisville School of Medicine, which had ties to the familiar Transylvania medical department. Missouri Medical College was absorbed by Washington University School of Medicine in St. Louis. Dr. Ellison's "certificate" came from the Board of Medical Examiners in 1877.

Also listed from Manchaca in Polk's 1886 directory, with no details, was Dr. W. J. Moore. Dr. Coleman cited a doctor with that name as a graduate of Jefferson Medical College of Philadelphia who arrived in Travis County in 1869.

A centennial history stated that "New Sweden was a bustling community center boasting of two doctors...two drug stores, and confectionery built by the doctors, and at one time a drug store operated by Theo Bloom." Polk's 1896 directory cited the presence of Dr. M. Carlsberg, with no details, and Dr. W. E. Gillespie, a regular physician and an 1890 graduate of the Medical College of Alabama, Mobile. The latter school evolved into the University of Alabama School of Medicine in Birmingham.

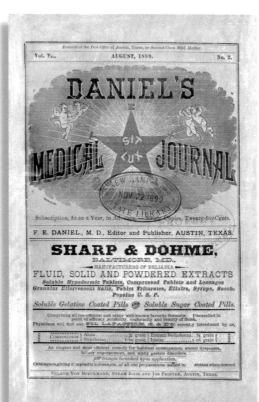

In 1871, Dr. T. O. Maxwell had arrived in Fiskville, the first stop for the stagecoach going north from Austin to Georgetown. He took a preceptorship with Drs. Wade A. Morris and J. W. McLaughlin, and in 1878 was certified by the Board of Medical Examiners. In 1882, he received his medical degree from Vanderbilt University College of Medicine. Dr. R. S. Shannon, Dr. Coleman writes, was certified by the Travis County Medical Society in 1875, and was practicing at Fiskville in 1886. Dr. Shannon likely was certified by the Travis County Board of Medical Examiners, which had been set up in 1874 after passage of the 1873 state law regulating medicine.

At Webberville, Dr. R. C. Moffett had arrived in 1853 as had Dr. J. B. Bacon. Dr. Bacon died in 1872. Dr. Lafayette D. Hill was a graduate of the University of Louisiana (which evolved into Tulane University). Arriving in 1853, he first practiced with Dr. T. J. Bennett, and later with Dr Robert Stewart, who arrived in 1861. He had joined Tom Green's Rifles, and chaperoned John Reagan's children from Richmond to Texas through the federal blockade during the Civil War. A member of the first medical examining board for the Sixteenth Judicial District in 1874, he practiced in Webberville from 1876 to 1885. A Dr. Rector also was in Webberville in 1876. Dr. John R. Simms had come in 1852, but retired from the practice of medicine in 1857. Instead, he ran for senator from Williamson County and owned a "tan yard" (for tanning hides) during the Civil War before selling it and moving to California in 1868. Also, Dr. H. P. Luckett had practiced in Webberville from 1867 to 1869, before moving to Bastrop.

Dr. W. T. Richmond began practicing in Manor in 1883, the year he graduated from the University of Louisiana (eventually Tulane University). Also in Manor were Dr. J. T. Carpenter, for whom Polk's 1886 directory had no information, and Dr. Richard S. Gregg who has been mentioned earlier. Arriving at Hornsby Bend in 1885 was Dr. Wayne Hamilton, a member of the Travis County Medical Society. Dr. J. B. Oatman practiced in Garfield from 1883 to 1884.

The *Texas Courier-Record of Medicine* cited the "Travis County Medical Association" in its February 1885 volume. "We are glad to report the reorganization of this important association, after a lapse of several months during which time they had no meetings. The members seem to have caught the inspiration of the spirit of organization and reform now stirring the Texas profession from Red river to the Gulf, and not wishing to be eclipsed by any more recent organization, have begun work again in earnest. At their last meeting, held on the 5th, [likely February 5, 1885] there was a good attendance notwithstanding the counter attraction of a grand Odd Fellows' ball going on."

The topic was "Pneumonia; is it an essential fever?" Drs. J. W. McLaughlin and T. J. Bennett had been "billed for the debate," but Dr. Bennett was ill and could not attend. Dr. McLaughlin responded that "It is of the greatest practical importance to discriminate between Pneumonia proper—*Croupous Pneumonia*—and other forms of inflammation of the lungs. Ordinary Pneumonia is an Inflammation attended with an indefinite amount of constitutional disturbance...," he said, then describing the ordinary type and noting that the "croupous" type was caused "by an unknown poison."

The *Courier-Record* also reported the organization of the Histological Society in Austin on February 5, 1885, with sixteen physicians. Members studied normal and pathologic histology using a microscope and the intentions were "to equip the society with microscopes of the best make and with all the necessary adjuncts for thorough study." The *Courier-Record* was published in Fort Worth, with Drs. W. B. Brooks and F. E. Daniel as editors. This preceded Dr. Daniel's move to Austin to start his popular "Red Back."

Travis County Medical Association, as cited in R. L. Polk's 1886 *Medical and Surgical Directory of the United States*, was meeting on the first Thursday of the month in the reading room of the Masonic Lodge in Austin. Its organizational date was listed as June 20, 1873. Officers were Drs. Daniel, president; Ralph Steiner, secretary; and T. J. Bennett, treasurer, all listed as M.D.s. [In October 1853, the original Travis Medical Society had been established as one of two district societies of the Texas Medical Association.]

The Texas Medical Association reported Dr. W. J. Burt, an M.D. from Austin, as secretary. The treasurer of the

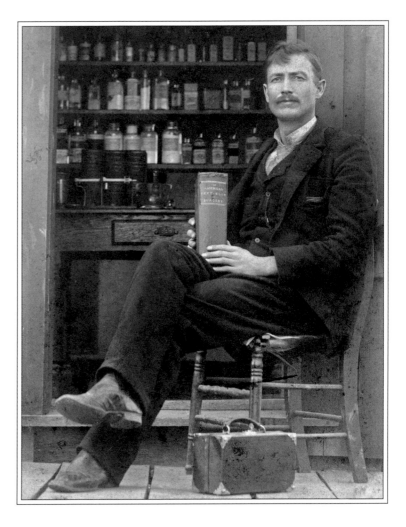

Dr. J. W. McLaughlin holding An American Textbook of Surgery, *ca. 1880s.*

Texas Homeopathic Medical Association, organized on May 1, 1884, was Dr. H. M. Bragg. The Texas Microscopical Association, organized in July 1885, cited Dr. McLaughlin as president and Dr. Daniel as secretary and treasurer.

Dr. Coleman writes that Austin's first black physician was Dr. Quinton Belvidere Neale who arrived in 1883 after earning his M.D. degree from Meharry Medical College in Nashville, Tennessee, in 1881. Also arriving was Dr. John F. McKinley, who had received his degree in 1879 from Meharry. He had undertaken postgraduate work at the University of Michigan Department of Medicine and Surgery (later the University of Michigan Medical School) in Ann Arbor in 1880 and taught physiology and histology at Meharry for three years. In Austin, he had an office at East Sixth and Brazos and specialized in ear, nose, and throat diseases. He became medical examiner for several Austin organizations, including life insurance companies, and reported that he was examiner for the state school for the mute and deaf. (It is not clear whether this was the "deaf and dumb" asylum or a similar school for colored youth. Regardless, both would be unified under the Texas School for the Deaf.) Dr. E. W. D. Abner, who graduated from Meharry in 1893, had an address in 1896 at 306 East Sixth Street in Austin. In addition to other work, he was physician for the Knights of Pythias and the Odd Fellows.

Dr. Abner also became a member of a new organization formed in Galveston in 1886, the Lone Star State Medical, Dental, and Pharmaceutical Association (at times referred to as the Lone Star State Medical Association). Drs. J. H. Wilkins and L. M. Wilkins, Galveston physicians and brothers, and Dr. J. S. Cameron, a San Antonio pharmacist, had invited all "Negro physicians" to meet with them. Twelve prospective members met during the Texas State Teachers Association meeting in Galveston. Dr. J. H. Wilkins became the first president. Only the Medico-Chirurgical Society of the District of Columbia, formed in 1884, had been organized earlier than the Texas organization. Polk's 1896 directory showed Dr. Abner as a member of the Lone Star association and Dr. McKinley as a past president.

Eighteen Austin physicians traveled to Galveston for the 1888 TMA meeting, which revealed a subtle change in membership—a "Miss" F. E. Collins of Austin, an 1886 graduate of Woman's Medical College of Chicago. She had been elected a TMA member in 1887, the first woman shown on the association's rosters. The roll also provided a picture of other Travis County members—their origins, ages, years of TMA membership, and medical education (the latter schools were all out of state).

Dr. F. E. Daniel also cited the election of "Dr. Florence E. Collins" in his *Texas Medical Journal*. "California is entitled to the credit for being the first State to recognize Lady Physicians," he said, "and Texas claims the honor of being the first to receive them into fellowship without a dissenting voice." He reported that Dr. Collins was accepted by a rising vote and was the first lady applicant the association ever had. She apparently was already the "very efficient Secretary and Treasurer" of the Travis County Medical Society and at its recent meeting had reported a case of urticario [sic]. Her state medical license was issued through Travis County on April 27, 1886. Born in 1861 in Wisconsin, she had graduated from Woman's Hospital Medical College of Chicago (later part of Northwestern University). On November 15, 1894, Dr. Collins married Dr. William J. Mathews, an 1867 graduate of the Royal College of Phy-

sicians and Surgeons in Edinburgh, Scotland. He was a widower with two sons, and his younger son, Claud Mathews, later also practiced medicine in Austin. Drs. Florence and William Mathews became the first physician couple to establish a joint practice in Austin, which continued after the birth of their daughter Florence. Dr. William Mathews also served as city health officer and president of the school board.

Dr. Ralph Steiner, the son of Dr. J. M. Steiner, served as the U.S. consul in Munich during the administration of President Grover Cleveland (1885-1889). An 1883 graduate of the University of Maryland School of Medicine, he attended many clinics and lectures in his specialty of otolaryngology while in Munich. He had practiced in Austin since 1885, served as aurist for the State School for the Deaf, and would become state health officer from 1911 to 1915. He also would be known as "The Father of the Sanitary Drinking Cup" and the "best known otolaryngologist in Texas," as Mrs. S. C. Red writes in *The Medicine Man in Texas*. In addition, he served on the University of Texas Board of Regents.

Dr. B. E. Hadra would be recognized nationally for his scientific work, particularly his method of repairing the pelvic floor. He published one of his two books, *Lesions of the Vaginal and Pelvic Floor*, in 1888. His work was "a signpost in the history of American gynecology" which marked "the beginning of modern operations for prolapse." Dr. Hadra reportedly became the first surgeon to "recognize the relationship of the diaphragm to rectocele and cystocele and to devise an operation for correction of these conditions."

Texas Medical Association leaders periodically tried to initiate a library and suggested housing it at the University of Texas or at the Capitol. Apparently, substantial association records were being kept in the hall of the Travis County Medical Society and in the office of the TMA secretary, Dr. Daniel of Austin. "It is extremely unfortunate," he told members in 1889, "that our committee failed to procure rooms in the Capitol for the use of this Association, since the accumulated archives and library have outgrown their quarters. No provision has ever been made by this society for them, and I would suggest that it would be well to authorize the secretary to purchase or have made a suitable receptacle for their preservation."

Also in 1889, two important events occurred: TMA sought a single state board of medical examiners appointed by the governor although it would be many years before this would see fruition and Dr. R. M. Swearingen became the first Travis County physician elected TMA president.

CHAPTER VI

UP TO DATE

B Y NOW MEDICINE IN TRAVIS County, Dr. James Coleman writes, was typical of that in America. Dr. J. W. McLaughlin served on a new Texas Medical Association Committee on Microscopy and Pathology formed in 1890 and chaired by the Osler-trained Dr. George Dock of Galveston. Dr. McLaughlin also presented a paper on immunity and contagion at the 1890 TMA meeting and in 1892 expanded on his concepts in a book, *Fermentation, Infection, and Immunity: A New Theory of These Processes, Which Unifies Their Primary Causation and Places the Explanation of their Phenomena in Chemistry, Biology and the Dynamics of Molecular Physics.*

Also at the 1890 meeting, Dr. Q. C. Smith of Austin, who, Dr. Nixon writes, "had an inventive turn of mind," once again demonstrated his surgical inventions, this time exhibiting obstetrical and rectal instruments. One doctor remarked that Dr. Smith "reminded him of a man who had an improved speculum which could be used at will,

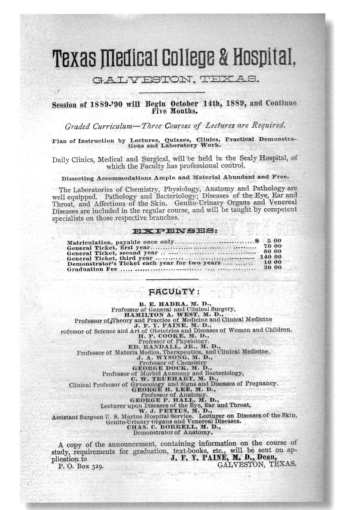

either as a speculum or as a tongue depressor." Dr. Smith was an 1868 graduate of the University of Nashville (a root school of the University of Tennessee Health Science Center College of Medicine). He reported that he was a life foundation fellow of the Society of Science, Letters and Art in London, a life member of the American Association for the Advancement of Science and the Texas Academy of Science, and belonged to many other organizations including the American Medical Association. He practiced at 617 Colorado in Austin.

Dr. Frances "Fanny" Elizabeth Daniel Leake (some sources spell her name without the final "e") became the second woman to practice regular medicine in Austin. An 1887 graduate of Woman's Hospital Medical College of Chicago, later a part of Northwestern University, she became superintendent of the Texas Department of Health and Hospitals. The mother of four daughters, she was one of the first women named to a state position. When seeking the support of a former professor for her application as

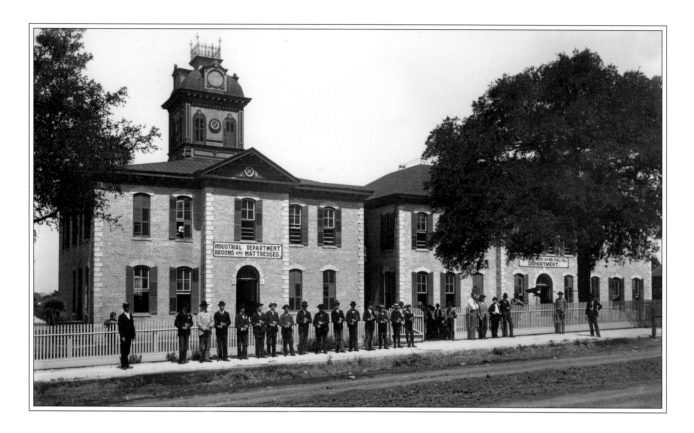

ABOVE: *The second location for the Texas School for the Blind. The building now is part of the University of Texas "Little Campus," Martin Luther King Jr. Blvd. and Interstate 35.* OPPOSITE PAGE: *Advertisement for Texas Medical College & Hospital, Galveston, 1889.*

superintendent, she had written a poignant yet gentle letter about the challenges she faced. "...owing to the South being so averse to accord anything to a woman, my political friends desired me to secure some testimonials from prominent Drs. in the North—Those we can string a lot of titles after names, members of the College faculty, if I could, as this they thought would go far toward removing prejudice from strangers and materially aid them in interesting other politicians in my cause."

The final decade of the nineteenth century brought great satisfaction to doctors who had pressed hard for a state medical school. In 1890, a teaching hospital, John Sealy, opened its doors in Galveston and in 1891 the long-awaited University of Texas Medical Department admitted its first students. Various admission requirements had been established to fill the school's first-year classes, and certain students meeting stiff requirements were able to enter as third-year students. Thus, a little more than a year after opening, in April 1892, the first state medical school in Texas graduated its first class. An Austin doctor, the "Honorable T. D.

Wooten, M.D., president of the Board of Regents," conferred the degree of doctor of medicine on three students. In 1919, the school acquired its designation as the University of Texas Medical Branch (UTMB), a familiar *alma mater* for many future Travis County physicians.

Only two months after its opening in 1890, John Sealy Hospital became the site of the John Sealy Training School for Nurses. With eighteen students, it was the first nursing school in Texas. Fort Worth Medical School—a medical department for the nonexistent Fort Worth University—also began classes in the 1890s and became the *alma mater* for a good number of Texas physicians.

Although limiting one's practice to surgery was not common, Dr. James E. Thompson of Galveston, UTMB professor of surgery, announced in 1891 that he was the first in the state to do so. In Austin, general surgery could be considered the first specialty, followed by the combined practice of ophthalmology and otorhinolaryngology. These self designations occurred long before the advent of a specialty board certification process. Long a topic of discussion, specialization had first been talked about by TMA doctors in 1869.

By 1892, Austin had forty-one doctors, including two oculist-aurist specialists, Drs. T. J. Tyner and W. H. Way. Most had offices along or near Congress Avenue and the state Capitol and two practiced in south Austin. Medical societ-

Geo. W. Hooton's
Medical Remedies,

if prescribed, will cure every case of Deafness, Rheumatism, White Swelling, Erysipelas, Cuts, Sprains, Burns, Scalds, Granulated Sore Eyes, Bad Blood. Skin Diseases, Scrofula, Sores, Coughs, Colds, Diphtheria, Stings or Bites of Insects or Reptiles, Congestion. Dyspepsia, Fever, Lung, Stomach, Bladder, Kidney and Spinal Diseases, by internal and external use.

MANY FRAUDS

have gone out and made men rich—don't think my remedies are also frauds till they have failed to cure you. This pamphlet notice may prove a blessing to you if you will give

Oil of Bloggettia

a fair trial. These remedies are made from a fusion of the finest drug oils in the world, and, though newly discovered, so many ailing and afflicted have been cured by them, upon whom all others had failed, that I am determined they shall find their way, as they have already largely done, into every part of the world.

Retail price or by mail, properly packed,

25 cents, 50 cents and $1.00 per bottle.

DRUGGISTS' ORDERS SOLICITED.

GEO. W. HOOTON,
Creedmoor, Travis County, Texas.

Advertisement for Geo. W. Hooton's Medical Remedies, 1893.

ies included the Austin District Medical Society, which met four times a year [the district society would have included physicians from surrounding counties]. The city directory indicated it had been organized on September 8, 1887; most recently had seventy-seven members; and met regularly at the medical hall, 513 Congress Avenue. Dr. J. W. McLaughlin was president; Dr. W. A. Ellison, first vice president; Dr. J. W. Hamilton, second vice president; and Dr. T. J. Bennett, secretary and treasurer. The board of censors was made up of Drs. A. N. Denton, A. J. Davis, T. O. Maxwell, S. E. Hudson, and F. R. Martin. [The "medical hall" cited may be the one to which Dr. Daniel referred in his complaint regarding the need for more space for TMA archives.]

The Travis County Medical Society had twenty-five members, and met on the first and third Thursdays of the month at the medical hall. Dr. B. F. Church was president; Dr. Frank Litten, vice-president; and Dr. J. Cummings, secretary and treasurer. The Texas Medical Association had 500 members and met the fourth Tuesday of each April. Dr. F. E. Daniel was secretary.

In 1894, a TMA study on county and district societies found that the Austin District Medical Society had 106 members with an average attendance of 35 and the Travis County Medical Society had 25 members with an average of 10 attending meetings. Only 13 of the 29 TMA-affiliated societies were active, and the vice president conducting the survey hoped for "an early resurrection day" when it would be discovered that societies "were not dead, but sleeping." TCMS may have been napping a little.

Polk's 1896 directory showed that Dr. H. B. Hill, Congress Avenue and Sixth Street in Austin, was secretary of the Travis County Medical Society and Dr. S. E. Hudson, 910 Congress Avenue, was secretary of the Austin District Medical Society. As district secretary, Dr. Hudson published a notice in the *Texas Medical Journal* (the "Red Back") that the thirty-sixth quarterly meeting of the district would be held September 24, 1896, in Austin. "An unusually interesting programme has been arranged..." he said, "We promise you a pleasant and profitable time."

Austin physicians' fees from this time revealed greater sophistication in the use of the microscope and laboratory examinations. They also seemed relatively high considering that Texas had suffered an economic depression in 1891 and, along with the rest of the country, the Panic of 1893. (Cotton had dropped to its lowest price at five cents per pound and corn was fifty-three cents per bushel.) Microscopic examination of urine was five to ten dollars as was the administration of anesthetics. A natural delivery (four hours) was twenty to thirty dollars; a laparotomy, $200 to $500; and capital operations from $100 to $1,000.

In 1894, again hosting the TMA, Austin physicians planned to see that guests were cared for in a "comfortable and elegant style," although at least two persons had to be lodged in a room. The Driskill Hotel offered board and lodging *per diem* at $2.50; the Hotel Salge and the Avenue Hotel, $2.00; the Hotel Orr, $1.50; and the Austin House,

$1.25. Dr. Daniel's "Red Back" announced that "Austin will have on her loveliest spring attire in April. Strawberries will be ripe, and roses in bloom. Our sweet south breezes will be laden with the breath of violets."

Dr. J. W. McLaughlin became the second physician from Travis County to serve as TMA president. Born near Springfield, Ohio, in September 1840, Dr. McLaughlin had taken a preceptorship with his uncle before attending a Cincinnati medical college. After serving in the Confederate Army, he received his M.D. degree in 1867 from what became Tulane University School of Medicine. Angry over the Civil War, he had started out for South America, but during a stop in Texas, he fell in love with his future wife. Practicing medicine first in Fayette County, he moved to Austin in 1870. In 1897, he filled a vacancy at the new University of Texas Medical Department after the first of the eight original professors resigned. Dr. McLaughlin also became the first instructor at UTMB to incorporate laboratory work into clinical teaching, and became chairman of the department of medicine. Active in numerous scientific and professional organizations as well as being a prolific author, he was president of the Travis County Medical Society and of the original Texas Academy of Science. He also became a University of Texas regent.

More specialized institutions were opening. The Hagey Institute of Austin, serving patients with addictions, was established in 1893. Dr. J. J. Tobin was president and treasurer and Dr. T. S. Petty had responsibility for therapy. In 1895, Drs. Hilgartner, McLaughlin, and Thomas Wooten, along with civic leader Alexander P. Wooldridge, incorporated the Texas Eye and Ear and Throat Charity Hospital.

Dr. Henry L. Hilgartner moved to Austin in 1891 and in 1896 founded the Texas Eye, Ear, Nose, and Throat Hospital. Born in 1868 in Baltimore, Maryland, he graduated from the University of Maryland School of Medicine in 1889 and interned at Presbyterian Eye, Ear, and Throat Charity Hospital of Baltimore. The *Texas State Journal of Medicine* described Dr. Hilgartner as "one of the foremost ophthalmologists in Texas. He was an original and advanced

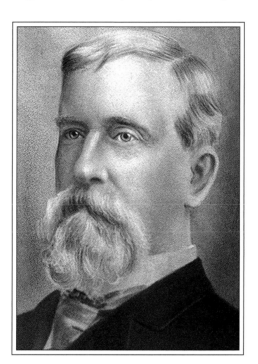

Dr. R. M. Swearingen was the first Austin physician elected as Texas Medical Association president.

thinker." Dr. Hilgartner also was an active participant and presenter at medical meetings, and in 1897, presented a TMA paper on "hypertrophy of the pharyngeal tonsil," stating that if general treatment and cod liver oil failed, there should be a "complete extirpation" of the tonsil.

Physicians whose service would extend into the next century were coming home to Austin. Drs. Goodall Harrison Wooten and Joe Sil Wooten, sons of Dr. T. D. Wooten, were among those returning and both would join their father's practice. Dr. Goodall Wooten had graduated in 1895 from what became Columbia University College of Physicians and Surgeons in New York. Born in 1869 in Paris, Texas, he earned a bachelor's degree in 1891 and a master's degree in 1892 from the University of Texas (UT). Dr. Joe Sil Wooten, who was born in 1871, also in Paris, Texas, graduated from UT in 1892 and also received his medical degree from Columbia University College of Physicians and Surgeons. Specializing in surgery, Dr. Joe Sil Wooten would serve as surgeon for the Missouri-Kansas-Texas Railroad Company and the International-Great Northern Railroad Company. The Wooten family had moved to the capital in 1876.

Only a few years after serving as TMA president, Austin's Dr. R. M. Swearingen, died in 1897 of glomerulonephritis.

In 1898, Dr. M. M. Smith of Austin was one of two TMA presenters on tuberculosis. "Sixteen years after Robert Koch had proved the contagiousness of the disease," Dr. Nixon writes, "there was still an alarming ignorance and carelessness as to its hazards. The old dogma of heredity was still abroad in the land. Both authors realized that prevention rather than cure was paramount. Both advocated education of the public and construction of state sanatoriums."

Also at the 1898 meeting was a new TMA member from Travis County, Dr. Joseph Gilbert, who had practiced briefly at Bastrop and Hornsby Bend before moving to Austin that year. Born in May 1873 at Hornsby Bend and first schooled there, he attended Austin High School in the 1880s and graduated in 1894 from the Agricultural and Mechanical College of Texas, later Texas A&M University. University of Texas Medical Department records show him as an 1897 graduate. Almost seventy years earlier, Dr. Joe Gilbert's great grandfather, Reuben Hornsby, had settled on a Stephen F. Austin land grant east of the future capital. Josiah Wilbarger's brother John had written that "a more beautiful tract of land can nowhere, even now, be found than the league of land granted to Reuben Hornsby." Dr. Gilbert, who later undertook postgraduate work in New York, Boston, Minnesota, Canada, and Europe, would have a long and distinguished history in Travis County and Texas medicine.

Great change was afoot. Rapidly expanding Texas railroads required surgeons along their routes and spawned group practices. In nearby Temple, Drs. Arthur C. Scott and Raleigh R. White, Jr., who had been physicians for the Santa Fe Hospital in Temple, formed the Temple Sanitarium, which became known simply as Scott and White. Austin had no railway hospitals, typically found in smaller Texas towns, but it had physicians who served the railroads. In addition, physicians were examiners for insurance companies.

In Minnesota, Dr. William W. Mayo and his sons, Drs. William J. Mayo and Charles H. Mayo, were leading the way toward group medical practice. The senior Dr. Mayo announced that it had become necessary "to develop medicine as a cooperative science; the clinician, the specialist, and the laboratory workers uniting for the good of the patient." He added that "Individualism in medicine can no longer exist." To Texas individualists, that probably was not a particularly comforting thought. On the other hand, Texas doctors had been forming partnerships for some time, if informally.

A new field of medicine was appearing in Texas. Andrew Taylor Still had developed the concepts of osteopathic medicine in 1874 as a frontier physician in Kansas and later in Missouri. In 1892, the first school of osteopathy was

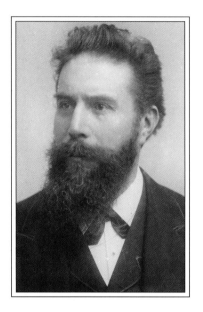

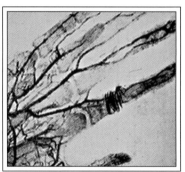

Dr. Wilhelm Roentgen (top) discovered the x-ray in 1895. Austin's first x-ray machine was built in 1897 (above). OPPOSITE PAGE: *City of Austin Physician's report, 1898-1899.*

established in Kirksville, Missouri, and an organization formed by students in 1897 evolved into the American Osteopathic Association. Dr. Mollie Baldwin, an osteopathic physician, was in practice in Waco by at least 1897, and in 1898, Dr. Rose Bathwick was in the *Austin City Directory*.

In San Antonio, Dr. Leonard Wood and Colonel Theodore Roosevelt trained the "Rough Riders" for the Spanish-American war. Texas physicians offered their services in the conflict, which saw seven times more deaths from disease (more than half from typhoid) than from bullets. Dr. Walter Reed and his commission, assigned the task of resolving the spread of typhoid in army camps, found that flies were the carriers, with dust and uncleanliness facilitating the spread. Meanwhile, Theobald Smith, Ph.D., and others demonstrated that ticks were vectors in the transmission of Texas cattle fever.

Wilhelm Conrad Roentgen had discovered the Roentgen, or x-ray, in 1895 and Antoine Henri Becquerel discovered radioactivity in 1896. Application of these discoveries had been rapid. Dr. Seth Morris, son of Dr. Wade Morris of Austin and a professor of ophthalmology at UTMB, became one of the first to have an x-ray machine in Texas, building one in 1897.

In less than a century, Travis County doctors had helped build a new republic, a new state, and a new capital. They had initiated a state medical association, established journals, and advocated laws for better health care. The Travis County Medical Society had seen Drs. R. M. Swearingen and J. W. McLaughlin elected presidents of the Texas Medical Association and had brought the first woman into the state association's membership. Austin was home to the long-awaited Main University (with its own medical department, albeit many miles from the city). More physicians now had formal education and some had become leading professors. Medical education standards, however, remained lax and although medicine had seen great scientific leaps, it had much more to learn.

Report of City Physician for month of December 1898

Hon. John D. McCall Mayor & City Council.

Number of Patients in Hospital December 1st 1898 — 22
Number of Patients Admitted to Hospital during
the month of December 1898 — 19
Number of Patients dismissed from the Hospital
during December 1898 — 12
Number of deaths in Hospital during December 1898 — 2
Cause of death Syphilis — 1 Malarial Fever — 1
Number of Patients remaining in Hospital
January 1st A.D. 1899 — 27
Number of visits made Pauper Patients in
city during December 1898 — 118
Number of Prescriptions written for Paupers
in city during December 1898 — 188
Number cases of Diphtheria reported in city
during December 1898 — 1
No other contagious or infectious diseases
reported during December 1898
The LaGrippe is prevailing to a considerable
extent throughout the city but generally in
a mild form. with this exception the general health
of the city is good.

Respectfully Submitted.
R. S. Graves M. D.
City Physician

CHAPTER VII

GOODBYE TO A FLAMBOYANT CENTURY

MEMORIALIZED AT THE SPRING meeting of the Texas Medical Association (TMA) was Dr. J. M. Litten, one of ten signers of the 1852 invitation from Travis County physicians to form a state organization. Only two signers remained alive, Drs. R. N. Lane and W. A. Morris. Dr. Morris died two years later at the age of ninety after practicing for more than sixty years. The date of Dr. Lane's death is not known. Dr. F. E. Daniel of Austin also eulogized Dr. R. M. Swearingen, Travis County's first TMA president, in an elegant six-page memorial.

Months later, the nation's most devastating natural disaster struck Galveston, home of the young University of Texas Medical Department. The Austin *Daily Statesman* recounted the night of September 8, 1900: "The storm which raged all across the gulf coast on Friday and yesterday was in evidence in Austin late afternoon and night. The

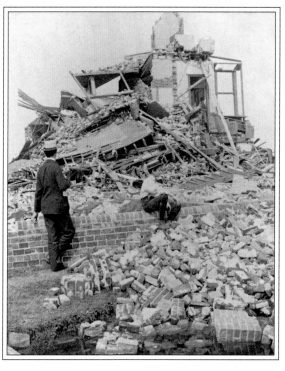

wind blew at a very high rate from dark on until an early hour this morning. The high wind was accompanied by a heavy rainfall filling all the gutters and waterways to overflowing.... During the day the reports reaching the city from Galveston were extremely alarming, and inasmuch as the telegraph wires were all down and there was no means of communicating with the Island City, none of the wild rumors could be confirmed."

Future Austin physician Zachary Thomson Scott, a medical student, was at St. Mary's Hospital in Galveston. Paul Lester, the author of *The Great Galveston Disaster*, reported that the infirmary was composed of a large brick building and several wooden structures, which housed nearly 200 patients "too sick and weak to battle against the elements and the raging storm, besides a score of sisters who were at the time acting as nurses." Scott left the brick building and began carrying each patient through waist-deep water. "Over 200 times he performed this feat, although before the task was completed the water between the two buildings was over six feet in depth," Lester writes. Even with debris flying, young Scott reportedly rescued everyone. The wooden structures were destroyed. "Such courage, devotion and heroism deserves a place side by side with that of the greatest heroes who ever lived," the author concluded.

The Medical Department did not escape—the old dome of the red brick building was gone, leaving a great gap in the roof. Inside was tangled rubbish. Even the "dead house" lost its roof, ruining cadavers. Estimates on the number of people who died during the storm range from six to eight thousand in the city of Galveston, with another two to four thousand deaths elsewhere on the island. Austin residents held a mass meeting, naming representatives of each ward to secure food, clothing, and cash. Dr. Ralph Steiner represented Ward 2 and Dr. V. O. King's wife Ward 11 in south Austin. More than $3,000 was collected and Dr. T. J. Jones of the state health department left for Galveston to render "any assistance in his power."

The *Daily Statesman* reported that Dr. J. W. McLaughlin, who had been appointed to the Galveston medical faculty in 1897, had telegraphed that he and his family were safe. On September 17, the newspaper reported that "Dr. Joe Gilbert and wife, who were married in Galveston last Thursday, have arrived in the city [Austin] and are guests of Mr. and Mrs. John W. Hornsby. Mrs. Gilbert had an almost miraculous escape from the fury of the storm. Her room alone of sixty in the large Lucas flats of that city remained intact when the building collapsed. Of the 100 people in the building at the time all were drowned with the exception of 22 with Mrs. Gilbert. After remaining until the next morning at 5 o'clock, they were rescued and carried to the Tremont Hotel, where Dr. Gilbert succeeded in

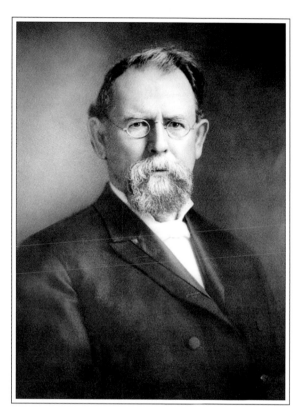

ABOVE: *University of Texas President William L. Prather supported education for the medical profession.* OPPOSITE PAGE: *Dr. Joe Gilbert's wife survived the destruction of the Lucas flats during the Galveston disaster.*

finding her." "I never expected to find her alive," he told a reporter, "but I intended to at least rescue her body. After reaching Houston I had some difficulty reaching Texas City, and after reaching there to secure passage to Galveston. However I succeeded in getting to Galveston and in locating Miss Thorne, and you may believe during all those harrowing times we lost no time in getting married and returning to Austin." "While worried almost wild myself, I could not help being shocked by the horrible scenes...." he added. "Though a physician and used to suffering and death, the sights there sickened me and I hope never to be so unfortunate as to view them again.... It is unquestionably the most horrible catastrophe that happened in the United States."

In addition to his private medical practice, listed in 1906 at 504 Congress Avenue, Dr. Gilbert served as surgeon for the Texas Confederate Home and as health officer for Austin and Travis County. He left Austin in 1906 to become the physician for Texas A&M, returning to Austin after two years. In 1909, he was asked to start the University of Texas student health service and, except for ten years, served as director until his retirement in 1946. During that period, he also served as physician for UT athletic teams. In 1914, as a new fellow of the American College of Surgeons, he began specializing in surgery. Polk's directory for that year listed him at the Scarbrough Building. In the 1920s, Dr. Gilbert became a member of the State Board of Health. He also was president of Travis County Medical Society and the Texas Medical Association, and became a founder of St. David's Hospital in Austin.

Although the cavalier issuance of medical diplomas through "diploma mills" was plaguing Texas, efforts were under way to build legitimate medical schools. A Dallas school affiliated in 1903 with Waco's Baylor University, from

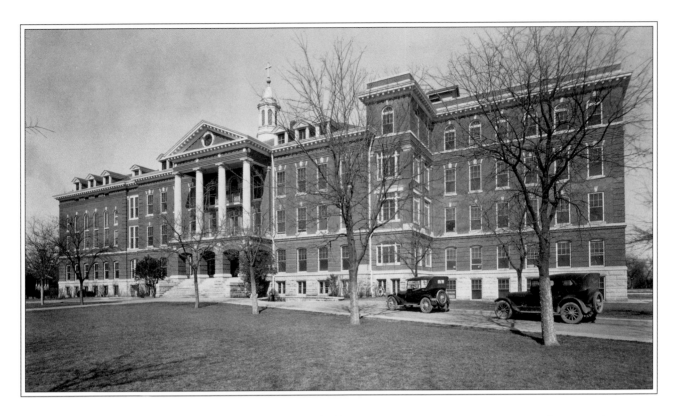

which Baylor University College of Medicine emerged. Baylor absorbed a second Dallas school and, in 1918, the old Fort Worth Medical School. In 1904, Southern Methodist University (SMU) opened its own medical school based upon one that had been formed nominally as Southwestern University Medical College. SMU graduated its last class in 1915.

Until the mid-1940s, Texas-educated doctors would come primarily from the University of Texas Medical Department (which in 1919 became the University of Texas Medical Branch) and Baylor University College of Medicine, including the schools it had absorbed. Out-of-state schools like Memphis Hospital Medical College and Tulane University School of Medicine, however, would have high numbers of applicants seeking licenses in Texas.

Texas doctors had attempted in the past to raise standards by seeking a single state medical licensure board. Instead, a 1901 compromise led to three separate boards for homeopathic, eclectic, and allopathic—or regular—physicians. Exempt were Christian Scientists, physicians practicing in Texas before 1885, and those who had recorded diplomas since 1891 with evidence that they came from medical colleges of respectable standing. Doctors from other states with equal requirements also did not have to be examined. Dr. M. M. Smith of Austin was appointed to the Board of Medical Examiners, which licensed allopathic physicians, and was elected secretary.

The loopholes in the three-board system caused dissatisfaction and a new fear was raised. Osteopathic physicians were arriving in Texas from the college in Kirksville, Missouri, and there were concerns they would obtain their own medical examining board. In addition, minor groups did not want to be absorbed by the regular profession. Meetings of constituencies resulted in the passage of the historic "one board" bill, which was signed into law in April 1907. Homeopaths, eclectics, osteopaths, physio-medicists, and allopaths now reported to the Texas State Board of Medical Examiners. The law—to become known as the Medical Practice Act—would remain the basis of the Texas medical system, although it would be amended many times. Dr. John F. Bailey, D.O., of Waco was the first osteopathic physician on the board.

Texas now required applicants to be "graduates of bona fide, reputable medical schools" that provided instruction of four terms of five months each. The new examining board cracked down on "diploma mills" and tried to enforce standards of licensees. Further, the American Medical Association had begun inspecting medical schools and recommended completion of a high school education as a prerequisite for entrance. It commissioned a study through the Carnegie Foundation for the Advancement of Teaching conducted by Abraham Flexner, which became a watershed for improvement of medical education in the United States and Canada. Published in 1910, it directly affected Texas schools; only one of four inspected, the University of Texas Medical Department, was deemed acceptable. Baylor University's medical program offered promise but suffered because of its "quite bare" laboratory and little assurance for supporting funds. Although prais-

ing the University of Texas Medical Department, Flexner offered constructive advice and criticism, including an opinion pertinent to Austin:

Meanwhile, to the outsider it seems a regrettable mischance that located the medical department away from the university. Were it placed at Austin, it would apparently gain in every way: the town is as large, and various state institutions there would strengthen its clinical opportunities; it would be easier to attract and to hold outsiders in teaching positions; the stimulus of the university would assist the growth of a productive spirit. Whether at Galveston the school will ever be creative is a question; should it become so, isolation increases the liability to slip back into an unproductive groove. Perhaps it is not yet too late for the people of the state to concentrate their state institutions of higher learning in a single plant.

In future years, this statement might hold special meaning for supporters of a University of Texas medical school in Austin.

Change also was stirring the nursing field. Student nurses had been trained in hospitals, but there were now efforts

to require more formal credentialing. In 1907, the Graduate Nurses Association of Texas, eventually the Texas Nurses Association, was formed and, in 1909, the Nurse Practice Act created the Texas Board of Nurse Examiners to examine and license nurses.

In 1902, a new hospital opened in Austin. St. Vincent's Aid Society had been concerned that Catholics were not receiving sacraments in hospitals and had appealed to the Daughters of Charity of St. Vincent de Paul. The Order agreed to open a new hospital if grounds and an appropriate facility could be provided. With the funds raised, the society purchased land on Twenty-sixth Street between Nueces and Rio Grande Streets. Named for Elizabeth Ann Seton, founder of the Sisters of Charity in America, Seton Infirmary was a four-story, red-pressed brick structure in southern colonial style. It had seventeen private rooms, eleven wards, and separate quarters for the sisters. Austin's first nursing school, with four students, also began on the top floor.

Polk's 1902 directory showed that the city- and county-owned hospital, called City-County Hospital had an ambulance service, and the 1906 directory showed that Seton also had an ambulance service. The first ambulances were horse drawn with the bodies of some ambulances later motorized before actual motor-driven vehicles became available.

In 1907, Travis County withdrew its support for the city- and county-owned hospital, which had a capacity of forty beds. Dr. Robert J. Brackenridge led the fight to pass bonds for a new hospital building, and in 1915, the forty-five-bed City Hospital, near the original hospital, was completed. Along with the new city hospital in Austin, a second nursing school also opened in 1915.

Dr. Brackenridge was named board chairman of City Hospital, serving until his death in 1918. On the board with him were Drs. S. E. Hudson, Joe Gilbert, Frederick Eby, and Margaret Holliday. In 1929, the Austin City Council renamed the hospital in Dr. Brackenridge's honor. Although he had earned a medical degree from Rush Medical College, Chicago, and practiced for awhile elsewhere, Dr. Brackenridge primarily was a businessman of wide interests. He came from a prominent family with ties to early American leaders; one of his brothers was George Washington Brackenridge, often known as Colonel Brackenridge, who

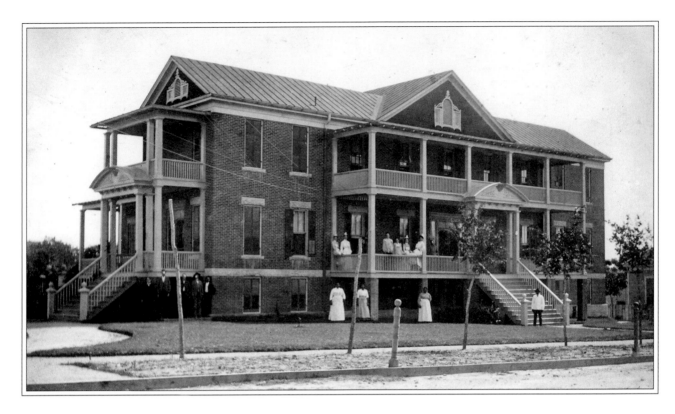

Austin Sanitarium was purchased by Thomas J. Bennett and Zachary T. Scott, ca. 1909.

settled in San Antonio and became a prominent banker, business, and civic leader there, and also a long-time member of the University of Texas Board of Regents. Brackenridge Hall, or Old B Hall, on the University of Texas campus was named for him. In 1874, Dr. Robert Brackenridge and brothers John Thomas Brackenridge and James Madison Brackenridge came to Austin, leaving the family home in Texana, Texas, a community in Jackson County, 130 miles southeast of the capital. The three brothers entered the banking business in Austin, establishing the First National Bank at Congress Avenue and Pecan (Sixth) Street. Robert discontinued the practice of medicine and became the cashier.

The first hospitals in Austin and Travis County had been private institutions run primarily by doctors. Fighting economic challenges, they had had a chameleonlike existence. Austin Sanitarium, however, at Fourteenth Street and Congress Avenue, had survived the previous century. In 1909, Drs. Z. T. (Zachary) Scott and T. J. Bennett had purchased the three-story brick facility, and in 1915, the Presbyterian Church bought it and renamed it the Presbyterian Sanitarium.

A view of Austin's medical and health organizations is seen through R. L. Polk's 1902 *Medical Register and Directory of the United States and Canada.* Dr. S. A. Harper was secretary of both the Austin Academy of Medicine and the Austin District Medical Society. The Texas Homeopathic Medical Association had three officers from Austin: William D.

Gorton, president; Julia H. Bass, secretary; and T. J. Crowe, treasurer. Polk's 1906 directory cited the Austin (Seventh) District Medical Association of the Texas Medical Association, with Dr. M. M. Smith as district president and Dr. W. A. Harper as secretary and treasurer. Dr. J. W. McLaughlin, Jr., was secretary of the Travis County Medical Society.

In 1903, the county medical society became the fundamental unit of the Texas Medical Association and the American Medical Association. This led to significant TMA membership increases and much greater influence in public affairs, including more legislative successes. Two Austin doctors served in the provisional TMA House of Delegates formed in 1903, with Dr. M. M. Smith representing "Austin Medical" and Dr. F. E. Daniel representing Austin District. Dr. T. J. Bennett of Austin became councilor for the new seventh district (succeeding the old Austin district) that comprised Travis and other Central Texas counties. The Travis County Medical Society, which apparently had stopped meeting again in the late 1890s, was revitalized in 1903.

Dr. Daniel's October 1905 "*Red Back*" reported on a district meeting in September 1905. Dr. W. Neal Watt had "a valuable paper on Tetanus"; Dr. W. J. Mathews discussed the ice pack in pneumonia; and Dr. M. M. Smith, the sanitarium treatment of tuberculosis. Dr. S. E. Hudson, who had been a TMA delegate to the AMA, reported on the recent meeting in Portland, Oregon. An "Editorialet" in this issue also substantiated that certain problems were being addressed out of state. The editor reported that Dr. B. M. Worsham, superintendent of the State Lunatic Asylum, had just recovered from an attack of appendicitis and "has gone to New York to have the thing cut out."

The Lone Star State Medical Association of Texas held its sixteenth meeting in Austin in June 1902, with fourteen members present. Nixon reports that the papers were similar to those at the Texas Medical Association meeting. Appearing before their "Negro brethren" were Dr. M. M. Smith, editor of the *Texas Medical News*, and a "Dr. Matthews." [The only member of the Travis County Medical Society with a similar name at the time was Dr. W. J. Mathews.] The association had met sporadically since its organization in Galveston, possibly because as late as 1901 no more than twenty African-American physicians were practicing in Texas. Two physicians, Drs. Edward W. D. Abner and James D. Daviss, were living in Austin. In 1898, Dr. Daviss practiced at 422 East Sixth Street. Another black physician who lived in Austin was Dr. John H. Stevens, born in Louisville, Kentucky, whose death came in the capital on June 15, 1932. Dr. Daviss had graduated from Meharry Medical College in 1891; Dr. Stevens in 1892; and, as reported earlier, Dr. Abner in 1893.

Dr. B. E. Hadra, twice an Austin physician and a past TMA president, was memorialized in 1903. Recognized nationally, he had also raised the level of scientific medicine in Austin and had diligently developed private hospitals, including a specialized "Ladies Infirmary."

This was a time of great advancement in basic science and clinical medicine. In 1905, Albert Einstein presented his revelations on time and space and Alexis Carrel sutured blood vessels and transplanted a puppy's kidney to another dog. Further, in 1901, the U.S. Army's Yellow Fever Commission, led by Dr. Walter Reed, resolved the question of the source of transmission of the disease that drove Texas coastal residents to Austin for respite. Dr. William C. Gorgas, who oversaw the eradication of mosquitoes in Cuba, soon eradicated them in Panama and also eliminated rats carrying bubonic plague.

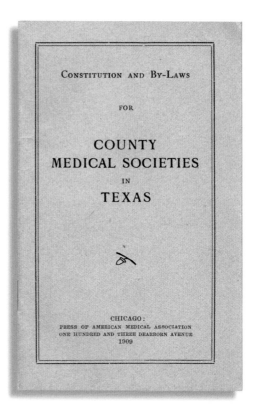

Constitution and By-Laws for County Medical Societies of Texas, 1909.

With 550 members attending, the 1904 Austin meeting was the largest in TMA history. One hundred and twenty-five county medical societies had been organized, among them the updated Travis County Medical Society. TMA members rode back and forth to the University of Texas on electric cars and walked to Brackenridge Hall, named for UT benefactor Colonel George Brackenridge, for fifty-cent dinners. One thousand people were present for a banquet at the Driskill Hotel as the music "rose with its voluptuous swell," and "the soft eyes looked love all right and the lamps shown bright over fair women & brave men." Dr. Daniel was elected TMA president, the third from Travis County.

The following year, Dr. Daniel opposed an effort by the TMA to establish its own journal. His publication had served—sometimes controversially—as the *de facto* association journal. He lost the fight, but continued his popular "*Red Back*" until 1920.

In July 1905, the first issue of the *Texas State Journal of Medicine* listed Travis County Medical Society members under "District No. 7, Austin." Other counties in this district were Bastrop, Burnet, Caldwell, Hays, Lee, Llano-Mason, San Saba, and Williamson. Travis had the most members, with forty-four, but Williamson was not far behind at thirty-four. Most Travis County members were from Austin, but from smaller towns came Drs. George S. Beaty, Manchaca; J. T. Black, Elroy; J. D. Fields and F. C. Gregg, both of Manor; J. R. Hunter, Hornsby; F. A. Maxwell, Del Valle; W. E. McCaleb, Webberville; and J. B. Sappington, Oak Hill. A number of familiar Austin names were listed. One physician, Dr. W. G. Webber of Merrilltown, had moved to Round Rock, and Dr. S. E. Lincoln, formerly of Manor, was living in Hutto. In 1908, Polk's directory cited as Pflugerville physicians Drs. James A. Gullette and B. F. Jones (both later practiced in the Norwood Building in Austin); Dr. Alexander Birge was in Manchaca; and—along with Dr. F. C. Gregg—Drs. Mathis G. Edgar and Victor D. Thomas were at Manor.

As outgoing TMA president in 1905, Dr. Daniel delivered his memorable address entitled, "Sentiment and Science," and with his "charming wife," led the "grand march." His health would begin to fail shortly after his term as TMA president. Three other Austin physicians spoke at the meeting: Dr. Henry L. Hilgartner reported a case on the correction of a facial deformity. In Vienna the previous summer, he had had the opportunity to see "paraffin and vaselin used in the correction of deformity. As the use of the latter is so much simpler, and the results seem to be equally as good," he said, "my opinion is that vaselin will come to be used exclusively...."

Dr. William J. Mathews described a successful amputation of the hip joint at City-County Hospital after another physician's repairs had not worked on a man who had fallen forty feet from a pecan tree. The operation was completed with scissors. "I learned this special use of scissors from Dr. Dawborn, the professor of surgical operations on the cadaver at the New York Polyclinic....All present were amazed and delighted at the small amount of blood lost during the operation....it was practically a bloodless operation, and the patient suffered almost no shock afterwards. It was remarkably easy to ligate all the arteries, almost as easy as on the cadaver, so thoroughly did Wyeth's method control the blood-vessels...." Dr. Mathews added that the patient left the hospital six weeks after the operation with the wound "perfectly healed."

Dr. J. W. McLaughlin, chairman of medicine at UTMB, urged physicians to become more clinical in diagnosis by using the microscope.

Osteopathic physicians in 1905 held their sixth session in Fort Worth with fifteen members present. They had organized in Sherman in November 1900 as the Texas Association for the Advancement of Osteopathy, the genesis of the future Texas Osteopathic Medical Association. The 1905 *Austin City Directory* also listed four osteopathic phy-

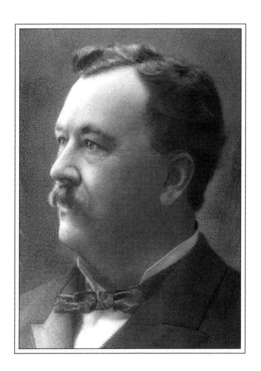

Dr. J. W. McLaughlin was a proponent of the use of microscopes in diagnosis.

sicians: Drs. Pratt L. and Rose Bathwick, Fairfax Fitts, and Mary Montgomery. Sixty-one allopathic physicians and thirteen dentists also were listed.

A member of Phi Beta Kappa, Dr. Margaret R. Holliday received a bachelor's degree in 1901 and a master's degree in 1902 from the University of Texas. Earning her M.D. degree from the University of Texas Medical Department in 1906, she was certified by the state on July 15, 1906. In February 1907, she was elected a member of the Travis County Medical Society. During 1906 and 1907, she served as an assistant superintendent in the state mental health asylum in Austin. She also became superintendent of Elm Grove Lodge which opened in 1906 to offer treatment for children and adolescents with nervous and mental diseases and physical deformities. "A Noble Work" in the *Texas Medical Journal* (the "Red Back") of September 1907 said that Dr. Holliday and Mrs. Dora McDaniel, who had been matron at the state asylum, established the institution. "There is no institution of the kind provided by the State, and none in Texas," the editor said. "Such an institution is greatly needed, and I am sure will be appreciated." He noted that, "Dr. Holliday, the superintendent, is a highly cultivated lady, who has had wide experience in this field." The twenty-five-bed hospital was closed by 1912. A member of the original Texas Academy of Science, Dr. Holliday was also a lecturer in abnormal psychology at UT. Her husband was Dr. Simon J. Clark, a 1907 UTMB graduate. The AMA recorded his specialty as OALR (ophthalmology, otology, laryngology, and rhinology). They had offices in the downtown Scarbrough Building.

The January 1907 issue of the *Texas State Journal of Medicine* reported that Travis County Medical Society officers were Dr. H. B. Granberry of Austin, president; Dr. J. T. Black of Elroy, vice president; Dr. G. M. Decherd, Austin, secretary-treasurer; Dr. J. R. Hunter, Hornsby, censor; Dr. W. J. Mathews, Austin, TMA delegate; and Dr. F. E. Daniel, Austin, alternate delegate. Because of its small number of physicians, Hays County Medical Society merged with the Travis society.

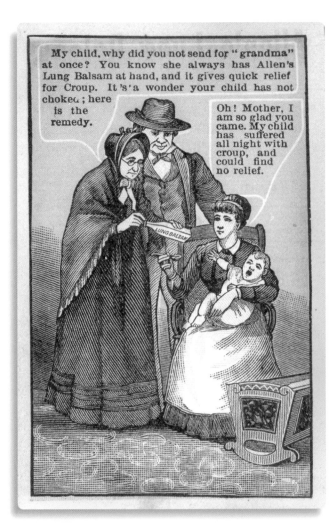

ABOVE AND RIGHT: *At the turn of the century children suffered from contagious diseases. This is an advertising card for a medicine to cure respiratory maladies.*

Physicians continued to survive by owning drug stores, contracting as life insurance examiners or railroad physicians, and by farming. A *Texas State Journal of Medicine* survey in 1907 reported that among 66 respondents from Travis County, 45 reported making more than expenses; 30 reported they were saving money; and 36 made a bare living. Annual expenses averaged $1,500, with an average yearly income of $2,000. Physicians were asking $2 for a home day visit; $4 for a home night visit; $1 for an office visit; $3 for a physical examination; and $25 for "obstetrical with forceps delivery."

The first two decades of the new century saw the passage of public health laws, often driven by doctors with their newfound political strength. In 1903, the Quarantine Department became the Department of Health and Vital Statistics, and in 1909, the State Board of Health, an entity long sought by the Texas Medical Association, was approved by the Legislature. The governor appointed Dr. W. M. Brumby of Austin to the board, where he was named president. Texas established many other important codes, including the Sanitary Code of 1910, which required physicians to report all contagious and infectious diseases. Included were Asiatic cholera, bubonic plague, typhus fever [sic], yellow fever, leprosy, smallpox, scarlet fever (scarlatina), diphtheria (membranous croup), epidemic cerebrospinal meningitis, dengue, typhoid fever, epidemic dysentery, trachoma, tuberculosis, and anthrax. Tuberculosis reports were to be kept "privately" and considered confidential, future state health officer Dr. George W. Cox writes. People with "pestilential diseases" like cholera, plague, typhus "fever" or yellow fever were to be kept in "absolute" isolation and the premises were to be under "absolute" quarantine. Those with dangerous contagious diseases like leprosy, smallpox, and others were to be placed in "modified" isolation, and those with non-quarantinable diseases, like typhoid fever and cerebrospinal meningitis (epidemic), epidemic dysentery, trachoma, tuberculosis, and anthrax were to be placed in "limited" isolation. A number of other state entities also would be formed, such as those on hookworm, anti-plague, and anthrax. In 1913, the Legislature called for public distribution of information on communicable diseases.

Smallpox vaccine was available and some help was provided for prevention of diphtheria. An antitoxin had been developed in the 1890s and the Schick test became available after the end of the first decade of the new century. Typhoid vaccine had been developed in the 1890s, and in the United States it was available for soldiers by the end of the first decade. In 1911, Texas also instituted compulsory smallpox vaccination in public schools, more than a century after the Spanish king first called for smallpox vaccination in the Province of Texas.

Most children experienced rubeola, whooping cough, mumps, rubella, and chickenpox. They were prevented from going to school for twenty-one days or longer. Children in a house with quarantinable diseases also could not go to school until they received a certificate from their attending physician, countersigned by the local health officer. Unpasteurized milk in this era caused considerable illness, among which was tuberculosis spread from cows. Infant diarrhea also was routine, especially in the summer, and not yet understood by all physicians. Babies often died of dehydration.

Diagnostic laboratories were becoming important in medical practice. In Austin, the Pasteur Institute of Texas had been established in 1903 at the State Lunatic Asylum to diagnose and treat rabies. Private laboratories run by individual doctors slowly began appearing in Texas, with the first in 1904 in San Antonio. Subsequently, other public laboratories were launched, including one for food analy-

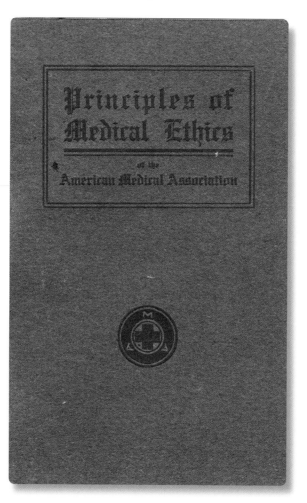

Booklet on Principles of Medical Ethics, *published by the American Medical Association, 1909.*

sis after the Pure Food and Drug Law was passed in 1906. The State Board of Health bacteriological laboratory was put in place in 1912. Significant findings on hookworm disease were also being made in Texas. Before long, there also was help in identifying and treating venereal disease, although the process was terribly painful. Antibiotic treatment was far in the future.

As an assistant to Dr. Worsham, superintendent of the State Lunatic Asylum, Dr. Jacob T. Wilhite with L. H. Kirk had helped establish the Pasteur Institute of Texas and soon after Dr. Wilhite was selected to run it. Known for his rabies research, he found new methods of diagnosis and treated 12,000 patients thought to have rabies infection, with only sixteen deaths. He also examined thousands of animals. Born in April 1876 near Creedmoor, Dr. Wilhite was the son of Travis County pioneers. Educated in Travis County public schools, he attended the University of Texas for two years. After receiving his M.D. degree from the University of Texas Medical Department in 1903, he interned at John Sealy Hospital. His obituary noted that he "had materially improved the method of staining the Negri bodies, and the formulae for his stains" became state property.

By 1912, besides tests on blood, water, and feces, laboratory tests at the state health department were primarily for diphtheria, typhoid, and malaria. In 1914, the state bacteriological laboratory also examined drinking water used on railway trains and in towns. It further conducted sputum studies (mainly for tuberculosis), hookworm examinations, and examined spinal fluid. By 1922, Wassermann tests and urinalysis were included. The laboratory also distributed diphtheria antitoxin, anti-meningitis sera, and typhoid vaccine, and in 1925 silver nitrate drops for the eyes of newborn infants.

The state combined its laboratories into the Bureau of Laboratories in 1928.

After Dr. J. W. McLaughlin died of cancer in 1909, Dr. H. L. Hilgartner memorialized him. Dr. McLaughlin "saw at once the necessity of bringing the laboratory work of the students in close connection with the teaching in hospital wards…for a time he and his assistant fitted up a room in the basement of the hospital, with simple apparatus, at their own expense, and it was only after bearing this burden for some years that the Regents of the University were able to provide funds.…"

On January 1, 1909, an Oklahoma City newspaper headline announced, "Five Colored doctors operate in this city—first major operation done in the history of Oklahoma solely by Colored Physicians." The article cited Dr. Charles R. Yerwood and carried his photograph. ". . . Dr. C. R. Yerwood of this city …last Saturday afternoon, demonstrated his ability as a surgeon. He is a talented young man, having completed his literary courses in Samuel Huston College, Austin, Texas, graduating with honors. He completed his medical course in Meharry Medical College, Nashville, Tennessee, from which school he graduated with honors. The young doctor has a brilliant future, and in short will prove himself among the best surgeons of the South, regardless of race or color." Dr. Yerwood was born March 7, 1882, in Austin where he attended public school and subsequently graduated from Samuel Huston College in 1902. He received his M.D. degree from Meharry in 1907 and practiced in Oklahoma City before returning to Texas to practice. He served as secretary of the Lone Star State Medical, Dental, and Pharmaceutical Association from August 1922 until his death in December 1940 in Fort Worth. His daughters, Drs. Connie R. and Joyce Yerwood, also became physicians.

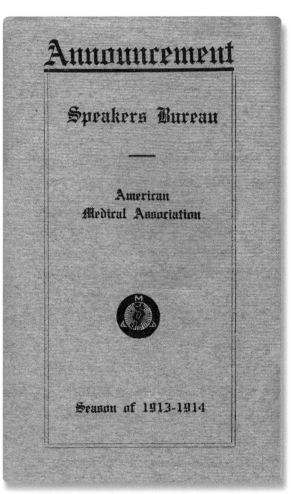

This American Medical Association 1913 booklet on speakers includes five doctors from Texas.

In November 1910, the Lone Star Medical Association again met in Austin—its twenty-fourth annual meeting—with forty-four attendees. Austin physician Dr. Walter H. Crawford was elected vice president. Born in 1875, Dr. Crawford had graduated from Leonard Medical School, which was the medical department of Shaw University in Raleigh, North Carolina, and furthered his studies at Illinois Medical College in Chicago in 1905. Absorbed by another school, the college eventually came under the aegis of Loyola University.

Three ambulance services operated in Austin in 1910. The *Austin City Directory* reported that Congress Avenue and Sixth Street had been paved; that 3,000 students were enrolled at the University of Texas; and that Austin remained a healthy place. "There is no local cause for disease, and Austin is known far and near as a health resort.… There were thirteen days during the past summer when there was not a single death in the city." The directory listed fifty-seven physicians and surgeons and three midwives.

Future physicians sometimes had to overcome extraordinary challenges to achieve their goals. Dr. Robert Vincent Murray, born in Fiskville, near Austin, in June 1889, was nine when his father died and he had to drop out of school. At age eleven, he began supporting his mother and brother by shoveling coal for boilers at the power plant for Austin's streetcars. Taking an examination for high school credentials at age seventeen, he went directly to medical school in Galveston, graduating at age twenty-one. He was the roommate of an older student, G. V. Brindley, Sr., a future surgeon and well-known leader of Texas medicine who became a partner at Scott and White in Temple in 1917. Dr. Murray returned to Austin in 1911 to practice medicine, serving for a time as city health officer. On the board of the Salvation Army, he also contributed services to the Children's Home of Austin. During World War I, he served with the military in France. His son, Dr. Robert Vincent Murray, Jr., recalled his father receiving patients at all hours at the family home in Austin, something his mother accepted as part of his work. Despite his father's lack of early formal schooling, he spoke "perfect English" and had "beautiful handwriting."

Addressing mental illness in 1912, the Texas Medical Association recommended a change in name for the State Lunatic Asylum to the Austin State Hospital. Committees supported remedial legislation for "the unfortunate insane of this State, and that without delay." Dr. F. S. White of San Antonio reported that in 1860 there had been sixty patients in the Austin hospital, a ratio of one to 1,007 of the population. By 1910, there were 4,808 in state institutions, a ratio of one to 810 people. A million dollars was being spent for their care. There had been progress, but Dr. White was concerned that too many individuals needing treatment were in county jails.

Dr. M. M. Smith of Austin was one of two doctors in 1912 discussing pellagra for the first time at the Texas Medical Association meeting. Since the first reported Texas death from pellagra in 1907, the number of cases was increasing rapidly. That the disease resulted from poor nutrition—often from a diet of corn or maize with little other food, leading to a niacin/tryptophan deficiency—still was not known. Another Travis County physician, Dr. W. A. Harper of Austin became a TMA officer in 1911, serving as one of two vice presidents.

In 1915, Dr. Matthew F. Kreisle opened his office for general practice in Austin, where he had been born in 1886. After attending schools there and graduating from UT, he received his M.D. degree from the UT Medical Department in Galveston in 1911. He became a lecturer in pathology and was an associate in pathology at John Sealy Hospital. Dr. Kreisle incorporated the tools of modern pathology—a microtome, stains, and a microscope—in his practice at a time when there were few pathology specialists in Texas. He also provided tissue studies for other physicians' patients, in effect becoming the tissue pathologist for Austin surgeons, continuing the service until he became too busy and other pathologists were arriving in town. Dr. Kreisle is recognized as the first internist in Austin and the first to have an electrocardiograph machine. He carried the bulky EKG equipment—which was moved around on rollers in hospitals—on house calls and lugged it back again. For several years, he also was the physician for Travis County. During World War I, he was a first lieutenant in the Army Medical Corps and during World War II was honored for his service with the military draft. He was elected twice as president of the Travis County Medical Society and considered a bibliophile of wide interests, especially in history and Texana. Two of his sons, Drs. James E. Kreisle and Matthew F. Kreisle, Jr., also became physicians.

Austin's first known Hispanic doctor, Dr. Alberto Gonzalo García, also established his practice in Austin in 1915, where he practiced medicine for forty-seven years. He became a long-time member of the state and county medical societies. Active in civic affairs, he founded *La Vanguardia*, Austin's first Spanish-language newspaper, with his wife Eva Carillo de García. Through it, he encouraged Hispanics to become active in local civic affairs. In later years, Dr. García worked closely with John Henry Faulk to expand the city library. Born in Guadalupe, Zacatecas, Mexico, in 1889, he was the son of a shoemaker. He and his sister were among forty-two children around the world adopted by Dr. John Kellogg, who helped and educated studious youth. Young García was sent to the American Medical Missionary College, an Adventist school in Battle Creek, Michigan, and then to Tulane University's School of Medicine. He first had established a private practice in Mexico but left in 1915 amid the unrest of the Mexican Revolution that had begun in 1910. His wife Eva was a missionary nurse selected for training by the Methodist Church.

Travis County doctors also were involved in the American Red Cross chapter in Austin, one of the earliest established by a county. Dr. Joe Sil Wooten, son of Dr. Thomas Wooten and brother of Dr. Goodall Harrison Wooten, was said to have organized the Austin chapter in 1916, and for seventeen years served as its chairman.

At the May 1917 meeting of the Texas Medical Association, Dr. Samuel Newton Key of Austin announced his pioneering work on "The Etiology of Winter Hay-Fever in Texas." He observed that "Certainly if there is any class of patients entitled to know the true nature of their complaint it is hay-fever sufferers." Little had been done in Texas, he said, to define hay fever localities and times of occurrence and duration in each area. "The usual conception of hay-fever is that it occurs twice a year, in the spring and autumn," he said, with a winter variety occurring in some portions of Texas. "As far as I know this winter hay-fever has never been previously described nor its cause ascertained. Coming as it does in mid-winter, the disease is frequently mistaken for a persistent 'cold.'" It typically appeared between mid-December and Christmas and lasted until mid-February and Dr. Key observed that it was more prevalent in Austin than spring or autumn types of hay fever. Assisted by Dr. M. S. Young at the UT Department of Botany, Dr. Key found that "only the male mountain cedar, *Sabina sabinoides*, is in flower during the winter hay-fever season." Following the suggestion of Dr. W. Scheppegrell, President of the American Hay-Fever Prevention Association," Dr. Key "exposed atmospheric pollen plates at various places in Austin." With an extract of the cedar pollen, Dr. Scheppegrell was able to induce a skin reaction in susceptible persons. Dr. Key concluded that the pollen of the mountain cedar caused winter hay fever and that this opened the road to pollen therapy, "which at present is our chief hope for the prevention and cure of hay-fever." "Hay" fever in central Texas became known as the annoying "cedar fever."

Born in Georgetown in September 1886, Dr. Key had come to Austin in 1895, after his father had become chief justice of the Texas Court of Civil Appeals. After attending the Whitis School in Austin and the University of Texas, he graduated from the UT Medical Department in Galveston in 1910. He interned at Philadelphia General Hospital and served a residency at Brooklyn Eye and Ear Infirmary. In 1914, he returned to Austin to practice ophthalmology and otolaryngology. He was certified by the American Board of Otolaryngology and was a fellow in the American College of Surgeons. He also worked as a bacteriologist for the Pasteur Institute. In 1924, he joined the staff of the old Physicians and Surgeons Hospital, from which St. David's Hospital emerged. In the early 1950s, Dr. Key served on the TMA Board of Trustees and briefly as secretary of the association. He also was president of the Travis County Medical Society in 1950.

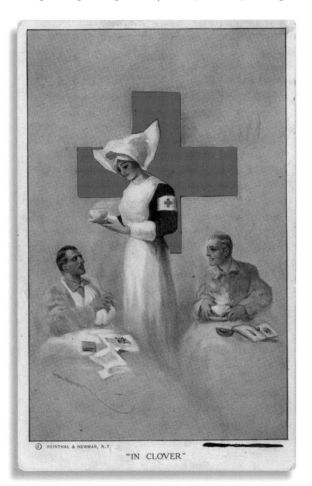

Postcard of a Red Cross nurse administering to wounded soldiers, ca. 1915.

Young Marie Correll's family had been in Austin since 1908 when her father came to teach electrical engineering at the University of Texas. News in those days arrived by telegraph or the newspaper and, long after she became Dr. Marie Tisdale, she vividly recalled her father coming in to inform the family about the start of World War I and the subsequent high emotions in Austin.

Many Travis County nurses and physicians served in the Army or Navy during the war, and two nurses, Alma Furr and Mamie Jones, died at camps in the United States. By the war's end, more than a fifth of Texas doctors and about a third of TMA members were in military service. Nearly 930 physicians from Texas had been commissioned, reported the president-elect in 1920, "a greater contribution than that of any other profession, except that of nursing." The president-elect added that "while those in uniform were doing their full part, the civil surgeon was doing his" part and more. "I know physicians over 65 years of age who during the war did not decline a single call."

A victim of poison gas weaponry during battle in World War I, Dr. Allen G. Heard was hospitalized in Rouen, Normandy, in northwest France. An assistant professor of medicine at UTMB when commissioned by the U.S. Army, he had been sent to France in October 1917. He returned to teach in Galveston, but, because of his injured lungs, moved to Austin to practice with his wife, Dr. Ethel Mary Lyon Heard. In 1922, both physicians returned to Houston, where Dr. Allen Heard died in 1926, unable to withstand an episode of pneumonia.

In addition to the atrocious injuries and deaths from gas weapons—especially mustard and chlorine—other maladies were treated during World War I. Trench fever was a significant cause of discomfort and morbidity as it spread

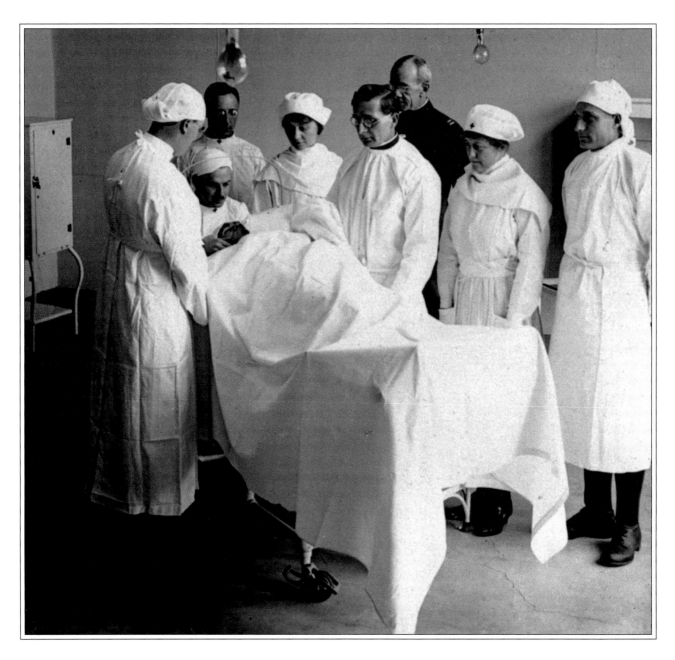

*Photograph of a wounded soldier about to
undergo an operation.*

rapidly in the crowded dugouts. The louse as a specific cause was not identified until the war was almost over. Also, a condition called gas gangrene—not related to gas weaponry, but the result of infection from *Clostridium perfringens* in battlefield wounds—was estimated to have caused hundreds of thousands of deaths.

The State Board of Health in July 1918 asked physicians and civic leaders to report on efforts regarding the new venereal disease law. Mayor A. P. Wooldridge declared that "five years ago Austin had abolished its red light district" and "those in a position to know" had told him that the venereal disease rate for the Austin Army camps was "less than other camps." The mayor said that Army reports also showed that prostitution had been "materially decreased."

Some medical progress came from the war. Dr. Nixon cited wound treatment, especially through the use of debridement, which became widely used, and the Carrel-Dakin method of wound irrigation, which likely controlled infections and saved many lives. Despite the infection rates on the battlefield, there were reportedly fewer deaths during World War I from disease than from battle wounds.

As soldiers were returning home, however, a devastating pandemic called the Spanish influenza spread rapidly. As early as March 1918, the disease struck around Fort Riley, Kansas. In October 1918, Austin was hit hard by the pandemic. Soldiers from three nearby military camps and students attending colleges in Austin also contributed to the rapid spread of influenza. Cots with patients filled corridors and surgery suites at City Hospital. Tents covered the lawn at Seton Infirmary. On October 10, the city closed public gathering places, schools, and churches. By mid-October, seventy-seven Texas counties reported an epidemic, and by November 11, Austin had more than 200 deaths. U.S. deaths would be cited at upwards of 600,000 and worldwide at twenty to fifty million. The *Texas State Journal of Medicine* lamented the lack of preparedness and funds and the November 1918 issue carried obituaries of eleven doctors lost to the illness. On December 26, Dr. George P. Smartt died in Austin following pneumonia after the flu. A graduate of Baylor University College of Medicine in Dallas, he had built a large medical practice in Manor and in the fall had moved to Austin to become the Travis County health officer, a position he held briefly before his death at age thirty-eight.

Dr. Tisdale recalled neighbors dying, doctors working day and night, and the shortage of nurses. Her entire family—parents and the four daughters—became sick, and her father developed asthma from which he suffered for the rest of his life. On Armistice Day, November 11, 1918, all family members were too miserably sick to participate in celebrations although they could hear the celebratory church bells ringing.

Ethel Parsons, R.N., of Austin, director of the Bureau of Child Hygiene and Public Health Nursing of the Texas State Board of Health and director of public health nursing for the American Red Cross (Texas), reported after the war that draft boards had found thirty-three percent of young men unfit for military service. She concluded that it was the duty of society to protect children from diseases to equip them for the "battle of life." She also observed that Texas was fortunate to have the Bureau of Child Hygiene and a growing number of public health nurses. On another matter, she addressed the state's high maternal mortality rate in 1918, reporting that 625 mothers had died in childbirth.

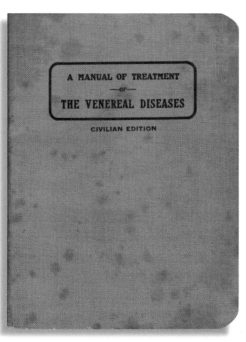

A Manual of Treatment of the Venereal Diseases, *published by the American Medical Association in 1919 and distributed by the Texas State Board of Health.*

The State Board of Health explained in a 1918 pamphlet on preventable diseases that tuberculosis was acquired by "indirect or direct contact with an infected person; by coughing, sneezing, kissing; by using infected linens, dishes, pipes, and toilet articles." Other diseases also were cited. Of unknown causes were smallpox, scarlet fever, dengue, mumps, German measles, and chickenpox. The cause of typhus "fever" was "not definitely determined"; of measles was "not yet discovered"; and of poliomyelitis was "by germ not identified." Trachoma was listed as being caused by germs; malaria by animal parasite; and hookworm disease by "a small worm about one half inch long and the size of a No. 30 sewing thread." Diseases cited with known causes were diphtheria, typhoid fever, epidemic dysentery, whooping cough, and spinal meningitis.

Austin lost an old landmark in 1918 when fire destroyed the Austin Sanitarium at Fourteenth Street and Congress Avenue. Fortunately, supplies were salvaged and moved to a house near Seventeenth and Rio Grande Streets. Later that year, Drs. R. W. Shipp, Joe Gilbert, Simon Clark, and W. E. McCaleb formed a partnership and took over the assets. When the partnership dissolved the next year, another group, with some of the former partners, was established under a new name, Physicians and Surgeons Hospital. The new partnership, with Drs. Gilbert, Clark, Sam Key, John C. Thomas, and Allen Heard, then oversaw the hospital.

Women had been able to earn licenses to practice medicine but could not vote in Texas until the Legislature granted them the right in the 1918 primary election, two years ahead of full suffrage following the federal constitutional amendment.

Born already were Travis County physicians whose lives would span all but one decade of the century and part of the twenty-first. That extraordinary journey, with all its fabled twists and turns, would lead to an amazing transformation in medicine.

CHAPTER VIII

A HOPEFUL START

M R. MATTHEWS' DRUG STORE AT Seventeenth and Lavaca Streets in Austin "had a mysterious medical smell, a pleasant aroma of flavorings and spices." Years later, when Marie Correll was Dr. Tisdale, she could almost smell the whiffs of that distinct synthesis in the pharmacy owned by her childhood friend's father, B. Bernard Matthews. "Medicines were compounded, then mixed to order as given in the doctor's Latin handwriting, individually made up for each patient. Pills were made by being mixed in a mortar and pestle, then rolled by hand into little balls. Powders were dispensed in little crisp white papers, each folded so as to compose one dose, sifted onto the surface of cold water in a glass when taken by the patient."

Marie had known a Travis County that few later could imagine. She had been born in September 1909 during a family visit back in Kansas. The family had moved to Neches Street in a new neighborhood three blocks east of the University of Texas. The gravel-graded streets passed through live oaks and cedar woods, and each morning Marie's mother drove their old black Buick to deliver her and her sisters to their schools. On the way home, Marie and a friend took the Rio Grande Streetcar to Sixth Street, changing to the Duval or the East Avenue car, and then walked the rest of the way, sometimes picking bluebonnets. When the University needed more space, the family left the beautiful house built by her Kansan grandfather.

About sixty miles east of the capital, near Carmine, young Kermit Fox knew a pleasant but challenging rural life. Dr. Paul E. Suehs had delivered him in 1913 in the house Kermit's grandfather, Lorenz Fuchs, had built on land acquired in 1855. Kermit's childhood on *La Bahía* prairie was embraced by historic Spanish pathways, the relatively fresh imprint of Stephen F. Austin's colonies, and the stamp of later German immigrants like his own family. A kerosene lamp provided light, and there was a wood stove for heating and cooking. There were no indoor toilets and running water came from a pitcher pump resting above the cistern or perhaps an outside cistern spigot. At first, the family traveled via its single buckboard over unpaved and ungraded roads. Cotton, corn, and hay were grown. Hogs had to be slaughtered and cattle dipped, especially after the arrival of the white-spotted tick, carrying Texas cattle fever. School terms lasted eight months and began in the fall after most of the cotton was picked. Work was done mostly on a blackboard or framed slate boards bound with reddish felt. Slate pencils were thin and bare, although some were encased in wood. Homework was done on wood pulp paper so coarse it would show small wooden splinters.

Dr. Paul Suehs, the general practitioner who had delivered the future Dr. Fox, had graduated from the University of Texas Medical Department in 1903. In 1914, he moved to Austin and became an eye, ear, and nose specialist. In the meantime, George W. Tipton, also born in 1913, had attended school at Troup, near Tyler in northeast Texas. He long remembered the terrible roads connecting those towns. At age six, he made a slide by standing a board

OPPOSITE PAGE: *Many Austin doctors had offices downtown in the Littlefield Building in the 1920s.*

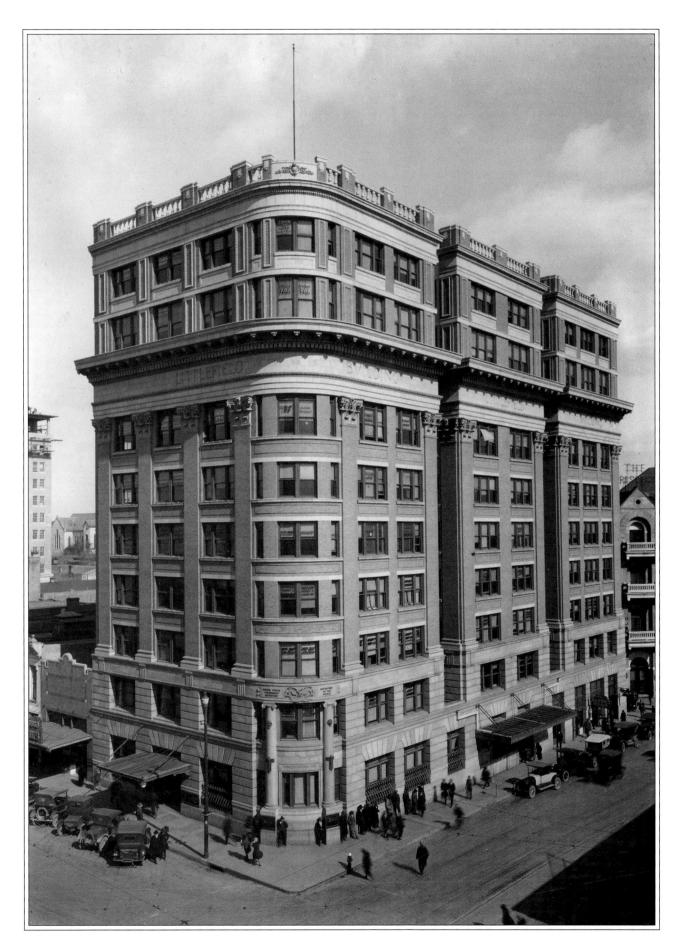

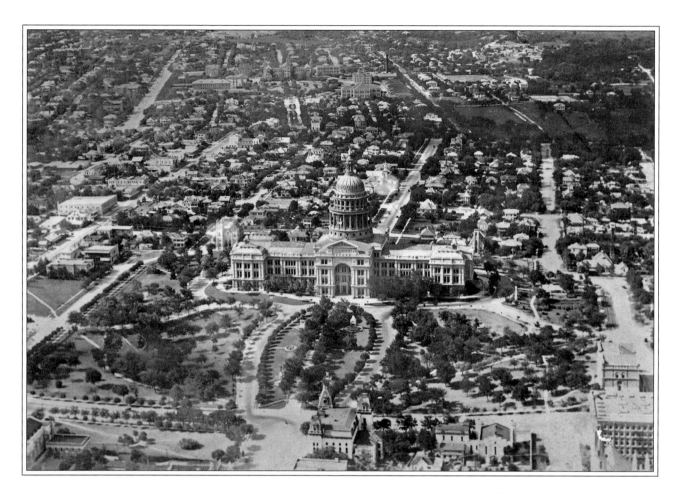

Texas State Capitol shortly before 1920.

against a fence and proceeded to descend it, thereby acquiring a large splinter. Fortunately, his physician uncle painlessly removed the foreign body, which quite impressed young George. His family later moved to the Highland Park area of Dallas because of the reputation of its schools, and a cousin, who came to live with them to attend school, developed appendicitis. The doctor treating her charged $150, which George also thought was magnificent. In addition, she got much better. George Tipton would face a circuitous route to his destination as an Austin surgeon.

A man in the future life of Marie Correll, Albert A. Tisdale, was a child of both country and city. In December 1906, Dr. Thomas J. Bennett drove his buggy from Austin to the family farm to deliver him. Then seven miles north of Austin, the farm some day would be encompassed by the city. Young Albert also learned about kerosene, wood stoves, and lye soap, and heard stories of hog-killing. On Sundays, the family rode in a horse-drawn buggy down Burnet Road to Alice Avenue (later Medical Parkway) to University Methodist Church. There also was a train, so friends from Austin, like the George Decherds, could buy tickets and visit them for the day. In 1919, the Tisdale family moved to 601 West Nineteenth Street (later Martin

Luther King Jr. Boulevard) in Austin, where Albert attended Austin High School. Dr. George M. Decherd, Sr., a 1905 graduate of the UT Medical Department, was known as a physician with a brilliant mind, and George, Jr., born in 1906, followed in his footsteps, becoming an outstanding physician and a professor of medicine.

In the fall of 1918, six months before the Austin birth of Georgia Felter, who would become Dr. Georgia Legett, her father had suffered devastating injuries in a motorcycle accident on Congress Avenue while on the way to work for the City of Austin. The ambulance driver had not wanted to pick him up but finally consented to take him to St. David's Hospital on Seventeenth Street. There, Dr. Joe Gilbert "worked with him for two days before he passed away." Mrs. Felter had made arrangements with Dr. Margaret Holliday to deliver the baby, but Georgia arrived without help in March 1919 at 900 Houston Street in Austin. A few months later her mother moved the family to its indebted farm at Webberville. With no life insurance, a toddler son, and a new baby, she had to make a living so she sold paper shell pecans, honey from the apiary she managed, and the cotton she raised. Fortunately also, she had earned a teaching certificate at age sixteen and had graduated from the University of Texas in 1910, so she began teaching school at Hornsby-Dunlap. For five years, the family lived with no electricity or plumbing. They had a kerosene stove, a fireplace to warm the house, a well for water, and a "three-holer" outside.

These future physicians had first-hand links to some of the best-educated physicians of the time. Eighty percent of prescriptions in the 1920s also required pharmacists to have a great deal of knowledge about preparation and compounding. There was promising science, including landmark discoveries of a few vitamins, and there were answers to treating pellagra and rickets through adding vitamins to food. Insulin, isolated in 1920, was being used to treat diabetes. Hormones had been named earlier in the century and a few new vaccines had been developed.

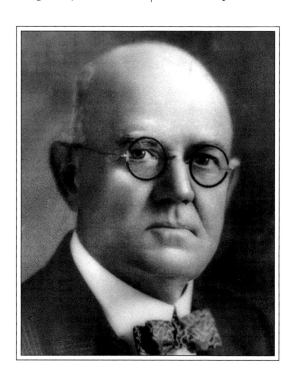

Dr. Thomas J. Bennett became the fourth Travis County president of the Texas Medical Association.

Science, however, simply had not yet found solutions for many diseases. A doctor's most important tool often was hope and reassurance. Calomel still was being given for fever, and paregoric was used for children in cases of colic or diarrhea and for mild pain. Blood counts and other laboratory analyses were not available immediately to practicing physicians. With lack of sterilization of milk, summer diarrhea was frequent. The importance of managing electrolytes during surgery was not recognized and intravenous fluids were not used by surgeons. Likewise, blood transfusions were crude. Cardiovascular diseases had become the leading cause of death, higher than influenza and pneumonia. Tuberculosis rates were high, and, at one point, cancer challenged influenza and pneumonia for a position close to the top. Childhood diseases remained fearsome with cases of measles, diphtheria, and pertussis exceeding half a million with 20,000 deaths yearly. Polio was prevalent in Texas in 1927, with forty-nine cases reported in Fort Worth. Despite the state's long history of smallpox vaccination, 2,059 cases of the old scourge also appeared in the first six months of 1927.

In 1921, the U.S. Congress had passed the Sheppard-Towner Act co-sponsored by Senator Morris Sheppard of Texarkana, Texas. Intended to reduce high infant mortality rates, the law provided states grants to develop health services for poor mothers. Some physicians were concerned that the law amounted to partial socialization of medicine.

Some form of prepaid insurance had long existed in Texas and had been a particular issue in the previous decade. It again was a major topic as was group practice and Dr. H. L. Hilgartner of Austin wrote his views in "A Criticism of 'Group Medicine'" in the *Texas State Journal of Medicine* of September 1922. He called for calm and critical consideration regarding the "current propaganda for 'group medicine.'"

In 1921, Dr. Thomas J. Bennett became the fourth Travis County physican to serve as president of the Texas Medical Association. Because of a "train of unavoidable circumstances" in 1922, he was unable to get to the distant El Paso meeting in time to deliver his outgoing presidential address, "A Plea for the Establishment of a State Psychopathic Hospital." The paper, however, was announced by title and later published in the *Texas State Journal of Medicine.* In it, Dr. Bennett spoke of the need for the diagnosis and treatment of mental diseases and mildly psychopathic conditions that were not "strictly within the domain of legislative enactments relating to the insane." In 1931, the Galveston State Psychopathic Hospital was established.

Since 1909, Dr. Z. T. Scott had been a partner in the Austin Sanitarium with Dr. T. J. Bennett, and also served as chief of staff of the institution when it became the Presbyterian Sanitarium. In the 1921 *American Medical Directory*, Dr. Scott indicated that his practice was limited to surgery. As early as 1911, he was a member of the Mayo Clinic's Surgeons' Club, attending periodic educational meetings in Rochester, Minnesota. From 1923 to 1926, he was president of the Texas Anti-Tuberculosis Association (eventually the American Lung Association of Texas).

He initiated the sale of Christmas Seals in Texas, borrowing $1,400 personally to buy the first made in the state. He also managed the Travis County Tuberculosis Sanitarium. His mother's death from the disease when he and his brother, Dr. Harper Anderson "Happy" Scott, were young had led to his deep interest in it. Born in Fort Worth in 1880, Dr. Z. T. Scott graduated from the UT Medical Department in 1903 and over the years did postgraduate work in New York, Chicago, and Vienna, Austria. During World War I, he organized a Reserve Naval Hospital Unit in Austin, which had been assigned to the Gulfport Naval Base in Mississippi. A lieutenant commander, he served with Dr. Frank Cousins Gregg, a 1900 University of Texas Medical Branch graduate and son of Dr. Richard S. Gregg of Manor, with whom he practiced. In 1922, Dr. Frank Gregg joined Dr.

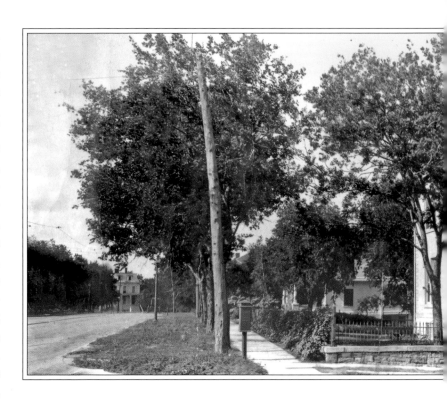

Z. T. Scott in Austin, where they were founders of the Scott-Gregg Clinic. Dr. Gregg also was the Austin city physician from 1935 to 1939.

Dr. Joe Gilbert continued to work with the Physicians and Surgeons Hospital, practiced surgery, and delivered many babies. He remained director of the UT Student Health Center. Dr. Gilbert and Dr. John Calhoun Thomas, who were running the hospital, soon recognized that their institution needed the community's help. They persuaded their church, St. David's Episcopal, to assume ownership, and in 1924, St. David's Hospital began as a charitable institution at Seventeenth and Rio Grande Streets. In 1929, the hospital moved into a new building on Seventeenth Street, remaining there until completion of the present hospital on East Thirty-second Street, which opened to patients on September 14, 1955.

Dr. Thomas was born in Rogers, Texas, in June 1884, and after attending public schools there and graduating from UT in Austin, he received his M.D. degree from the UT Medical Department in 1908. He was a member of Alpha Omega Alpha honorary fraternity. Practicing first in Temple, Texas, in 1914 he moved to Taylor to build and operate the Taylor Sanatorium. He was called into military service during World War I and served in France as a captain in the Army Medical Corps from 1917 to 1919. He returned to open a private practice in Austin. A "charter member of the present Travis County Medical Society," he served as secretary in 1921 and as president in 1943. He

ABOVE: *Nurses standing outside St David's Hospital at 610 West 17th Street.* OPPOSITE PAGE: *In 1929, St. David's Hospital moved into a new building on 17th Street.*

———————————

became a fellow of the American College of Surgeons. An "avid supporter of and worker for the new St. David's Hospital in Austin," he died in 1954.

Another long-time Austin practitioner, Dr. George Horace Gilbert, brother of Dr. Joe Gilbert, limited his practice to radiology. Born in November 1879 in Hornsby, he was educated in Austin public schools and at the University of Texas. Graduating from the UT Medical Department in 1903 and completing an internship at St. Mary's Hospital in Galveston, he set up an office in his Austin home. It remained there until his death in 1945. As a member of the U.S. Navy Medical Corps during World War I, he served as an assistant post surgeon at the Naval Hospital in Gulfport, Mississippi. Like his brother, he was held in high regard by medical associates and by Austin citizens.

Dr. Ethel Mary Lyon Heard, licensed in Texas in 1910, had been on the UT Medical Department faculty. She established her practice in Austin in 1920 in the Littlefield building, providing services to women and serving as the UT women's physician. Born in Ohio in 1876, she earned her M.D. degree in 1905 from Woman's Medical College of Pennsylvania in Philadelphia. During World War I, she was in charge of the Red Cross maternity hospital for refugees in France, where her husband, Dr. Allen Heard, was

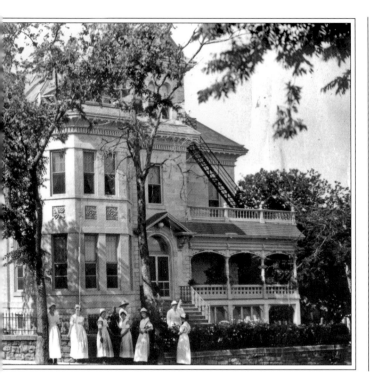

serving in the U.S. Army. The *American Medical Directory* of 1921 cites her specialty as gynecology but does not indicate that she limited her services to the field. She remained in the city for only two years.

A native of Hearne, Texas, Dr. Jesse John Brady had come to Austin for his premedical training at the University of Texas, subsequently graduating from UTMB in 1922. Returning to the capital, he served an internship at Seton Infirmary. Austin would claim him as a physician and a valued surgeon for the next forty-eight years.

Arriving in 1926, Dr. Carolyn Crowell was one of two physicians at the University of Texas. During her earlier years, she also was a night resident physician at Brackenridge Hospital. Born in 1893, she had received a B.A. degree from Bryn Mawr College in Pennsylvania and a B.S. degree from Pennsylvania State University. During World War I, she had taken a job as a chemist in a munitions factory and was hospitalized for treatment of carbuncles. She decided to become a physician and graduated in 1925 from the Uni-

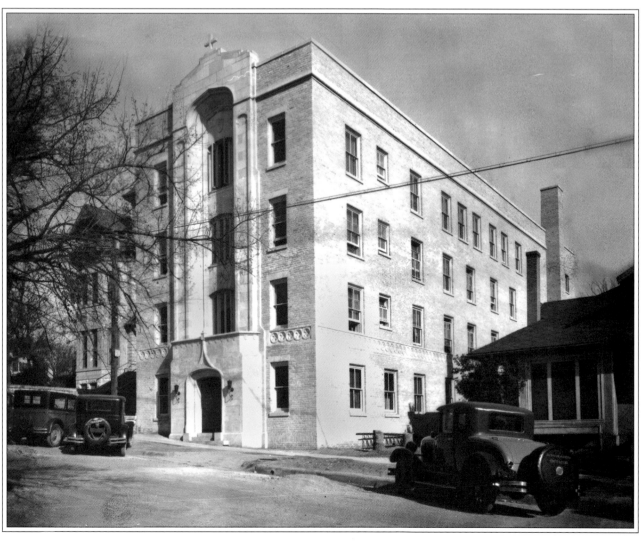

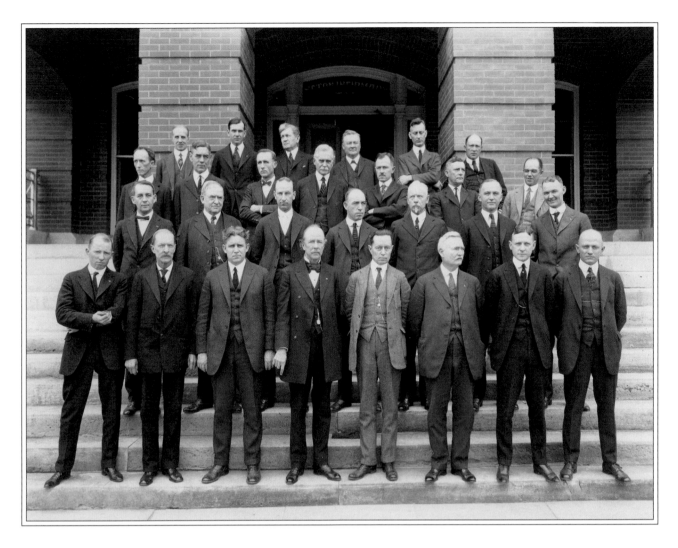

versity of Pennsylvania School of Medicine, followed by an internship at Woman's Hospital of Philadelphia. In Austin, her first visits to men's dormitories caused a stir—a male patient once hid beneath the sheets, refusing to let her examine him for suspected appendicitis.

There was a growing recognition that children were not merely "little adults," and in 1927, Austin welcomed its first physician trained specifically for a pediatric specialty. Dr. Thomas D. McCrummen had grown up in the capital after his birth in Paris, Texas, in 1898, and had graduated from the University of Texas in 1921. He received his medical degree from UTMB in 1923. After serving an internship at Philadelphia General Hospital until May 1925, he became chief resident physician at St. Christopher's Hospital for Children in Philadelphia. In Austin, he became highly respected and extremely busy. He also served as president of the Travis County Pediatric Society and the Texas Pediatric Society.

In late December 1926, Austin honored Dr. William Neal Watt after his death. Born in Steel Creek, North Caro-

lina, in December 1856, he was educated in the common schools there. He received his M.D. degree in 1877 from the Medical Department of the University of New York (which eventually merged with other schools including Bellevue Hospital Medical College). Practicing first in North and South Carolina, he moved to Burton, Texas, in 1880, and in 1892 relocated to Austin. An active and beloved physician, he was in general practice until paralysis struck in 1925.

Dr. William E. Watt had joined his father's practice in 1916. He was born in November 1891, attended Austin schools and then Ford's Academy, receiving his M.D. degree in 1915 from the University of Tennessee College of Medicine in Memphis. He was appointed to the Texas State Board of Medical Examiners by Governor Miriam Ferguson, serving until Governor Coke Stevenson transferred him to the Texas Fish and Game Commission. In addition to membership in his county and state medical societies, Dr. Watt became a fellow of the American College of Surgeons and a member of the Southwestern Surgical Congress. During World War I, he was a captain in the U.S. Army Medical Corps.

His brother, Dr. Terrence Neal Watt, born in Austin in October 1905, attended Texas A&M for premedical studies and graduated from the University of Tennessee College of Medicine in 1931. After a rotating internship at Memphis General Hospital (also called John B. Gaston Hospital) from 1931 to 1932, he returned to Austin where he was a general practitioner and surgeon until 1956. As a member of the U.S. Army Medical Corps from 1942 to 1946, he served in the United States and Europe, becoming a lieutenant colonel.

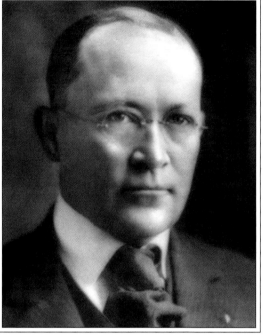

Dr. Joseph Gilbert was president of the Texas Medical Association in 1927-1928 and founder of the University of Texas Student Health Center.

After an unfortunate incident in which the previous city physician had shot the city manager, Dr. Lee Edward Edens in 1926 was appointed city health officer. Born in Bertram, Texas, in February 1894, he attended Southwestern University in Georgetown, was a 1921 UTMB graduate, and interned in Ohio at Cleveland City Hospital (later part of University Hospitals of Cleveland). He became Travis County Medical Society president in 1931. Dr. Edens went to New York in 1936 and returned to Austin in 1938.

When Travis County lost its beloved Dr. Thomas J. Bennett, Dr. Alonzo A. Ross of Lockhart delivered a memorial at the 1927 TMA meeting. He called him one of nature's noblemen, "kind, gentle and considerate at the bedside, faithful, honest, ethical and sincere in his professional relations, and modest.... courageous and fearless...."

Dr. A. Fitzhugh Beverly of Austin nominated Dr. Joe Gilbert as president-elect of the Texas Medical Association and he was elected unanimously. At the end of his 1927-1928 year as the sixtieth TMA president, Dr. Gilbert proposed that the State Board of Medical Examiners be given authority to enforce medical law with funding from an annual physician registration fee. In the absence of a state

disciplinary function, TMA had assumed a law enforcement role. Most physicians were not TMA members, however, and it was thought that a universal fee would lead to all doctors sharing disciplinary responsibility. The new process went into effect in 1932.

At the close of Dr. Gilbert's term and only four years after the Travis County Woman's Auxiliary was formed in 1924, Daisy Thorne Gilbert, his wife, became the tenth president of the TMA Auxiliary. She served from 1928 to 1929. The formation of the Dallas County Medical Society's Auxiliary in 1917 had led to the establishment of the TMA Auxiliary in 1918 and the AMA Auxiliary in 1922. Physicians' wives, who previously had helped at meetings, wanted to extend the goals of the medical profession and to offer community service. They further worked to advance health and education and promoted acquaintanceship among doctors' families. The early activities of the Travis County Auxiliary included support of pasteurization to assure a pure milk supply for children and helping the Texas State Department of Health with its program to register all births in the county. The Auxiliary also promoted vaccination of school children against smallpox. Over the years, it would undertake countless health-related programs.

On July 1, 1928, Dr. Sidney Bohls succeeded Dr. Jacob T. Wilhite, director of laboratories at the State Health Department, who had died of bronchopneumonia following influenza. Born in 1898 in Pflugerville, Dr. Bohls graduated from UT in 1921 and UTMB in 1925. Completing an internship at Santa Rosa General Hospital in San Antonio in 1926, he undertook postgraduate study at the Rockefeller Institute in New York and at Harvard Medical School in Boston. During World War I, he served in the U.S. Army. His laboratory pioneered research on relapsing fever, typhus, and smallpox vaccines. The state also during this time made available the first production of typhoid vaccine and diphtheria toxoid, and conducted research on rabies. Tests were developed for the most common fevers. Dr. Bohls authored numerous scientific papers and organized the schools of medical technology at Brackenridge and Austin State hospitals.

In 1929, Dr. Truman Nicholas Morris became a general practitioner in Austin. Born in Bakersfield, Missouri, in April of 1903, he attended public schools in Mammoth Spring, Arkansas; earned a B.A. degree at the University of Arkansas, Fayetteville, in 1922; and graduated from Jefferson Medical College, Philadelphia, in 1927. He served a rotating internship from 1927 to 1929 at Jefferson Medical College Hospital. In 1936, he returned to school for specialty education, first taking a three-month seminar in gynecology at New York Post-Graduate Medical School. He entered a residency in gynecology and obstetrics at New York City Department of Hospitals (Lincoln Hospital) for thirty-three months, finishing his work in 1939. He would be considered Austin's first specialist in obstetrics and gynecology, although Dr. Ethel Heard had provided women's services briefly in the early 1920s. Dr. Morris was president of Travis County Medical Society in 1934 and 1942 and of the Seventh District Medical Society.

After interning at Kansas City General Hospital, Dr. Charles P. Hardwicke became a member of the Travis County Medical Society in 1928. Born in Abilene, Texas, in 1902, he attended Southern Methodist University and the University of Texas, and received his M.D. degree from UTMB in 1926. He returned for postgraduate education at Cook County Postgraduate School, Chicago, in 1937, at Harvard University in 1940, and at the University of Pennsylvania in 1943. He also served as director of the UT Health Service. Active in medical organizations, he was president of the Travis County Medical Society in 1930 and 1946. In 1953, he was certified in colon and rectal surgery. Dr. Hardwicke's office initially was located in the Capital National Bank Building and later on East Thirty-second Street.

Adventure still could be found in the hill country. Four University of Texas students in 1929 encountered more than they expected while exploring a shallow limestone cavern near the mouth of Fall Creek—as would an Austin pathologist, Dr. George Malcolm Graham. At the base of a 104-foot fall was a clear pool from a "spring-fed creek plunging over a fern-covered cliff to the river bottom." After investigating the pool, three students developed chills and fever, and Dr. Graham and UT physician Dr. Burford Weller found spirochetes in one student's blood. Collecting ticks (*O. turicata*) from the cavern, Dr. Graham was able

to transmit the infection to animals. A week later, he also developed relapsing fever.

In 1932, Dr. Graham received a telegram from Dr. E. Brumpt, a professor of parasitology at the University of Paris, who wanted Dr. Graham to accompany him to the cavern and collect ticks for his laboratory studies. Vernon T. Schuhardt, Ph.D., who had worked at the state laboratories, recalled the escapade. "Since I had isolated spirochetes from another patient into white mice at the State Department of Health Laboratory, Dr. Graham asked the director of the laboratory, Dr. Bohls, and me if we would care to go along....Apparently the thought of a noted parasitologist from Europe coming to visit a country-boy doctor from Texas was too much for Dr. Graham. When we picked him up he was pretty well inebriated and continued to nip at his bottle on the way to the cavern." He was considered immune because he'd already suffered relapsing fever, so he was asked to crawl in to gather the ticks. A week later he again came down with the fever.

"With some humor," Dr. Schuhardt wrote, "he later proclaimed he had proved two things: an attack of relapsing fever didn't result in immunity, and alcohol in the system didn't protect against the infection." Dr. Schuhardt also demonstrated how the spirochetes could cause repeated relapses through antigenic mutation and, through his research, also acquired a severe, prolonged case of the fever. Dr. Schuhardt, who organized and directed the Biologics Division at the state health department, became a long-time UT professor.

Drs. Graham's and Weller's findings were published in the *Journal of the American Medical Association* in 1930, one of the early reports on relapsing fever in Texas. Dr. Graham was a charter member of the Texas Society of Pathologists in 1921 and was listed by the AMA in its 1929 *American Medical Directory* in a then-new section on "Pathologists Conducting Approved Laboratories."

Dr. Ralph Emerson Cloud, born on a plantation in Del Valle in January 1876, attended Travis County schools, the Minnie Carrington University Preparatory School in Austin, and the University of Texas. Graduating from UTMB in 1907, he took postgraduate courses in neuropsychiatry in New York City. Dr. Cloud established the Oaks Sanitarium in 1916 and remained as a director until 1940. He became president of the Travis County Medical Society and the Seventh District, and a diplomate of the American Board of Psychiatry and Neurology. An author and speaker on many psychiatric issues, especially schizophrenia, he became superintendent of the Austin State Hospital in

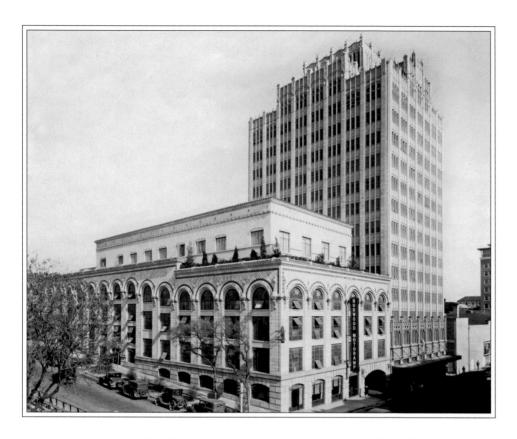

The Norwood Building, completed in 1929, would become an important medical hub.

1943. When a new title was being considered for City Hospital in the late 1920s, Dr. Cloud was among committee members recommending that it be named for Dr. Robert J. Brackenridge.

Marie Correll had graduated from Austin High School and secretly chose a premedical degree plan at the University of Texas, where she was one of two young women in a premedical German class. Albert Tisdale was one of the males in the class and they became good friends before he left for UTMB in the fall of 1928.

Dr. Charles R. Yerwood, who had practiced in rural Gonzales County, opened an office on 421 East Sixth Street in Austin, having moved to provide better educational opportunities for his daughters Joyce and Connie. Their mother had died before they could get to know her. Although they sometimes rode with him as he saw patients, he had discouraged them from entering medicine because he thought it too hard. The future Dr. Joyce Yerwood remembered, "Daddy was an old fashioned family doctor whom we swore we would emulate. He loved this adoration until the time came for medical training—then he balked like an old Texas mule! He had tried to divert us long before medical years, by having us trained to be

'ladies' in Eliza Dee Home and by giving us courses in music and the arts...."

Joe Thorne Gilbert, son of Dr. Joe Gilbert, was preparing to become a physician. Born in Hornsby Bend in August 1905, he attended Texas A&M, and graduated from UT with a B.A. degree in 1926, where he was a member of the swim team. After studying medicine at UTMB for two years, he transferred to the nation's first medical school, the University of Pennsylvania School of Medicine. He received his M.D. degree in 1929 and was a member of Alpha Omega Alpha honorary scholastic fraternity. In 1929, he started a two-year internship at the Hospital of the University of Pennsylvania in Philadelphia.

In 1928, Alexander Fleming observed that a mold had inactivated staphylococcus bacteria left uncovered in a Petri dish. Identifying it as one from the *Penicillium* genus, he reported his finding in the *British Journal of Experimental Pathology* in 1929. Its true value awaited future discovery.

On Friday, October 28, 1929, the American stock market crashed, sending the country into deep economic depression. Hospital donations dropped and physicians would see more diseases of nutritional deficiency; they also would relay tales of being paid in syrup, peaches, eggs, and other commodities. Meanwhile, a former school superintendent, now an administrator at Baylor University Hospital in Dallas, arranged for teachers to pay fifty cents monthly to a fund that guaranteed hospital care for twenty-one days. The plan evolved into Blue Cross and Blue Shield of Texas. Such programs helped hospitals remain solvent and facilitated growth. More babies also would be born in hospitals than at home.

In downtown Austin, the fourteen-story Norwood Building, completed in 1929 at 114 West Seventh Street, would become an important medical hub. With the capital's first self-parking ramp, it also became the city's first air-conditioned office building.

CHAPTER IX

A DESPERATE TIME

DR. JOE THORNE GILBERT looked back on life in the 1930s before penicillin and other antibiotics, and before discovery of the Rh factor, isotopes, tranquilizers, and vitamin B12. There were no specialty boards. He knew little of lung cancer and congenital heart disease and never recommended surgery for them.

"The actual specific medications could practically be counted on one hand. Digitalis was available for the failing heart, insulin for diabetics, and thyroid extract for metabolic disorders; early syphilis could be controlled with mercury and arsenicals; malaria could be treated with quinine, and the illness had to be suspected in every patient because insecticides of the future were not available to con-

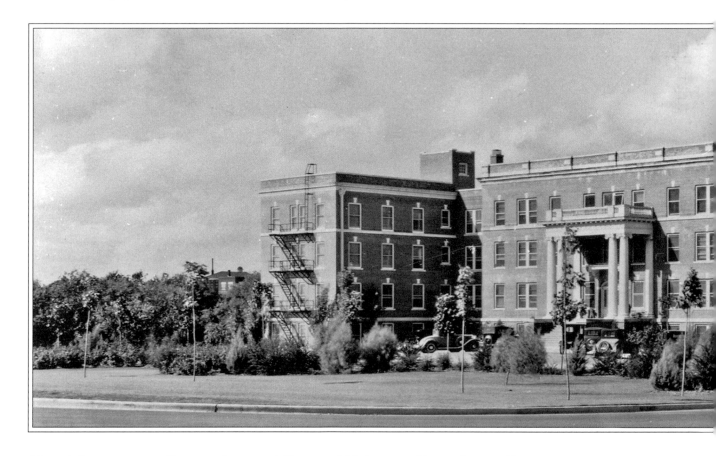

trol mosquitoes. For anesthesia, the main agents were nitrous oxide and ether, and they were administered by nurse anesthetists, with brief training at a larger hospital, or a doctor performing the service as a sideline.... relaxation was practically nil. One was accustomed to 'fighting' the extruding bowel throughout an abdominal procedure. The fairly recently introduced spinal type of anesthetic provided...the blessed relaxation.... This was considered hazardous, however, and had very poor patient acceptance. It was given by the surgeon and the patient was monitored perhaps by a nurse and perhaps only by a student nurse. Control of the level of anesthesia was poorly understood. We did use it and the good Lord looked after us.... He was also with us on those occasions when a hastily placed wet sheet was all that separated a live cautery from a semi-closed anesthesia of highly explosive ethylene."

"Typhoid fever was still prevalent...treated by starvation and the so-called supportive treatment," he remembered, "with a four-to-five week acute phase, weeks of recuperation and perhaps re-growing of hair....One sat by and hoped that a Peyer's patch in the small intestine would not blow out producing a fatal peritonitis. It had a 25 percent mortality. Pneumonia, too, had a 25 percent mortality, in spite of the recently introduced technique of sputum typing of the disease into one of the four types and then giving the specific serum. Septicemia, meningitis, and scarlet fever also took their heavy toll."

"Home deliveries were frequent; a bag containing home delivery essentials, even forceps, was kept at the hospital, available for a small fee. For a ten-day, all-inclusive OB package deal, the hospital charged fifty dollars."

Major operations had a fifteen to thirty percent mortality rate.

"Pleural empyema or pus in the chest," he said, "was a rather frequent complication of pneumonia. Chest surgery was limited to draining these, after they had become walled off. A few thoracoplastics were being done to collapse or rest the diseased lung. Ping pong balls were also put in the chest cavity for this same purpose by some. No one knew anything about anesthesia under pressure or of even seeing a pulsating heart through the chest cavity, much less operating on it."

Osteomyelitis or bone infection was feared. Middle ear disease and surgical mastoid drainings were everyday affairs for the ear, nose, and throat specialists. After a tooth extraction, a patient might develop a hopelessly extensive facial cellulitis and cavernous sinus thrombosis.

After City Hospital got a south wing, a west wing, and landscaping, it changed its name to Brackenridge Hospital.

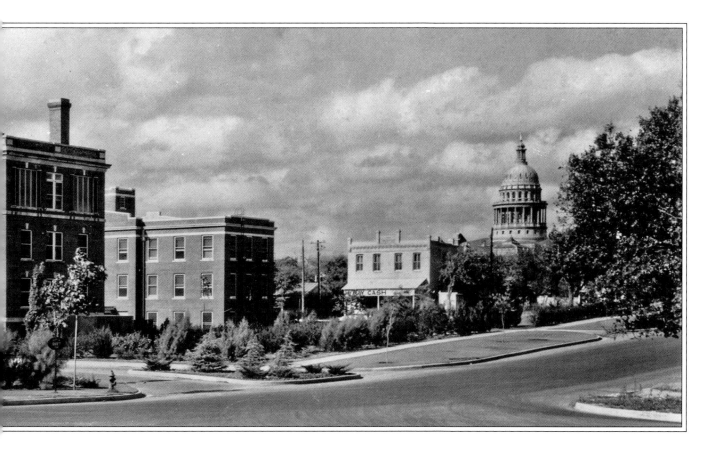

"It was maddeningly frustrating and saddening to attend the child dying from scarlet fever complications. Or to sit all night with the patient dying of pneumonia—the mother of one of your close friends—listening futilely to the chest for the sound of the rale called *crepitus redux*. This audible physical sign indicated possible impending recovery."

Physicians were taught to expect bad results, he recalled, and patients were aware of the dangers, but seemed to understand and appreciate that doctors were doing everything possible. "I shall never forget one of the dramatic results observed in one of our beloved coaches at the University of Texas.... He had typical lobar pneumonia, fever was 106, and he was cyanotic; in an oxygen tent. He was unable to retain the then available oral sulfa drugs. Word came to us that some one had another form of sulfa—sulfapyridine—for experimental use that had been given successfully in a few instances, by injection. We had some of this flown in from another city—it was a powder. Despite all of our efforts we could not get it into solution and the solution remained cloudy but we gave it anyhow...under the skin as hypodermoclysis. Within eight hours there was a dramatic improvement and ultimate recovery. This, to all of us, was an unforgettable medical milestone."

Like his father, Dr. Gilbert served as a surgeon for the UT Student Health Center. He became a fellow of the American College of Surgeons and the Southwest Surgical Congress, president of the Texas Surgical Society in 1966, and in 1973 was appointed to the Texas State Board of Medical Examiners. He also served as chief of staff at St. David's Hospital. Twice, he was president of the Travis County Medical Society and in 1947 he became a diplomate of the American Board of Surgery. He also authored papers in *The American Surgeon*, *The American Journal of Surgery*, and the *Texas State Journal of Medicine*. Active in

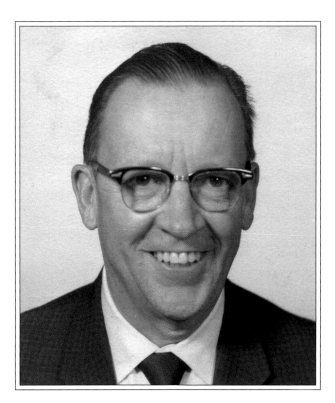

Dr. Joe Thorne Gilbert, like his father, served as surgeon at the University of Texas Student Health Center.

community affairs, he was a founding member of Good Shepherd Episcopal Church.

At basic levels, science was progressing. The earliest sulfa drugs—offering great hope as antibiotics—were trademarked as Prontosil and Neoprontosil, with the latter almost specific for gonorrhea. In the 1930s, Mayo Clinic researchers, led by Edward C. Kendall, isolated cortisone from adrenal glands, leading to the first available steroid drug, although it was not used clinically until 1948. Dr. Philip S. Hench in 1948 and 1949 successfully used it in arthritic patients. Elmer V. McCollum and others at Johns Hopkins distinguished the roles of vitamins A and D, concluding the latter was the controlling factor in preventing rickets, and thus showing why cod liver oil was valuable. In this decade of the nineteen thirties, there were also discoveries in the world of physics with ramifications for medicine.

Travis County physicians continued their education through society meetings. In 1932, Dr. Happy Scott encouraged physicians to use tact to reduce the "fear of complicated labor induced by the usual harrowing experiences related by well-intentioned women." He condemned using quinine to induce labor because of the risks of stillbirth but believed a Roentgen examination before labor could help determine "the exact position of the child and the presence of any skeletal abnormalities." A Dallas physician's paper on the etiology and pathogenesis of hypertension was discussed. Noting that "hypertensive types" would be recognized at an earlier stage in the future, the author observed that the "old concept that age plus 100 makes the correct blood pressure is changing, and it is becoming accepted that there is no standard normal blood pressure for persons of various ages."

Tuberculosis was the leading cause of death among Texans aged fifteen to forty-five at this time, and in 1935 Dr. Z. T. Scott spoke before a state symposium on tuberculosis. He hoped for "vaccination, early diagnosis, and treatment to completely eradicate the Great White Plague."

Dr. H. W. Newman moved to Austin in 1933, having been a missionary in China and with the Red Cross in Siberia during World War I. With the assistance of the American Association of University Women, he opened the first free clinic for children at Brackenridge Hospital. He kept his private office until 1956, but remained in charge of a clinic for one day a week in the "Negro" housing unit of the City-County Health Unit. Born in Rochester, New York, in December 1878, Dr. Newman held a B.A. degree from McMaster University in Toronto, and had received his M.D. degree from the University of Michigan Medical School in 1908. He also had studied at UTMB. Dr. Newman had a personal tie to Austin physician Dr. Frederick Eby, his sister's husband.

Dr. Robert E. Bratton, a Round Rock native and UT graduate, came to Austin in 1930 to practice general medicine. He had received his M.D. degree from Tulane University School of Medicine, interned at Charity Hospital of Louisiana, New Orleans, and undertaken surgical residencies at Shreveport Charity Hospital and in Monroe, Louisiana.

Also arriving in 1930 was Dr. Hugo Alfred Auler. The son of Dr. Edwin Brunelle Auler of Elgin, he attended Elgin High School and the University of Texas. In 1927, he graduated from Tulane University School of Medicine, followed by an internship at Charity Hospital of Louisiana and a residency at Shreveport Charity Hospital. He became a fellow of the American College of Surgeons.

Dr. Ben R. Eppright probably was the first dermatology specialist in the city. Born in Manor in September 1900, he was a 1925 UTMB graduate and first practiced in his home town before moving to Austin. He was a 1930 dermatology graduate of the New York Skin and Cancer Hospital. He became the 1932 president of the Travis County Medical Society. Margaret Schoch, a psychology major at the University of Texas, was the daughter of Dr. Eugene Schoch, a UT professor who had founded the discipline of chemical engineering there and was active and influential in many other realms. After graduating from the university, Margaret had gone to UTMB in Galveston to study medical technology. While training among the medical students, she told her father she had decided to enter medical school. After receiving her M.D. in 1932, she returned to Austin and worked with Dr. Eppright in his dermatology practice. The two physicians later were married.

Dr. Eppright also brought Dr. C. H. "Hal" McCuistion into his dermatology practice in the Norwood Building.

Born in March 1913 in Valley View, Texas, Dr. McCuistion graduated from high school in Gainesville, Texas. After finishing his work at UT, he left for Galveston, and received his M.D. degree from UTMB in 1938. He interned at the Robert B. Green Hospital in San Antonio and briefly practiced in Austin. In the 1940s, he twice undertook postgraduate work at the Mayo Foundation in Rochester, Minnesota. During World War II, he served as a major in the U.S. Army Air Corps (the future U.S. Air Force) on the continent and in Guam. He returned to Austin to practice and became president of several organizations, including the Texas Dermatological Society, the Texas Mayo Clinic Alumni Association, and the Travis County Medical Society.

Austin already was home for others or they had come to UT for their education. In 1936, Dr. Judson Harriss Williams, a Giddings native, resumed a private practice as a surgeon and family practitioner in Austin, having been an associate professor of surgery at UTMB in Galveston. He had received his B.A. degree from UT in 1922 and his M.D. degree from UTMB in 1927. His internship was at St. Mary's Infirmary in Galveston, after which he practiced medicine in Smithville and then in 1928 at the UT Student Health Service.

In 1931, Dr. William M. Gambrell arrived from Belton, where he had been in general practice since 1920. Born in Waco in August 1890, he was educated in the Lockhart public schools and in 1910 entered Southwest Texas Normal College (eventually Texas State University). With a certificate, he taught first grade one year and after college graduation taught science at Lockhart High School. Becoming superintendent of Lockhart schools, he took correspondence courses and attended UT the summer before entering the Medical Department in 1916. He worked nights, attending classes during the day, and received his M.D. degree in 1920. He was a member of Alpha Omega Alpha. His graduate training was at the New York Lying-In Hospital (later consolidated under Cornell Medical Center). In future years, he limited his practice to surgery, obstetrics, and gynecology. Dr. Gambrell would be of great significance to the Travis County Medical Society and TMA. One son would practice medicine in Luling, Texas.

A graduate medical education landmark was set in June 1931 when Brackenridge Hospital received its first intern. Dr. George Edmund Bennack, born in Pleasanton in April 1900, had attended UT from 1924 to 1927, and had graduated from UTMB in 1931. Before undertaking his medical education, Dr. Bennack had been a master railroad machinist to help put two younger brothers through dental school. They had then helped him through college and medical school. With the city health officer, Dr. Lee Edens, as his supervisor, Dr. Bennack spent his year in a typical rotating internship, completing his training in mid-July 1932. There was no division of services and he was always on call. He also worked in the clinics. Dr. Ben Eppright was in charge of the skin clinic and Dr. Henry Hilgartner, Jr., typically staffed the eye clinic. Dr. Claud Miears of the ear, nose, and throat clinic performed the tonsillectomies. Dr. Bennack was paid fifty dollars a month—five times more than the average in other institutions across the country—plus room, board, and laundry. The hospital had fifty beds, with "white" patients in the main hospital and the "Negro" patients in the annex, which could be reached through a breezeway. Dr. Caroline Crowell, a general practitioner and physician at the UT Student Health Center, assisted Dr. Bennack with emergencies at night. "She lived in the hospital and had a room on the second floor over the emergency room," Ms. Mary Micka reported. "When an emergency came in, she would hear it and go down to help out. She and Dr. Bennack played tennis when he got a break. The courts were across the street, and when he was needed, someone would come out and call him."

Dr. Bennack was a captain in the U.S. Army Medical Corps for four years during World War II, stationed on the continent and in the Pacific theatre, including Japan. He practiced primarily in Raymondville in south Texas, where he became president of the Cameron-Willacy Counties Medical Society in 1949. One of his sons, Gene, became an orthopedic surgeon and another son, a dentist.

Dr. Claud Martin, also a 1931 UTMB graduate and classmate of Dr. Bennack's, was the first resident at Brackenridge, serving a one-year term beginning in 1932. He had interned at John Sealy Hospital in Galveston. In Austin, he also earned fifty dollars a month. Most of his year was spent in surgery and thus his training was designated as a surgical residency. Dr. Martin remained in Austin to practice medicine. In 1991, Ms. Mary Micka of the Central Texas Medical Foundation interviewed Drs. Bennack and Martin for the *TCMS Journal* when both physicians were in their nineties. Both had vivid memories of their years at Brackenridge Hospital.

Travis County doctors like Dr. Thomas McCrummen, who had been in Austin since the 1920s, continued their civic service along with their busy practices. Dr. McCrummen had been a delegate to the White House Conference on Child Health and Protection during Herbert Hoover's administration and served on the board of the Austin Community Guidance Center, which he had helped to launch. In 1934, he was certified by the American Board of Pediatrics during the program's first year. With an office in the downtown Norwood Building, he was the only pediatrician in Austin until Dr. Thomas J. McElhenney arrived in 1933.

Born in February 1897 in Atlanta, Georgia, Dr. McElhenney was a University of Alabama graduate and received his medical degree from Tulane University School of Medicine in 1922. He had begun the practice of medicine in Bessemer, Alabama, after serving in the U.S. Army Chemical Corps during World War I. From 1921 to 1923, his internship and subsequent pediatric residency were at the Employees Hospital (later Lloyd Noland Hospital) of the Tennessee Coal and Iron Railroad Company in Fairfield, Alabama. He had established the first well-baby clinics in Alabama and in 1934, with the help of the Junior League, opened the first such clinic in Austin. He also had participated in the White House Conference on Child Health and Protection in 1930, and was state chairman of the White House Conference on Children and Youth in 1960. Dr. McElhenney was certified as a pediatric specialist in 1935 by the American Board of Pediatrics. In 1939, he had an office on Nueces Street and was chief of pediatrics at Brackenridge Hospital. He was also president of the Travis County Pediatric Society and the Texas Pediatric Society. A long-time member of the board of the American Academy of Pediatrics, he also was chairman of the American Legion's child welfare committee for fifteen years.

After completing a scholarship for advanced public health work at the University of Michigan, Dr. Connie Ralstine Yerwood returned to Austin in 1936. She joined the Texas State Department of Health, the first black physician known to have been employed there. Among her early duties as a field medical consultant was helping to raise the educational level of midwives in east Texas. Reportedly the first "second-generation" black physician practicing in Travis County, she faced and would overcome many challenges because of her race. She was born in 1907 in Victoria, Texas, while her father, Dr. Charles Yerwood, practiced in rural Gonzales County. After graduating from Samuel Huston College (later Huston-Tillotson) in Austin, she earned her medical degree in 1933 from Meharry Medical College in Nashville, Tennessee, as did her sister Joyce.

She recalled filing her medical license with the Travis County clerk. The man waiting on her said, "Oh, a lady doctor. Where did you go, Galveston?" She responded, "Now you can look at me and tell that I didn't go to

Galveston, can't you?" She explained, "None of us could go to Galveston in those days...." but people took it for granted that if one went to medical school it was there. Because they were women, the Yerwood sisters also had difficulty finding a residency, but a friend of their father's helped find them positions at General Hospital in Kansas City, Missouri. Joyce married a physician, moved to Connecticut, and became a family physician in Port Chester, New York. Her father, who once discouraged her, gave her equipment to start her practice. Joyce also praised Connie for her support. "YOU carried me through that first year of practice, morally and financially," she wrote, "for the depression was for real."

Dr. Sandy (often recorded officially also as Sandi) Esquivel was an outstanding athlete at the University of Texas in multiple fields—track, cross country, and basketball—and was inducted into the University of Texas Hall of Honor. As the individual cross-country champion in 1924 and 1925 in the Southwest Conference, he led his UT team to titles in both years. In 1925, he set a conference record in the two-mile run that stood for twenty-four years. He was a member of the championship track team in 1925 and 1926, and was named an All-American in 1925. In addition, he was captain of the 1926 basketball and track teams and played on the unbeaten conference championship team in 1924.

In 1935, Dr. Esquivel arrived as the first orthopedic specialist in Austin. In praising him, Dr. Kermit Fox observed that Dr. Esquivel encountered many hurdles, but "having been a superb athlete he hurdled over most." In the early years, "broken hips were not yet treated by nailing"; there were no formally trained anesthesiologists and probably no trained physiotherapists. "It was necessary for Dr. Esquivel to furnish most of his own orthopedic operating instruments and equipment." The future Dr. Robert N. Snider also recalled that Dr. Esquivel spent long hours before antibiotics were available treating patients with osteomyelitis by curettage and drainage. Born in El Paso in 1904, Dr.

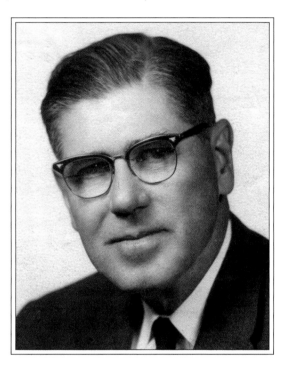

Dr. Henry Hilgartner, Jr., staffed the eye clinic at Brackenridge Hospital.

Esquivel graduated from UT in 1926 and from UTMB in 1930. He served an internship at King's Daughters Hospital at Temple from 1930 to 1931 and from 1933 to 1935 he trained at what became the New York Orthopaedic Hospital in New York City, one of the oldest orthopedic training programs in the country. After he opened a free orthopedic clinic at Brackenridge Hospital, other hospitals offered needed ancillary systems such as physical therapy and x-ray equipment. Dr. Esquivel also was associated with Shriners Hospitals for Crippled Children. With an office in the Norwood Building, he remained in private practice until his death in 1969.

Dr. Elizabeth Paterson began a general practice in Austin in 1932, with an office in the Norwood Building. Born in June 1900 in San Antonio, she received a bachelor's degree from Newcomb College of Tulane University, New Orleans, and an M.D. degree from Tulane University School of Medicine. She undertook an internship at Children's Hospital in San Francisco from 1929 to 1931. In Austin, she practiced some anesthesiology, along with her general practice. In later years, at the encouragement of Dr. David O. Johnson, Austin's first formally trained anesthesiologist, she underwent a residency in anesthesiology at UTMB, completing it in 1950, and returned to practice with the Austin Anesthesiology Group. Dr. Paterson was known affectionately by operating room and hospital staff as "Dr. Pat."

State government and higher education largely sustained Austin during the Great Depression. Federal programs supported public works and a home for student nurses at Brackenridge, allowing the hospital to expand nurse training. Away at school, future Austin physicians had jobs with the National Youth Administration (NYA), a government education assistance program. Practicing physicians were brought into federal programs, like the Federal Emergency Relief Administration, and were expected to furnish medical services to indigent patients for reduced fees. At first, doctors considered the effort laudable but grew concerned about the dangers of socialized medicine. In this era also the Social Security Act of 1935 was passed.

In 1937, Dr. H. L. Hilgartner, Sr., died in Atlantic City, New Jersey, one day after presenting a paper with his son to the organization that became the Association for Research in Vision and Ophthalmology. Dr. Kermit Fox understood from Dr. Henry Hilgartner, Jr., that his father had performed the first cataract operation in Texas.

Dr. James M. Coleman arrived in Austin in 1937 to become director of maternal and child health and later director of public health, welfare, and hospitals at the Texas State Health Department. Born in November 1906 in Brinkley, Arkansas, he was a graduate of Ouachita Baptist University at Arkadelphia, Arkansas. He received his M.D. degree in 1930 from Baylor University College of Medicine in Dallas, where he became a member of Alpha Omega Alpha. Dr. Coleman served an internship and residency at St. Louis City Hospital, and then undertook further graduate work, acquiring a master's degree from Harvard University School of Public Health in 1939. In addition, he studied at Vanderbilt University School of Public Health, the University of Wisconsin, and the University of Chicago. He was certified by the American Board of Pediatrics in 1940. Dr. Coleman had begun his medical career in 1934 as a Plano general practitioner.

After practicing at Mexia and Amherst, Texas, Dr. Barth Milligan, Sr., moved to Austin in 1939 to practice. Born in Thomaston, Texas, in October 1897, he attended UT and graduated from UTMB in 1924. In 1924 and 1925, he served an internship at John Sealy Hospital in Galveston and followed that in 1939 with postgraduate study at Tulane University School of Medicine. Dr. Milligan was known for delivering numerous babies at home and helping midwives in trouble. His office adjoined his home and he saw many patients long after most doctors' offices had closed for the day. His son, Dr. Barth Milligan, Jr., also would later practice in Austin.

Dr. Edward L. Roberts, a 1931 graduate of Meharry Medical College, arrived in Austin in late November of 1932, where he opened a clinic in East Austin. In 1935, he was listed at 1174 Navasota Street. He interned at John A. Andrews Hospital in Tuskegee, Alabama, and was considered a pioneer in Austin in making "clean, comfortable and sanitary hospital rooms available to his race." His clinic on Navasota Street was said to be the only one "of its kind in the southwest, owned and operated by Negroes."

In 1936, when the Reverend Francis R. Weber founded Holy Cross Catholic Church for black parishioners, he learned that one of their chief needs was medical care for the needy. With the Missionary Franciscan Sisters of the Immaculate Conception, he opened Holy Cross Hospital in July 1940 at 1106 Concho Street, near the 1600 block of West Eleventh Street. Dr. Weber served as architect and did much of the carpentry work. The institution was considered the first black Catholic hospital in the state. An August 1940 *Austin American-Statesman* article reported that Holy Cross had twenty-four beds with a special ward of nine "small beds" for infants. Fees were to be low, as little as $1.50 per day. Seven other beds in a separate room were to be reserved for staff. The hospital's most valuable piece of equipment, at $700, was a "violet ray machine," donated by a San Antonio physician. Pressure cookers and kitchen pots were used to sterilize instruments. Sister Celine Heitzman, a 1938 graduate of George Washington University School of Medicine, became the resident physician in 1942 and would be credited with improving the institution. Cited as the first Catholic nun in the United States to become a physician—she was an M.D.—she would deliver nearly 4,000 babies during her twenty-four years at the hospital. Born as Margaret Heitzman in Paterson, New Jersey, she had undertaken graduate studies in Baltimore and at Children's Hospital, in Washington, D.C., with an additional three months spent at Margaret Hague Maternity Hospital in Jersey City, New Jersey. During the 1940s, Sister Celine fostered a racially mixed hospital staff at Holy Cross Hospital. Initially, Holy Cross was the only hospital in Austin allowing black physicians to treat their own patients. A new modern masonry hospital with fifty beds was built in 1951 on East Nineteenth Street (later Martin Luther King, Jr. Boulevard), followed by another expansion in 1964.

Arriving in 1939, Dr. Beadie Eugene Conner helped raise funds for Holy Cross Hospital and was among the first physicians to practice there. Born in Texarkana, Texas, in July 1902, Dr. Conner earned a B.A. degree in 1926 from Fisk University in Nashville, Tennessee, and a medical degree from Meharry Medical College in 1930. His internship was at Kansas City General Hospital Number 2 in Kansas City, Missouri. (Until 1957, Kansas City had two general hospitals—one for white and one for black patients. They were later combined and replaced by Truman Medical Center.) Dr. Conner also undertook postgraduate work at Flint-Goodrich Hospital in New Orleans in 1936 and 1937. He became a co-organizer of the Austin Negro Chamber of Commerce in 1940 and highly prominent in the Austin community. He served as secretary of the Lone Star State Medical Association and in 1957, after black

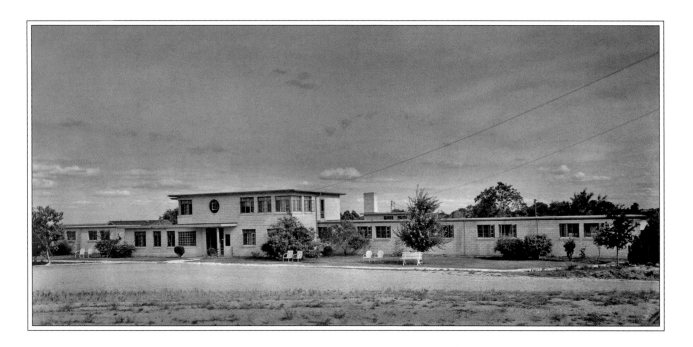

Travis County Tuberculosis Sanitorium opened in 1940.

physicians became eligible for membership, he became a TMA member.

Among the large array of drug store names listed in the 1937 city directory were Ransom's Drug Stores, White Pharmacy, five Renfro Drug Company Stores (including The Rexall Store), the Prescription Laboratory, Beck's Drug Stores, Kelly Everette Pharmacy, Kuhn's Pharmacy, Matthews Drug Store, the University Drug Store, Varsity Drug Store, Grove Drug Store, and Walgreen Drug Company of Texas.

On South Congress Avenue was Brown's Rest Home; the East Sanitarium was on 1206 East Avenue; the Marguarete Home and the Austin Convalescent Home on Lafayette Avenue; and the Oaks Sanitarium on the Upper Georgetown Road. The city had homes for children, "old ladies," "old Negro" women, Confederate men and women, and the Travis County Poor Farm. It also had the Travis County Lighthouse for the Blind, founded in 1934 by Dr. H. L. Hilgartner.

Tuberculosis remained a problem, and in 1940, the Austin-Travis County Tuberculosis Sanatorium opened east of Austin on Webberville Road. On the site of a camp set up in the 1920s, it later was dubbed Brackenridge East.

Prospective physicians struggled during the Depression. Marie Correll graduated from UT in 1930. Her friend Albert Tisdale returned to summer school in Austin after his first year of medical school and received his bachelor's degree from UT. With funds tight, however, he had to drop out of medical school. Marie's family was experiencing a

pinch, so she took a social worker position at the San Antonio State Hospital. After she and Albert were married in August 1932 at her parents' home in Austin, they left for medical school at Tulane University in New Orleans. Finding odd jobs, they nourished themselves ingeniously—such as by using milk samples left from tests in the biochemistry laboratory and a large piece of beef steak that had been used experimentally in the physiology laboratory. With invitations to eat and gifts of crabs from Lake Pontchartrain, they survived. Walking everywhere, they put cardboard in their shoes when the soles wore through.

When the Depression worsened in 1933 and 1934, Marie dropped out of school and returned to work as a social worker, this time among the black unemployed in New Orleans. She raised green flies in sterile cages for the surgery department and was an assistant in the anatomy department's laboratory. When he graduated, Dr. Albert Tisdale started his internship at Charity Hospital and had to move into intern quarters. Marie found jobs to support herself and a small place with another intern's wife. It was a year of "bitter poverty." Interns in 1934 had no pay, but did have room, meals, and seven-to-ten dollars a month from an insurance fund. In the evening, she sat on a curb outside the hospital, hoping her husband could bring his meal leftovers in a paper napkin. "If he couldn't bring my 'sandwich,' I went without," she said. Happily, if the food arrived, "the bread was freshly baked French bread, or hard French rolls with soft centers, and the meat was French daube, seafood, or chicken.... home cooked New Orleans style food...."

In 1935, Albert went to Shreveport for a residency and Marie returned to school, graduating in 1937, the year her father died. Dr. Joe Gilbert back in Austin had attended her father and reported the cause of death as coronary occlusion. Although Marie was at the top of her class, she had to arrange for her own internship because no hospital wanted a woman. The old Medical and Surgical (later Baptist) Hospital in San Antonio, although not a teaching hospital, accepted her. Her husband meanwhile worked as a medical officer at a Civilian Conservation Corps camp in Tennessee and, as an Army reservist, spent two weeks in officers' training in Pennsylvania. After Marie finished her internship in June 1939, she and Albert headed to Lafayette, Louisiana, where he opened an office. Life was pleasant, but with Hitler's advances in Europe, Albert was ordered to active duty.

Other young people also delayed their dreams. David O. Johnson dropped out of high school and, like Dr. Bennack, worked on the railroads. He would return to school in his twenties.

Georgia Felter graduated from Austin High School in 1935 and received her bachelor's degree with high honors from UT in 1938. Dr. Margaret Schoch Eppright had advised her that if she could make a B grade in physical chemistry at UT she would have no trouble in medical school. Also serving as young Georgia's mentors were Dr. Eugene Schoch (Margaret's father) and UT physician Dr. Caroline Crowell. Dr. Eugene Schoch, Jr., remembered that his father encouraged women to go into medicine. Most professors discouraged women, he recalled, especially one "tough old professor." Georgia was accepted into UTMB where she worked with the National Youth Administration helping with a study on clotting in rabbits. She also oversaw nurses at their residence, basically as a chaperone, and maintained the switchboard at night. She also met her future husband, Carey Legett, Jr., at UTMB. Planning to be a medical missionary, she also wanted to prove that marriage, family, and a career in medicine were possible.

Carey Legett, Jr., was born in January 1918 at Port Lavaca, Texas. At age six, he began picking cotton on a friend's farm. The payment was one dollar for one hundred pounds of cotton picked. At age eight, working from sunrise to sunset, he picked his first one hundred pounds of cotton. Graduating from high school in the coastal city, he attended Victoria Junior College and proceeded to UT. After one year he was accepted at UTMB. He, too, held a National Youth Administration job and became a student intern at the U.S. Marine Hospital in Galveston.

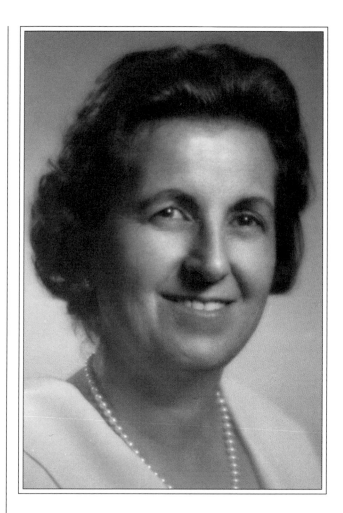

Dr. Marie C. Tisdale.

A class behind Georgia Felter at UTMB was Ruth M. Bain, whose life would be guided by something her mother told her. Born in Normangee, Texas, in 1919, she had grown up in Centerville, Texas and graduated as high school valedictorian in 1936. As she and her mother shelled black-eyed peas on their front porch, her mother said, "Ruth, you have this idea that you want to be a doctor....you have a great deal of determination and I feel that if you really want to do this, and you persist, in this great country of ours, doors will be opened for you." Ruth attended Texas State College for Women (later renamed Texas Woman's University) in Denton and, lacking six hours for her chemistry degree, entered UTMB in 1939. In those days, it was typical to begin medical school before completing one's undergraduate degree, but she earned credit for science courses at UTMB and in May 1940 received her B.A. degree in chemistry.

After graduating from the two-year Blinn College in Brenham, Kermit Fox, with his valedictorian's scholarship, headed toward Austin and the University of Texas in 1931. His future wife, Jewel, a native of Giddings, took her nurse's training in Austin, staying at the Seton Infirmary nurses' home on Rio Grande Street. After finishing at UT, Dr. Fox received his M.D. degree from UTMB in May 1936, and was commissioned as a first lieutenant in the U.S Army Reserve. He took a bus to New York for a rotating internship at Rochester General Hospital, and developed an interest in orthopedics. After practicing briefly in Rochester, he returned home in 1939 when his father died and in August of that year opened an office in Bryan, Texas.

George Tipton graduated from high school in 1931, earned a B.S. degree from the University of Texas in 1935, and an M.D. degree in 1938 from UTMB. Army recruiters were waiting for his graduating class, too, and he agreed to be sworn into the Army Reserve, expecting to serve one year. In the meantime, he took an internship at UTMB from 1938 to 1939, followed by another at Jefferson Davis Hospital in Houston from 1939 to 1940.

Identical twins Clifford and Lansing Thorne were born in 1921 in El Paso where they grew up, but after their father lost his job during the Depression, they moved to Austin to live with relatives. It was a good place to acquire their college education, and in 1938, the future Austin pediatricians began their studies at UT. In 1944, their younger brother, Milner Speer Thorne, a future Austin anesthesiologist, also graduated from UT.

Robert N. Snider's father in Brownwood also lost his job during the Great Depression and young Robert, observing the prosperity of his out-of-state radiologist uncle, decided he also wanted to become a radiologist. After graduating from Brownwood High School in 1939, he arrived in Austin in 1940. The only radiologist agreeing to teach him for a hundred dollars was Dr. Rabun Thomas Wilson. With the funds earned working for him, he paid his way through a premedical course at UT. He also worked at Brackenridge Hospital for about two years doing whatever he could to earn money—x-rays, orderly work, running electrocardiograms, and mopping floors.

Dr. Wilson, an 1884 native of Belton and a radiologist, had moved to Austin in 1936. He had attended Belton public schools and Wedemeyer Academy in Belton, receiving his M.D. degree from the UT Medical Department in 1911. His internship was at the state hospital in Abilene and he served residencies and practiced at the Santa Fe and Scott and White hospitals in Temple. A charter member of the Texas Radiological Society, he was certified by the American Board of Radiology and authored many published papers. In addition to civic activities, Dr. Wilson was a member of the TMA Board of Councilors.

Dr. Snider recalled that the kilovoltage for the therapy machine in Dr. Wilson's office was set by two stainless steel balls. "One served as the anode and the other the cathode. As these were brought together—whenever a spark jumped from one to the other—that was the kilo voltage." Laura Weed, "the nice lady who taught me, jumped every time this happened.... There was always the smell of ozone in the air...there was no good way to determine how much x-ray was given to a skin cancer. Skin dose was measured as 'erythema dose' signifying how red the skin got after so much radiation." Electrocardiographs were done on paper strips that had to be developed to see the image. Produced from a bright light shining on a galvanometer wire, he said, they vibrated as the examination was performed. The fragile wire frequently broke.

Gowns, gloves, and masks were reused. From her nurse's training at Seton Infirmary in the early 1930s, Jewel Fox recalled that torn gloves were saved for patching. Dr. Snider remembered the recycling of needles. "After use, they were washed and placed in a sterilizer or boiled in water or soaked in antiseptic solutions. They were wrapped in a cotton cloth and that was it." There were no standards for sharpness, so even after much sharpening there were many blunt needles.

Dr. Oliver W. Suehs, son of Dr. Paul E. Suehs, returned to Austin in 1941 to join his father's practice. Born in Carmine, Texas, in November 1911, Dr. Suehs graduated from Austin High School in 1928, from UT in 1932, and from UTMB in 1936. He completed a two-year rotating internship at the Graduate Hospital of the University of Pennsylvania and a three-year residency in bronchoesophagology and otolaryngology at Jefferson Medical College Hospital in Philadelphia. Dr. Suehs became known as an outstanding physician and a gentleman.

As war clouds darkened, military service ensnared more doctors. In February 1941, Dr. George Tipton left for Camp Barkley near Abilene, Texas, and soon headed overseas. Dr. Kermit Fox forgot about signing up for the Army Reserve, but on July 29, 1941, he and other medics were sworn to secrecy and left San Antonio by train for Camp Murray near Fort Lewis, Washington, and by boat to the Alaska Defense Command.

In 1940, British researchers isolated and purified penicillin after rediscovering Fleming's 1920s work and in 1941 sought help from the U.S. government, which made production a priority. The antibiotic would be available to the military but not to civilians, with rare exceptions, until after the war.

CHAPTER X

WARTIME: SACRIFICES AND SHORTAGES

SOPHOMORE RUTH BAIN WAS IN THE bacteriology laboratory at the University of Texas Medical Branch at Galveston (UTMB) on Sunday afternoon, December 7, 1941, "making agar and listening to the radio. That was how I learned the shocking news that Pearl Harbor had been bombed....We students remained glued to the radio, knowing full well that the war would impact our lives." Near New Orleans, Dr. Marie Tisdale was trying to get a residency. At a pediatric faculty social, she learned about Pearl Harbor and went home to wait for her husband, Dr. Albert Tisdale, but he was confined to the Army base.

In the spring of 1942, Drs. Georgia and Carey Legett, Jr. graduated from UTMB. Carey began his internship at Jefferson Davis Hospital in Houston, but, as an Army Reserve lieutenant, was called to active duty in July. Training at the Medical Field Service School at Carlisle, Pennsylvania, before transferring to the Army Air Corps, he completed his training at the School of Aviation Medicine at San Antonio's Randolph Field, with further training in Nashville, Tennessee. He was sent "red alert' overseas as a flight surgeon for the 2nd Troop Carrier Squadron and became organizational group surgeon of the 3rd Combat Cargo Group. He spent two years in China, India, and North Burma, including flying over the "Himalayan Hump." He became a major and completed thirty missions in Douglas DC-3 airplanes, the Army's C-47s.

Ruth Bain and her classmates received their degrees from UTMB in December 1942 rather than in the spring of 1943, "virtually pushed through," with no summer breaks.

Joining the Army Air Corps in 1942, Dr. Joe Thorne Gilbert also became a flight surgeon and a hospital commander, rising in rank to lieutenant colonel. Dr. Oliver Suehs became chief of the otolaryngology department with the 127th General Hospital Unit, staffed by UTMB faculty and students, in the European theatre. Dr. Charles P. Hardwicke entered the Army Medical Corps in 1942, becoming a major, and Dr. Robert Bratton joined the Navy. These are examples of many others to come.

Physicians were acquiring knowledge they would bring home to Austin. Dr. George Tipton, who had signed up for one year of military service, served for five years, three of them in North Africa, Sicily, and Italy with the U.S. Army's Fifteenth Evacuation (Surgical) Hospital. In 1943, he learned a term new to him from French troops in North Africa—triage—a process for sorting casualties after catastrophic battles. At the Anzio beachhead in Sicily, a 400-bed portable hospital could be split so that half could be moved forward at a time. Dr. Tipton and his fellow medics used whole blood generously to replace blood loss but, when needed in some situations, they rehydrated plasma usually to increase volume, mixing it with whole blood. Most wounded had suffered blast injuries from artillery shell fragments. If a soldier bled out, he was administered

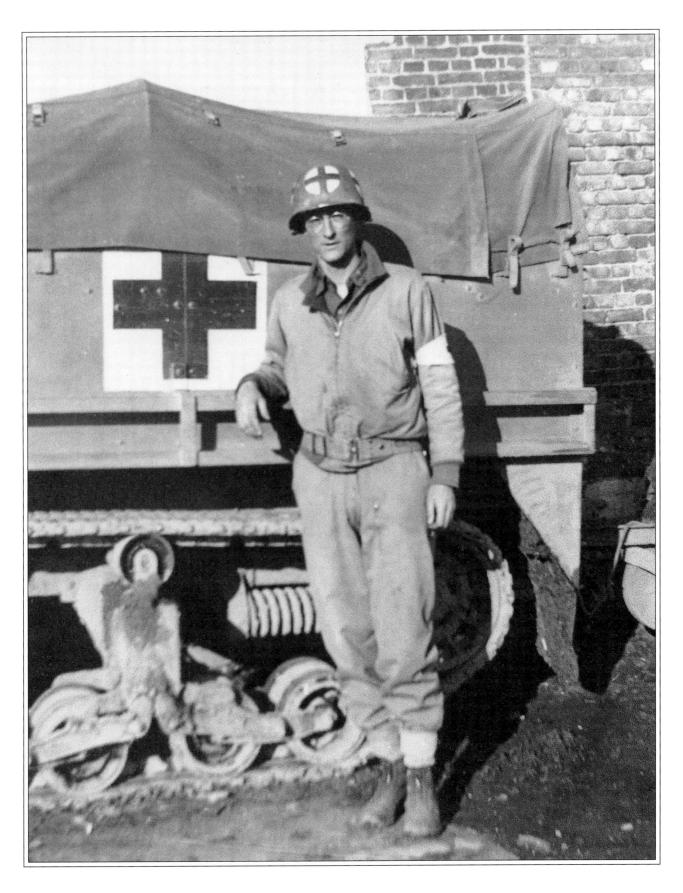

Dr. Jim Kreisle served as surgeon for the 32nd Mechanized Cavalry. He commanded the medical detachment behind the front lines during the Battle of the Bulge.

low titer O type blood that had not been crossmatched. In medical school, there had been no heart or vascular surgery, but on the battlefield, Dr. Tipton operated on big arteries, closing them with good results. He learned that three times as many soldiers were diagnosed with psychoneurosis as with other wounds. In 1944, he used the new miracle drug, penicillin, experimenting to get the right dosage.

At Fort Raymond, Alaska, Dr. Kermit Fox commanded a 150-bed hospital. He, too, used penicillin for the first time, although each time a committee's approval was necessary. In 1943, he was sent to Camp Wolters at Mineral Wells, Texas, and became orthopedic section chief. Rationing—from shoes to sugar to meat—was in place, and the Fox family was typical in "making do." Jewel Fox swapped coupons and stamps to get diaper material for baby Kermit, Jr., and made him a coat with her old nurse's caps.

No one knew how long the war would last, and in Austin Dr. Sidney Bohls processed blood plasma for civilian emergencies.

Dr. S. H. "Bud" Dryden had been called to active duty with the Army Air Corps after completing an internship at City-County Hospital in Fort Worth. Born in February 1914 in Abilene, Texas, he had attended Abilene Christian College and graduated from Baylor University College of Medicine in Dallas in June 1940. He was a flight surgeon for the 64th Carrier Group in England, North Africa, India, Italy, and France. In 1945, he would join the Scott-Gregg Clinic, inheriting Dr. Z. T. Scott's patients.

Dr. David O. Johnson interned from 1942 to 1943 and then began his residency, but soon left for the U.S. Army's 109th Evacuation Hospital in Europe. On the battlefields, Dr. Johnson directed the "administration of more than 11,000 anesthetics," writes Dr. James Prentice of his mentor. He would leave the service as a major in 1945. He also would become "a medical history scholar." Serving in the Army's Thirty-sixth Division was Dr. Benjamin M. Primer,

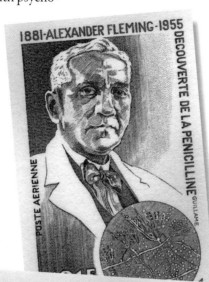

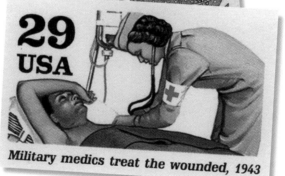

Military medics treat the wounded, 1943

TOP: *Commemorative stamp for Sir Alexander Fleming's discovery of penicillin. Penicillin was the "wonder drug" during World War II.* ABOVE: *Commemorative World War II stamps illustrating military medics treating the wounded.*

Sr. He had graduated from UTMB in 1924 and earned a master's degree in public health at Harvard Medical School. He became director of public health in Austin.

Dr. Morris D. "Mac" McCauley was in the Army Medical Corps with the Fifty-sixth Evacuation Hospital, attached to the Forward Fifth Army active in Naples, Foggia, the Po Valley, Sicily, the Northern Appenines, Rome-Arno, and the Anzio Beachhead. Born in 1911, he graduated from Wayne State University College of Medicine in Detroit and completed an internship and a residency in obstetrics and gynecology at Detroit Receiving Hospital and Herman Keifer Hospital. In Austin, he taught in the nursing schools at Brackenridge, Seton, and the University of Texas, and also in UT Special Education Programs.

Dr. Raleigh Ross, born in Lockhart in 1913, was the son of Dr. Alonzo A. Ross, the 1933 president of the Texas Medical Association. A 1935 graduate of UTMB, he was an intern and a resident in thoracic and general surgery, and was also chief resident, at the Hospital of the Protestant Episcopal Church in Philadelphia until 1941. A lieutenant colonel in the Army Medical Corps, Dr. Ross would be acknowledged as the first board-certified chest surgeon in Austin, earning his surgery certification in 1943 and in thoracic surgery in 1949.

Dr. Walter Donald Roberts, a Burkburnett native, received his M.D. degree from UTMB in 1943. He was an intern at the U.S. Naval Hospital at Corona, California, from 1943 to 1944; did a pathology residency at UTMB from 1947 to 1948; trained in internal medicine at Scott and White, in Temple, from 1948 to 1949; and trained at Harvard (Boston City Hospital) in 1952. From 1943 to 1947, he was in the Navy Medical Corps, serving at Texas A&M and in California, and was with the Second Marine Division in Saipan, Okinawa, and Japan.

Born in Dallas in 1912, Dr. William White Kelton graduated from Highland Park High School and attended Southern Methodist University. He received his M.D. degree from Baylor University College of Medicine, Dallas, in 1936. His internship and residency were at Charity Hospital, New Orleans. He began practicing in Austin in 1939 and left in 1942 for the Army Medical Corps, where he became a captain. He received board certification in pediatrics in 1942.

After earning his M.D. degree from the University of Oklahoma College of Medicine in 1931, Dr. Joe C. Rude interned at Parkland Hospital, Dallas, followed by residencies in radiology at Cornell Medical College and Harvard Medical School from 1937 to 1939. He was with the 131st General Hospital and the 802nd Hospital Center.

Dr. James Edwin Kreisle, son of Dr. Matthew F. Kreisle, Sr., became a UT Phi Beta Kappa graduate. He graduated from Harvard Medical School in 1942, and after a year's internship at Massachusetts General Hospital in Boston, was commissioned in 1943 as a lieutenant in the Army Medical Corps. In the European theatre, Dr. Kreisle commanded the medical detachment behind the front lines during the Battle of the Bulge.

Dr. Garland Zedler, a radiologist at Seton Hospital, was born in Yorktown, Texas. A UT graduate, he received his M.D. degree from UTMB in 1938, served a rotating internship at St. Joseph Hospital, Kansas City, Missouri, and was a junior resident at Brackenridge Hospital. He was in the Army five and a half years, three in the South Pacific, and became a major. His radiology residency, 1946-1949, was at the Edward Mallinckrodt Institute of Radiology at the Washington University School of Medicine in St. Louis. He would earn board certification in radiology.

Dr. Kermit Fox was a founding partner of Austin Bone and Joint. Commanding a hospital at Fort Raymond, Alaska, during World War II, he made use of penicillin for the first time. A committee had to approve each use of the drug.

Some who served in the war were not yet doctors. Robert Snider was away from Austin between 1943 and 1946 and was a line officer in charge of a Navy landing craft control boat in the first wave on the beaches in the Philippines.

Another prospective physician became a pilot. Born in Sanger in Denton County, Texas, in September 1919, J. Nelson Sanders had attended schools in Rosenberg and Gal-veston while his father was at UTMB and briefly in Denton before the family moved to Caspiana, Louisiana. He graduated from Louisiana State University in 1940 with four years of premedical education and was accepted into its medical school. With three siblings in college or medical school, he felt his family could not afford it, however, and joined the Army Air Corps. He served five and a half years, becoming a pilot in the new B-29 airplane. Sent to fight the Japanese in 1944, he was stationed first in India and China—where he flew over "the Hump"—and then at Tinian Army Air Force Base in the Northern Marianas. In one of his many close calls, his plane nearly rammed into another that had crashed on takeoff. Proceeding with their mission, the crew soon found that their Bombay tanks did not work and, without extra gas, all four engines shut down over the Indian Ocean. Pilot Sanders ditched the airplane and the British Navy rescued him and six other crew members, including the gunner whom he had freed after he was trapped with a broken hip. He had to return to destroy the plane that was in the path of big ships. Bodies of four other crew members were found later, one floating in the water 140 miles away. After thirty-seven missions, he left the South Pacific on July 4, 1945, having flown 3,500 hours, including 650 combat hours. Retiring as a major, he applied to commercial airlines but no pilot positions were available.

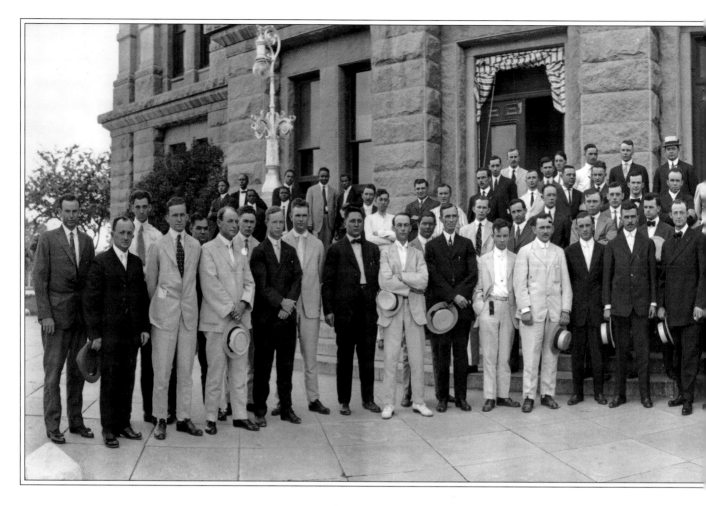

He opted to use his premedical education and entered the University of Tennessee College of Medicine in Memphis, whose quarter system would allow him to graduate faster. Offered a pilot's job for Trans World Airlines two weeks after his medical school acceptance, he instead became an M.D. in early 1949.

Homer R. Goehrs, born in Houston, graduated from Lamar High School there and in 1943 entered the Navy as an enlisted corpsman through its V12 program.

Premedical students also had accelerated schedules. Clift Price's father had been a government civil engineer and the family lived in several north Texas locales before he graduated from Woodrow Wilson High School in Dallas. They moved to Austin so he could attend UT, where he was rushed through his premedical course. He left in mid-1943 to attend UTMB.

By January 1943, Texas was fifty-seven percent over its quota of military volunteers. A third of the state medical association was in military service and although efforts were made to shift civilian doctors to needy areas, physicians at home were spread thin. For three years—from 1943 to 1946—Dr. Z. T. Scott was chief of staff at Brackenridge

Hospital. Dr. Thomas McCrummen's son recalled that his father's already heavy load was exacerbated, with the telephone ringing twenty-four hours daily and his father working twelve to fifteen hours a day. Despite this pressure, Dr. James Prentice would remember his childhood pediatrician as a gentle, good doctor, with "great toys" and "fun to go to." Dr. McCrummen also was careful to write specific dietary and other instructions for James's mother. Dr. Eugene Schoch, Jr., also had special memories of Dr. McCrummen as his pediatrician.

Dr. James Coleman began as a resident surgeon with the state health department in 1941 and served as city health officer at Brackenridge from 1943 to 1945. He was chief of pediatric services at Brackenridge and Seton Hospitals and director of health and welfare for Travis and Bastrop Counties. He also directed residency training at Brackenridge Hospital.

In 1943, Dr. Bain was at St. Louis City Hospital in Missouri for her rotating internship. One brother was to land at Normandy shortly after D-Day and another was in the Southwest Pacific for the invasion of Tawara Atoll in the British Gilbert Islands, and had not been heard from in

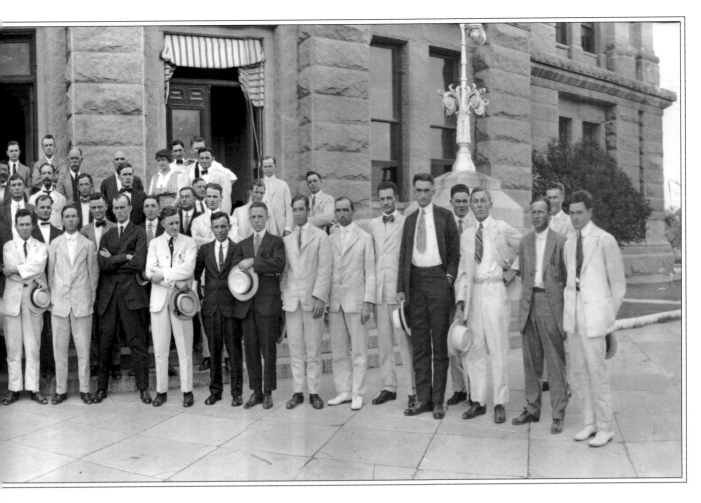

Texas State Board of Medical Examiners standing outside the State Capitol.

months. With her mother at home alone managing the Centerville Hotel, Dr. Bain returned to Texas and sought work in Austin. Dr. Coleman's chief resident had received greetings from Uncle Sam and, expecting new interns, he needed a resident with some training. He offered her $125 a month plus room, board, and laundry—a big raise over St. Louis, where she had earned $10 a month plus room and board. She completed what amounted to a family practice residency, including six months of straight surgery, and taught in the Brackenridge School of Nursing.

Because doctors were so short-handed, she said, "If I saw one of the physicians' patients in the emergency room, the doctors often advised me to admit them, stating they would see them later. These same physicians helped with our program at Brackenridge by volunteering to supervise interns and residents." In one instance while she was a surgical resident in 1945, a profusely bleeding man was brought to Brackenridge. Ordering him to surgery, she called Dr. Banner Gregg, a respected general practitioner who did much

surgery. He was on a house call but gave her explicit emergency instructions, and she completed the operation successfully. The patient, however, was in irreversible shock and died shortly thereafter. Intravenous fluids then were in glass bottles, which could not be squeezed, she recalled, and "there was no way to force the fluids into the body rapidly except by raising the bottles higher."

Dr. Gregg's son, Dr. Frank H. Gregg, recalled that his father "really worked, refining his interest in general surgery. I think I perceived the respect and devotion he had for his patients, his willingness to put in long hours. Even after he retired from private practice, he worked as medical director of Travis State School and as Staff Physician at Austin State School before definitely retiring." As the city physician, his father had performed surgery for charity patients at Brackenridge.

Two other individuals helped keep things going at Brackenridge Hospital during the war. One was Dr. Revace O. "Sam" Swearingen, described as a "a prince of a guy," by Dr. Robert Snider. He "covered during the shortage of doctors—he ran the hospital." A man called "Swede" was "very, very smart and could learn by watching others—before long

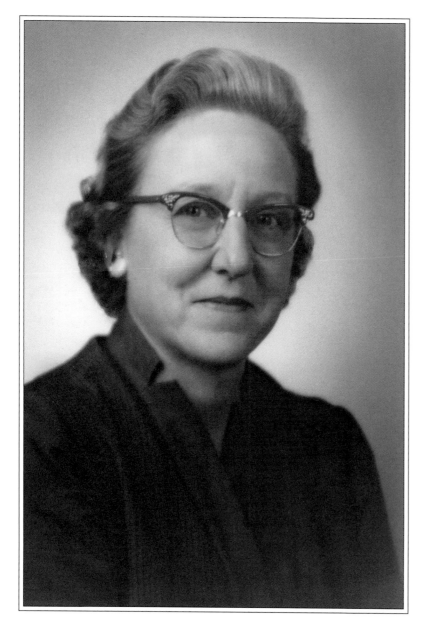

Dr. Ruth Bain returned to Austin and completed a residency that included six months of surgery. She also taught at Brackenridge School of Nursing.

he was in the operating room doing the work of the scrub nurse." Dr. Kermit Fox recalls also that orthopedists considered "Swede" a major asset. He knew him during the 1950s as "the affable and able Carl Sundberg," who had an innate sense of how broken bones should be set, splinted, or cast.

With the war in Europe heating up, Dr. Albert Tisdale was transferred to Fort Knox, Kentucky, with orders to England, which was to become the staging area for the invasion of Europe on D-Day, June 6, 1944. Dr. Marie Tisdale returned to Austin with their adopted daughter. Licensed

under Louisiana's Napoleonic law, which gave women considerable rights, she discovered in 1944 that a married woman in Texas could "not buy or sell or sign any legal paper without her husband's permission and signature." She tried to lease an office for a medical practice. "No one would even discuss a lease with me. I should have my husband come to see about it—oh, he is overseas, do you have anyone to represent you?" She could not even get an office telephone. "Can you see how necessary it was," she would reflect, "that I should want equal rights for women?" She applied to the Travis County Medical Society, however, and "with great satisfaction to myself, I was voted in as a member."

Overburdened with work, Dr. Thomas McElhenney offered Dr. Tisdale a position. Realizing it was the only way she could work, she accepted it and quickly became as busy as any doctor. On Saturdays, when fathers could get off work to take the family to the doctor, she often had fifty office appointments after making morning rounds at Seton, St. David's, and Brackenridge hospitals. After office hours, she made telephone calls and evening hospital rounds before going home. Dr. Tisdale later marveled that doctors were able to treat many illnesses in this era, because civilian doctors did not have access to penicillin until 1945 or 1946, and even when available, it was very expensive.

Dr. Glevis W. Cleveland of Winters, Texas, graduated from UT and received his M.D. degree from Baylor University College of Medicine in Dallas. After interning at Shreveport Charity Hospital from 1941 to 1942, he took a residency at Brackenridge in 1942 and 1943, and remained in Austin for twenty-nine years as a general practitioner. He was on the TMA executive board, and served as president and board chairman of the Texas Academy of Family Physicians.

Arriving in 1943 was Dr. Leonard C. Paggi, an internal medicine specialist. A native of Port Arthur, he received a B.A. degree from UT in 1936 and an M.D. degree from UTMB in 1939. His two-year internship and two years of residency training in medicine were at Charity Hospital of Louisiana in New Orleans. From 1942 to 1943, he was assistant director of medicine and subspecialties, and took postgraduate courses at Louisiana State University Medical Center.

Dr. Robert B. Morrison was born in his Austin family home on Carrington's Bluff, 1900 David Street, in December 1912. He graduated from Austin High School and UT, and was a 1939 honors graduate of the Louisiana State University School of Medicine. Interning at Hillman Hospital in Birmingham, Alabama, he trained in chest diseases at the Texas Sanatorium for the treatment of tuberculosis. He also served a residency at Union Printers Home and Hospital in Colorado Springs, Colorado, and undertook postgraduate work in bronchoscopy at Temple University in Philadelphia. In Austin, Dr. Morrison directed the Brackenridge Tuberculosis Clinic. He became president of the Texas Tuberculosis Association (later the American Lung Association of Texas) and the Travis County Tuberculosis Association. He was on the board of governors of the American College of Chest Physicians.

Carl Sundberg in the Brackenridge cast room.

Before coming to Austin in 1943, Dr. David Wade was superintendent of the State Psychopathic Hospital in Galveston until a hurricane led to its closure. He became superintendent of the Austin State School for Mental Defectives and then superintendent of the Rusk State Hospital. In 1945, he opened a private practice in psychiatry and in 1947 established the Oak Ridge Sanitarium for nervous and mental diseases in Austin. Born in Jacksonville, Arkansas, in 1910, he graduated from the University of Arkansas School of Medicine in 1938 followed by a residency at St. Vincent Infirmary in Little Rock. He completed a residency at the State Psychopathic Hospital in Galveston in 1942 and took a visiting residency at New York Psychiatric Institute. He was certified by the American Board of Psychiatry & Neurology in 1944 and in mental hospital administration in 1952. An Army major during the Korean Conflict, he was in charge of psychiatric facilities for the Fourth Army at Brooke Army Medical Center in San Antonio.

Dr. J. Edward Johnson arrived in Austin in 1944 as an internal medicine specialist. Born in November 1892 in Thalia, Texas, he earned his B.S. degree from the Univer-

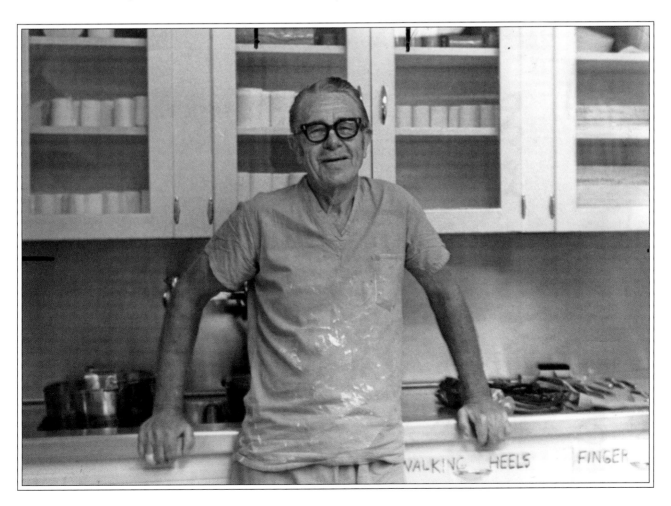

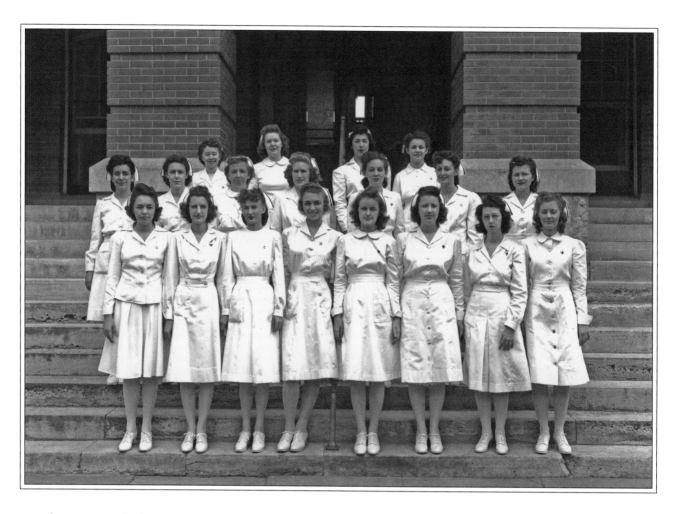

Seton School of Nursing, graduation class, 1944.

sity of Virginia in Charlottesville, and his M.D degree from UTMB in 1925. After interning at John Sealy Hospital, he was a general practitioner in several locations. He was active in state and national medical societies and authored many articles and editorials in the *Texas State Journal of Medicine*. He served as TCMS president in 1949 and was also president of the Texas Tuberculosis Association.

In 1943, a mild revolution altered plans for some future Travis County physicians. Texas had only two medical schools—UTMB in Galveston, the state-funded school, and Baylor University College of Medicine in Dallas, a private Baptist institution. The latter was receiving an increasing amount of money from the Southwestern Medical Foundation run by a former dean. A philosophic disagreement regarding services to the city of Dallas erupted between the Foundation and the Baylor trustees. Thus, when the Houston-based M. D. Anderson Foundation offered Baylor a site in the planned Texas Medical Center there, the Baylor trustees decided to leave Dallas. A month later, in May 1943, Baylor graduated its last Dallas class and in July opened in a converted Sears, Roebuck & Company building in Houston. Meanwhile, Southwestern Medical

Foundation formed Southwestern Medical College and found temporary quarters. After the split in "old Baylor," students and faculty made difficult decisions. Most seniors remained in Dallas, but the war also affected their options. The Navy ordered students enrolled in its V12 College Training Program to Houston whereas the Army assigned its ASTP (Army Specialized Training Program) students to the unit at Southwestern.

Charles F. Pelphrey graduated with the first Southwestern class in March 1944. He interned at Baylor University Hospital in Dallas and started surgery training. Cognizant that a good surgeon should know pathology, he took a residency under Dr. Joseph M. Hill who was working on the Rh factor in blood, and manufacturing typing serum. Dr. Pelphrey witnessed the death of a patient whose blood had been hemolyzed, which may have brought about routine Rh typing. Dr. Hill made such typing mandatory, and Baylor became the first nongovernmental hospital to routinely do typing for the Rh negative factor. Dr. Pelphrey also soon learned that pathologists could diagnose cancers from cells and about George Papanicolaou's test to detect cervical cancer.

Lansing Thorne had started at Baylor, but remained in Dallas, graduating in December 1944 from Southwestern Medical College. He undertook a rotating internship at Wisconsin General Hospital in Madison in 1945, and a residency in pediatrics at Texas Children's Hospital (later Children's Medical Center) in Dallas from 1945 to 1946. From 1946 to 1947, he served with the Army Medical Corps at Fort Hood, Texas, and at Fort Ord in California, becoming a captain. Completing his pediatric training at Cincinnati Children's Hospital, he arrived in Austin in 1949. From 1951 to 1952, during the Korean Conflict, he was a senior assistant surgeon in the U.S. Public Health Service in Alaska. His twin brother, Dr. G. Clifford Thorne, also graduated from Southwestern Medical College in 1944. He interned at Duke University Hospital in Durham, North Carolina, from 1945 to 1946; undertook a fellowship at Texas Children's Hospital, Dallas, in 1945; and served a residency in pediatrics from 1946 to 1948 at Cincinnati Children's Hospital, Like his brother, he also arrived in Austin in 1949. The brothers maintained separate pediatric practices but shared a building and facilities. Each thus could practice according to his own personality. Both were certified by the American Board of Pediatrics in 1951.

When Dr. Sam Wilborn joined the Drs. Thorne, they moved into another building at Medical Arts Square, sharing the structure but maintaining separate practices. Born in Snyder, Texas, in 1923, he received his M.D. degree from UTMB in 1941 and interned at John Sealy Hospital, Galveston from 1941 to 1942. His rotating residency was at Brackenridge Hospital where he was Courtesy Staff. In the Army, he became a captain and at Children's Medical Center, Dallas, he became chief resident from 1946 to 1948. In 1953, he was certified by the American Board of Pediatrics.

Many Travis County physicians would continue to have military obligations.

Spouses also contributed to the war effort in many ways. Married in 1944, the former Eugenia Worley and Eugene Schoch, Jr., left for Galveston during a time of forced blackouts and the US patrolling the Gulf Coast for German submarines. He had begun his medical education at UTMB in 1943 and would continue his studies. A 1942 UT graduate, she had worked with the US Weather Bureau in Washington, DC, charting weather maps to help determine their value in forecasting. She was prepared to teach general science and biology, but took a job with a dermatology professor studying a substitute for quinine. With the delicate insertion of a needle in a leg vein, new drugs were tried on malaria-infected canaries. The study led to the future use of Atabrine.

In mid-war, Dr. George Cox, state health officer, reported a rise in poliomyelitis. Sadly, Dr. Bain's eleven-year-old niece was among those admitted to Brackenridge Hospital's iron-lung unit. "My niece's family and I...hovered over her, watching almost helplessly as the ravages of bulbar polio took her young life in 1944."

Physicians clearly were focusing on specialties. Dr. Oliver Suehs, who became chief of staff of St. David's Hospital and president of Travis County Medical Society, was a co-founder in 1945 of the Texas Association of Otolaryngology-Head and Neck Surgery. Dr. Georgia Legett completed an internship at Jefferson Davis Hospital, Houston, and practiced family medicine briefly in San Antonio. She then undertook residencies in obstetrics and gynecology and in anesthesiology at the Margaret Hague Maternity Hospital in Jersey City, New Jersey, followed by a gynecological residency and an appointment as service as attending staff at Jersey City Medical Center from 1946 to 1949. After two years in the Far East, Dr. Carey Legett returned to the U.S. for training in psychiatry to care for stressed air crews. After completing his military service, he joined his wife in New York, training in ophthalmology at Jersey City Medical Center and at New York Eye and Ear Infirmary. He also studied basic sciences in ophthalmology at New York University School of Medicine and was house surgeon in the infirmary.

With the war over in 1945, troops began returning home, and Travis County physicians were among those bearing decorations for valor and service. A *New York Times* reporter observed, however, that "There is little glory in the Medical Corps. It is just hard, dirty work and mighty dangerous.... They are proud to have saved 97 out of every hundred wounded...that their miracle drugs and blood banks send from 50 to 80 back to fight again...nobody in our whole vast Army, not even the foremost combat crew or the deadliest flying wing, has done a finer job than the Medical Corps."

Scores of veterans returned to college under the Servicemen's Readjustment Act of 1944—the GI bill—bringing unusual medical problems, recalled Dr. Bain, who served at the UT Student Health Center. They included "malaria (the most frequent war-related disease), intestinal parasites, stress-related problems, and old injuries that caused difficulties."

CHAPTER XI

READJUSTMENT AND MOVING FORWARD

PHYSICIANS RETURNING FROM THE military brought new skills and concepts, including experience with specialization. Some had received advanced formal training and others returned to school. Medical societies helped doctors relocate and adjust to civilian life, and Austin specialists established the Journal Club for hospitality and to facilitate participation in hospital staffs.

In 1946, Dr. Sam N. Key, Jr., returned to practice ophthalmology with his father. Born in Austin in 1916, he graduated from the University of Pennsylvania School of Medicine in Philadelphia. He followed that with a clerkship at the Mayo Clinic, an internship at Robert Packer Hospital in Sayre, Pennsylvania, and a residency in ophthalmology at the University of Iowa.

In 1946, Dr. Edward L. Zidd began practicing surgery in Austin. In 1947, he joined the staff of Holy Cross Hospital and was instrumental in developing its facilities. A native of Hartford, Connecticut, he graduated from Adelbert College in Cleveland, Ohio (later Adelbert College of Western Reserve University) and received his M.D. degree in 1950 from Western Reserve University School of Medicine in Cleveland. His internship and residency were at St. Alexis Hospital in Cleveland.

During the war, Dr. Sandy Esquivel had taken care of orthopedic patients, including sports teams and athletes. Both Dr. Albert Tisdale and Dr. Frederick C. Lowry joined

his practice in 1946. Born in Cedar Rapids, Iowa, Dr. Lowry attended the State University of Iowa (the University of Iowa) in Iowa City for premedical education and received his M.D. degree from its College of Medicine in 1937. He was an intern at Harper Hospital in Detroit, Michigan, and at Kings County Hospital in Brooklyn, New York, and a resident at the Brooklyn Cancer Institute. In 1942, 1946, and 1947, he was an orthopedic surgery resident at University Hospital in Iowa City, Iowa. In the interim, he had been a captain in the Army and in 1966 would become a volunteer physician in Vietnam in 1966.

In 1946, Dr. James Coleman left the state health department to organize a private group practice, Children's Medical Center, at 108 West Thirtieth Street, with Drs. Ralph Hanna and William White Kelton. Dr. Hanna, a native of Tularosa, New Mexico, studied at the University of Arizona and the Texas College of Mines and Metallurgy (later UT El Paso). He received his M.D. degree from the University of Texas Medical Branch (UTMB) in 1937 followed by a pediatric residency at the Institute of Pediatrics in the College of Medical Evangelists in Los Angeles, California.

Making Austin home in 1947 was Dr. Morris Polsky. Born in a village outside Kiev in the Ukraine in 1908, he came with his parents to the United States and was educated in Kansas City, Missouri. He received his M.D. degree in 1929 from Kansas University School of Medicine and trained in dermatology and syphilology at the New

York Skin and Cancer Hospital, earning board certification in 1932. He first practiced in Kansas City. He also served in the Civilian Conservation Corps and was a major in the Army Medical Corps during the war, stationed in the occupied Philippine Islands. The author of numerous published articles, he also was editor of the *TCMS Journal*.

Thinking the war was behind him, Dr. George Tipton returned to Galveston for a residency in general surgery. While making rounds at John Sealy Hospital, however, he was stunned by an explosion on April 16, 1947. Two old liberty ships had been docked at the Monsanto Chemical Company in Texas City and ammonium nitrate, a volatile fertilizer, had erupted into fire on the *Grandcamp*. Another ship, the *High Flyer*, also containing the fertilizer plus sulfur, was evacuated and set adrift. Dr. Tipton and other staff quickly found themselves treating warlike mass cas-ualties—wounds from blasts, burns, fragments, and breaks. He saw the ball of rotating fire that rose after the *High Flyer* exploded. In the end, thousands were injured and an estimated 600 were killed. The fate of many could not be determined. There was an overwhelming need for blood, and the experience spurred the founding of the American Association of Blood Banks, which set up a nationwide network of blood banks and regional clearinghouses.

In Austin, physicians organized a blood bank committee of Drs. Sidney W. Bohls, Happy Scott, John F. Thomas, Revace O. (Sam) Swearingen, and E.K. Blewett. Chaired by Dr. Bohls, the group discussed the concept of a blood bank with the city and others. Finding interest, but no financial commitments, they recommended that Travis County Medical Society take the lead.

Dr. Morris Polsky practiced in Austin from 1974 to 1994 and served as editor of the TCMS Journal.

A former Austin resident returned in the fall of 1946 to become director of the UT Student Health Center. Dr. George M. Decherd had been a UTMB professor of renown, and many of his students were practicing in the capital. At his request, Dr. Ruth Bain joined him at the old "B" Hall health facility on the UT campus. Dr. Decherd had attended Austin public schools and in 1926 received a bachelor's and a master's degree from UT. He earned his M.D. degree from the University of Minnesota Medical School, followed by postgraduate work. In 1933, he became an instructor in medicine at UTMB, left to teach at the Louisiana State University School of Medicine, and returned in 1938 "to enliven an era of active cardiovascular investigation" with Dr. George R. Herrmann. In 1946, he was appointed a full professor of medicine at UTMB and moved to Austin. A diplomate of the American Board of Internal Medicine, he authored many scientific articles. He also was chief of staff at Brackenridge Hospital.

By now, Austin had a growing number of well-trained diagnosticians, and among them were Drs. William (Bill) P. Morgan, Horace Cromer, George Clark, Lang Holland, and Walter K. Long.

In 1947, Dr. Raleigh Ross, not long out of military service, led a new impetus to enhance the physician training program at Brackenridge Hospital, with Seton and St. David's hospitals also participating. He instituted daily rounds throughout the units and recruited interns and residents from medical schools. A broad-based rotation system was established in specialty fields and the emergency room was covered around the clock. Although the training program was not integrated formally with a medical school, students wanted the hands-on training of Austin doctors, who donated their services as part-time faculty. Students "could learn by doing, and we could help them establish a practice," recalled Dr. Ross. By the 1950s, the program was accredited by the American Medical Association, the American College of Surgeons, and the American Hospital Association.

Austin's midtown area around Fifteenth Street, close to the Capitol and UT, was becoming a new medical hub that was about equidistant to Seton, St. David's, and Brackenridge hospitals. Dozens of physicians rented or bought houses—often half of a house—sometimes in conjunction with other practitioners. They converted living rooms into reception areas, other areas into examining rooms, kitchens into laboratories, and porches into equipment rooms. The air conditioning, if it existed, usually was an evaporative cooler.

Dr. James M. "Jimmy" Graham arrived in 1949 as a general practitioner, setting up practice at 1402 Nueces and later at 1504 Guadalupe Street. Dr. Otto Brandt, Jr., had an office at 1506 Guadalupe Street. They shared a reception room and an x-ray machine. Born in Cisco, Dr. Graham grew up in Sweetwater, Texas. He attended Texas Technological College (later Texas Tech University) in Lubbock and graduated from UTMB in 1944. He completed his internship at Jefferson Davis Hospital in Houston. In the Army Medical Corps, he became train surgeon to the Red Cross hospital and commander for a train that carried wounded soldiers in cars marked with red crosses to military hospitals closest to their home towns. He ran a battalion aid station on Kyushu Island, Japan, and a military hospital for the 24th Infantry Division, becoming a captain. He also saw the aftermath of the atomic bombs at Hiroshima and Nagasaki. On his return to Texas, he took a rotating residency at Robert B. Green Memorial Hospital in San Antonio, moving to Austin in 1947 for a surgical residency at Brackenridge Hospital. He held many positions in the Travis County Medical Society and the Texas Medical Association, where he was a member of the Board of Trustees.

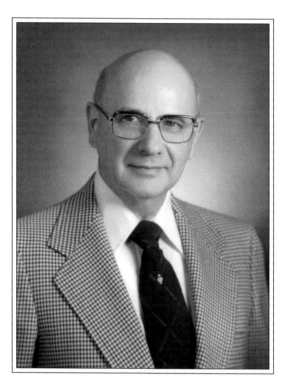

Dr. Charles T. Pelphry was the first physician in Austin to perform Rh testing.

Dr. Otto Brandt was born in Brenham, Texas, where he attended Blinn College. After earning his UT degree, he graduated from UTMB in 1942. He did an internship and a rotating residency at St. Paul's Hospital in Dallas. A captain in the Army, he served from 1944 to 1946 in the United States and in the Pacific. After training in internal medicine at Jefferson Davis Hospital in Houston, he came to Austin in 1947 to take up a two-year obstetrics-gynecology residency at Brackenridge Hospital.

In 1948, Austin welcomed more formally trained specialists, including physicians trained in fields that were new to the city.

After graduating from Southwestern Medical College, Dr. Charles T. Pelphrey completed his service with the Navy. He was asked by Dr. Sidney Bohls, who had left his post at the State Department of Health, to join him in his private laboratory in Austin. Dr. Pelphrey soon had an opportunity to apply his advanced training when he learned that Rh testing was not being done. Ordering typing serum, he became the first physician to do the testing in Austin. Reports on histology examinations required several days at that time and he wanted specimens processed over night and reported the next day. He bought tubing at a plumbing shop and copper screening at a hardware store to solder little carriers for tissue. After completing his gross tissue work in the office laboratory, he pulled a string through everything, dropped the tissue into a solution, and took his contraption home to an oven he had installed in his tool house. His alarm clock woke him through the night so he could move specimens from one solution to another. Placing them in paraffin and wrapping them in paper towels early the next morning, he delivered the specimens to technicians to cut tissues. Later, an Auto-Technicon allowed the work to be done automatically. When he became head of the pathology laboratory at Seton, Dr. Pelphrey at first had only a single light bulb and one refrigerator, but the hospital later built a modern laboratory. As "the fellows began returning from war, they wanted better and more," he said, and he was happy to oblige them.

Dr. Albert A. La Londe, Austin's first neurosurgeon, and Dr. David O. Johnson, its first fully trained anesthesiologist, arrived in the city in 1948. During his first year, Dr. La Londe performed the first intracranial surgery in the city at Brackenridge Hospital. Born in Denison, Texas, he was the youngest of eight children of an engineer for the Missouri, Kansas, and Texas (the Katy) Railroad. The family home was situated across from the birthplace of President Dwight D. Eisenhower whose father also worked for the railroad. Graduating from UT in 1938, he received his M.D. degree from UTMB in 1942, followed this with an internship, and then practiced briefly as a family physician in El Paso. During a fellowship in general and neurologic surgery at the Cleveland Clinic Foundation, he studied with pioneer neurosurgeon Dr. W. James Gardner. They discovered a new way to treat chronic intramembranous subdural hematoma as they cared for a patient whose spinal fluid pressure was extremely low, causing him to lose consciousness. After the subarachnoid injection of saline, the hematoma flowed out and the patient regained consciousness. Although still a fellow, Dr. La Londe was the lead author on their report, "Chronic Subdural Hematoma. Expansion of Compressed Cerebral Hemisphere and Relief of Hypotension by Spinal Injection of Physiologic Saline Solution," published in the *New England Journal of Medicine* in 1948. It was the first report using this method

Construction photo of the new Student Health Center at the University of Texas at Austin, 1950.

in the world literature and was cited in the history of neurologic surgery edited by Johns Hopkins University professor A. Earl Walker in 1951. Dr. La Londe and his future partners routinely used the procedure.

Arriving as a board-certified neurosurgeon, Dr. La Londe formed the Austin Neurosurgical Association. For many years he was the only neurosurgeon between Dallas and San Antonio, on call at all times. On Saturday mornings he held a neurology clinic to treat patients with problems such as Parkinson's disease. Serving Brackenridge and Seton hospitals, he carried his own instruments in a leather suitcase. They were sterilized at each hospital to be ready at the next. In the early days, Dr. La Londe recalled, the only treatment besides surgery was radiation but diagnostic studies rapidly improved.

The arrival of ventriculography allowed the neurosurgeon to see a mass on the x-ray; likewise, pneumoencephalography permitted a view of distortions, or shifts, of the ventricles and thus provided indirect evidence of the presence and location of any mass. A subsequent advance was arteriography in which dye was injected into the carotid arteries and multiple x-rays were taken as the substance coursed through them. Blood vessels could be seen and, if they were not in the proper location, the surgeon knew there was a space-occupying lesion, aneurysm, or hydrocephalus because the vessels were stretched.

Since Austin had no trained neurologist, Dr. La Londe also cared for poliomyelitis patients—usually those with the bulbar type, which disabled the brain stem. They were

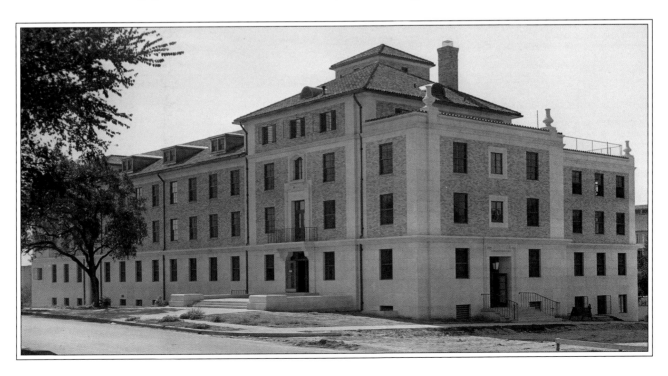

placed in a respirator and he visited them and checked their fluids, but there was no real treatment for patients with this type of poliomyelitis. Patients who did not have to be in an iron lung could be treated with the Sister Kenny method, which involved the use of hot moist towels; it alleviated pain but did not help with recovery.

Dr. La Londe practiced alone until Dr. Robert G. Farris, a 1949 graduate of UT Southwestern Medical School, joined him in 1956, followed by Dr. William R. Turpin, a 1951 graduate of Bowman Gray School of Medicine.

Dr. David O. Johnson, Austin's first formally trained anesthesiologist, was born in Philadelphia and graduated from Jefferson Medical College of Thomas Jefferson University in 1942. He interned at Presbyterian Hospital, Philadelphia, from 1942 to 1943, and was a resident in anesthesiology at Presbyterian Hospital, Philadelphia, in 1943 and from 1945 to 1947. In the interim, he served in the Army. He would be certified in March 1952 by the American Board of Anesthesiology and credited with changing the way anesthesia was practiced in Austin. In 1950, he assembled the Austin Anesthesiology Group—perhaps the first anesthesiology group practice in the United States—beginning a partnership with Dr. Glen J. Radcliffe, the first to join him. Dr. Radcliffe later left to become a Houston practitioner. Others joining Dr. Johnson in the first decade were Drs. Earl L. Yeakel, Jr., James W. Lassiter, Darrell Faubion, Elizabeth Paterson, and Robert Umstattd.

After military service, Dr. Kermit Fox served a residency in orthopedic surgery in Iowa City, Iowa, and in Memphis, Tennessee, at the Campbell Clinic, where he met an old acquaintance, Dr. Lawrence L. Griffin of Beeville, Texas. They decided to establish an orthopedic practice in Austin. Arriving in 1948 and borrowing $2,000, they began the "Drs. Griffin & Fox" practice on August 1, 1948, in an old house at 409 West Fifteenth Street. Dr. Fox assigned an insurance policy as collateral. They crammed in a reception area, examining rooms, equipment, and a developing room for x-rays. Initial funds were used as a down payment on a $7,000 General Electric x-ray machine, its tube the "state-of-the-art rotating-anode type." It could take "good x-ray pictures of backs, even of heavily-built patients." Utilities were not expensive, but air conditioning and central heat were not common and they had neither. In summer, the small reception area could be stifling.

They were the fourth and fifth orthopedists in Austin and they shared equal income, expenses, and duty hours. The concept of a fifty-fifty partnership, including expenses, duty hours, and evenly split vacation time was a "bit new"

in Austin. Some patients also had a hard time accepting that one physician might be off call. This eventually became the norm. The first six months' receipts did not reach the amount of the rent—one hundred dollars per month—but made them eligible for GI bill assistance. "I remember how helpful this seemingly small subsidy was," Dr. Fox recalled. The partners worked hard to build the practice, including making calls to neighboring towns like Georgetown, Taylor, Giddings, La Grange, Burnet, Bastrop, and Smithville.

Medical societies frowned on "self-aggrandizement," thus card announcements and signs were to be understated and small. Dr. Fox recalled a bit of criticism from the county medical society because of the sign that he and Dr. Griffin erected so that patients would not miss the narrow, recessed entrance to their small office. Austin hospitals had few orthopedic operating instruments, thus they assembled their own, as had Dr. Esquivel before them. They kept the instruments double-wrapped in heavy ducking in stainless steel pans, and carried larger items in a canvas overnight traveling bag. Physicians previously relied on plaster splints and casts, sometimes ordering custom-made braces from the Lux Artificial Limb and Brace Company in San Antonio or from Marlin, Texas. Dr. Fox recalled that until 1949, "when Woody Hargroves with the able assistance of Obie Hess, opened the first brace shop in Austin, local orthopedists had to do without the services of a bracemaker." Until 1951, when Dr. John A. Lambert opened a limb prosthesis shop, that service was sporadic. Having been cross-trained in plastic surgery and neurosurgery at the Campbell Clinic in Memphis, Drs. Fox and Griffin performed some surgery in these areas. They also did some skin grafts and disk surgery.

Brackenridge Hospital was the center for polio victims in Central Texas and Dr. Clifford Thorne was among the physicians treating them. Cited in the history of Brackenridge, he said "About all you could do was prescribe bed rest....We could minimize the muscular damage to speed up the recuperative process. We could assist with respiratory muscular paralysis. We constantly performed lab tests to check the patients' electrolytes...so they stayed in chemical balance." He had great empathy for polio patients. He had broken his arm in a bicycle fall at age six, and was left with a damaged nerve which contracted and drew his arm up to a ninety-degree angle.

Preventive help was on the way in 1948. At Harvard Medical School, researchers John F. Enders, Thomas H. Weller, and Frederick C. Robbins learned how to grow polio virus in the laboratory, setting the stage for the development of future vaccines.

Becoming a physician after graduating from UTMB in 1950, Dr. Robert Snider interned at Garfield Memorial Hospital in Washington, DC, followed by a residency with a group of physicians. He returned to Austin in 1954 as the first full-time radiologist for Seton Hospital, succeeding Dr. Zedler. In 1956, he began offering radiology services in a remodeled house on Rio Grande Street. Equipment included a diagnostic x-ray unit with fluoroscopy and two state-of-the-art radiation treatment units. In 1968, the group became the Austin Radiological Association.

Dr. James Kreisle completed a residency at Massachusetts General Hospital in 1947 and took a one-year fellowship at the Mayo Clinic where he saw Dr. Philip S. Hench administer the first cortisone injection in the world to an arthritic patient. In 1950, Dr. Hench was one of three recipients of the Nobel Prize in Physiology or Medicine for discoveries regarding hormones of the adrenal cortex, their structure, and biological effects—including his discovery that cortisone could reverse the inflammation of rheumatoid arthritis. In 1949, Dr. Kreisle joined the practice of his father, Dr. Matthew Kreisle, Sr. His younger brother, Dr. Matthew Kreisle, Jr., a general surgeon, joined them later.

Dr. William P. "Bill" Morgan earned his internal medicine certification in 1942. Born in 1904 in Lockhart, Texas, he had graduated from Baylor University College of Medicine in Dallas, in 1927. He received a Master of Science in Medicine degree from the University of Pennsylvania in 1932, interned at Baylor University Hospital in Dallas, from 1927 to 1928, and undertook postgraduate training

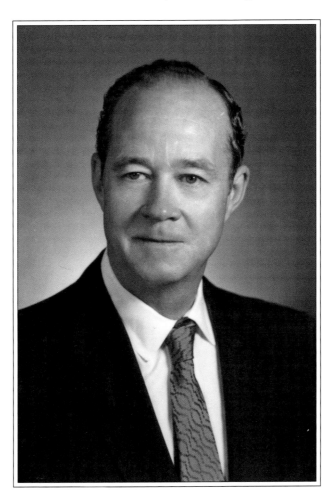

Dr. Robert N. Snider was the first full-time radiologist for Seton Hospital.

at the University of Pennsylvania from 1930 to 1932. Dr. Virgil Lawlis recalled that Dr. Morgan had a special interest in heart disease.

Dr. George Clark, a native of Des Moines, Iowa, was certified in internal medicine in 1946. He had received his M.D. degree from the University of Iowa College of Medicine in 1937 and served his internship and residency at Geisinger Memorial Hospital in Danville, Pennsylvania, from 1937 to 1939. He also undertook a fellowship at The Cleveland Clinic, Ohio, from 1940 to 1942. He became a captain in the Army, serving from 1942 to 1945.

Born in Austin in 1919, Dr. Walter Long received his M.D. degree from Harvard Medical School in 1943. Serving an internship and residency at Boston City Hospital from 1943 to 1945, he became a research assistant in cardiology in the Thorndike Memorial Laboratory there from 1945 to 1948. In 1945 and 1946, he was an assistant in medicine at Harvard. A captain in the Army Medical Corps, he served during the Korean Conflict and became chief of cardiology at William Beaumont Hospital at Fort Bliss, El Paso. He was certified in internal medicine in 1953 and his first practice in Austin was at 503 West Fifteenth Street.

When Dr. W. Donald Roberts, a UT physician, found a satisfactory office for a private practice, he knew that he could not afford it alone with a wife and children to support. He asked Dr. Ruth Bain to join him and the two rented a "one-man" office in the 1400 block of San Antonio Street. Each worked half time at UT. At the private office, each had one side of a desk for files and, for two years, one physician worked mornings and the other afternoons. When Dr. Roberts returned to an internal medicine residency, Dr. Bain took over his practice, leaving her university post for her now full-time practice.

Like their predecessors in 1853, a few Austin physicians in 1948 had a plan. They wanted the Texas Medical Association to come home, basing their position on the 1901 charter, which stated that the corporation "shall have its principal office and place of business in the City of Austin, Texas." It had operated primarily in Fort Worth during the combined tenures, lasting almost half a century, of two physician executives and editors, Drs. Ira C. Chase and Holman Taylor. The desire for relocation was more than sentimental, with some members believing that the Texas Medical Association needed an official Austin presence to better monitor legislation.

Dr. Hardwicke hosted a gathering of Travis County Medical Society officers and others to discuss the possible move to Austin. Present were Dr. Joe T. Gilbert, president, and Drs. H. L. Klotz, M. Allen Forbes, William M. Gambrell, Sam N. Key, Sr., and Gabriel F. Thornhill. Attendees included Mr. Walter E. Long, secretary of the Austin Chamber of Commerce, and other civic and business leaders. The Chamber of Commerce pledged cooperation and an Austin bank promised financial aid. Soon afterward, the regular monthly TCMS meeting was held, with Dr. Joe T. Gilbert presiding and Dr. Key reporting the recent activities.

"Interest was enormous, and all decisions made were unanimous," Dr. Hardwicke recalled in memoirs left for the TMA library. A Medical Service Committee was appointed to spearhead the project, with Dr. Gambrell as chairman. Members were Drs. E. K. Blewett, Sidney Bohls, G. W. Cleveland, James M. Coleman, J. E. Johnson, Sam N. Key,

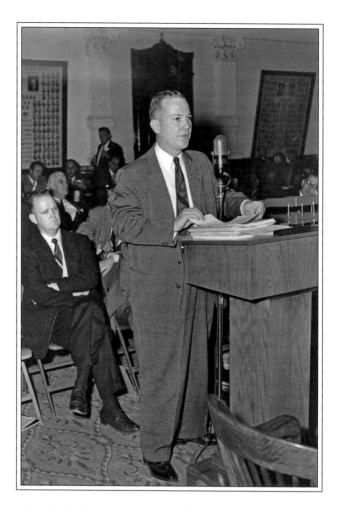

Dr. E. K. Blewett appearing before the Texas legislature.

Sr., David Wade, Raleigh Ross, M. D. McCauley, and J. T. Robison. The committee also included Travis County delegates to the Texas Medical Association, the Seventh District councilor, and society officers. The public relations firm, Syers, Pickle, and Wynn, was hired. J. J. "Jake" Pickle of Austin, a principal, later became a long-time Congressman.

Dr. Sam Key, Sr., suggested that the Travis County Medical Society offer a suitable place for the new building and a temporary home for the library and staff. Interim arrangements were made for the Victorian John Bremond home at 700 Guadalupe. A campaign was launched to attain TMA approval and a large Travis County contingent established headquarters at the annual meeting held from April 26 to April 29, 1948, at the Rice Hotel in Houston. Dr. Gambrell informed the House of Delegates of the plans and the city's support, and by a vote of 106 to 40, delegates in a secret ballot approved the move to occur before the next legislative session. Austin doctors were appointed as a building committee, with Dr. Sam Key, Sr., as chairman. Members were Drs. David Wade, William M. Gambrell, and C. P. Hardwicke. Two TMA trustees, Drs. F. J. L. Blasingame and Merton M. Minter, were consultants. The Travis County Medical Society arranged purchase of a $15,000 lot, assessing each member $90, and later donated to TMA the site at the southeast corner of Nineteenth Street (later named Martin Luther King Jr. Boulevard), which fronted on North Lamar Boulevard. The Texas Medical Association board bought adjoining land at a cost $17,500 and construction began in early 1951. Dr. Key devoted extraordinary time to the project, visiting "fine buildings" and selecting the building stone, many furnishings and draperies, and central air conditioning.

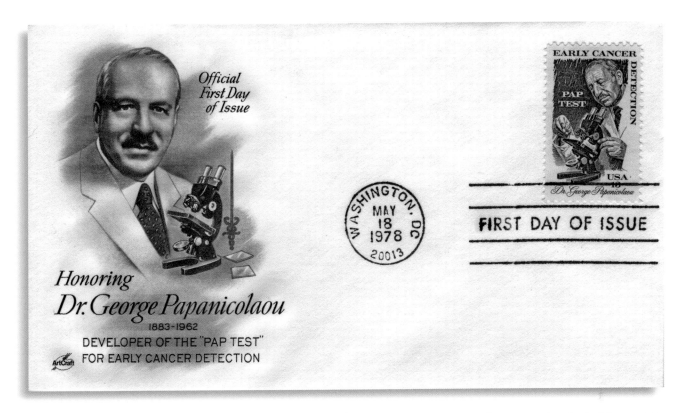

Commemorative envelope honoring Dr. George Papanicolaou who developed the "Pap" test for early cancer detection.

Drs. Georgia and Carey Legett returned to Austin in 1949 to open offices at 1707 Colorado Street, each forming separate solo practices in their specialties. Later, Dr. Georgia Legett also practiced with Dr. Milton Turner, a long-time Austin obstetrician-gynecologist. Dr. Legett recalled that she brought the "Pap" smear test to Austin five years ahead of others. One of her professors at Cornell University Medical College was Dr. George Papanicolaou, whose work on a vaginal smear was published in a 1943 monograph, *Diagnosis of Uterine Cancer by the Vaginal Smear*. Dr. Legett had also studied continuous caudal anesthesia at Philadelphia Lying-in Hospital with the renowned anesthesiologist, benefactor, researcher, and inventor, Dr. Robert A. Hingson. The Drs. Legett had four children and shared responsibilities for rearing them. For instance, she looked after them the first half of the night and he watched over them the second half. The Legetts became enthusiastic supporters of the blood and tissue banks of the Travis County Medical Society.

Milner Speer Thorne, the younger brother of Drs. Lansing and Clifford Thorne came to Austin to practice anesthesiology. He had studied at Baylor University College of Medicine in Houston, graduating in 1948. Interning at Shreveport Charity Hospital from 1948 to 1949, he served an anesthesiology residency at John Sealy Hospital in Galveston from 1949 to 1953.

Dr. Darrell B. Faubion was born in 1916 in Llano, Texas, graduated from UT Austin in 1940, and from Southwestern Medical College, Dallas, in 1944. He interned at the Robert B. Green Hospital, San Antonio, and from 1948 to 1949 was a resident at University Hospital in Minneapolis, Minnesota. The Army Medical Corps claimed him in 1945 and 1946. Drs. Milner Thorne and Darrell B. Faubion joined the Austin Anesthesiology Group and later formed a group at the new Seton hospital in 1975. Their partnership merged with the Capitol Anesthesiology Association in the early 1980s, and the Seton and Brackenridge groups also merged then.

Dr. John F. Thomas, son of Dr. John Calhoun Thomas, was born in Taylor, Texas, in 1916. He graduated from UT in 1936 and from the University of Pennsylvania School of Medicine in Philadelphia in 1940. After interning in the university's hospital, he was a fellow in surgery at the Mayo Foundation in Rochester, Minnesota, from 1942 to 1944 and from 1946 to 1947. He also served in the Navy. Certified by the American Board of Surgery in 1949, he was the president of the Travis County Medical Society in 1953. While serving as president of the Texas Division of the American Cancer Society, Dr. Pelphrey recalled that Dr. Thomas discussed Pap smears with Austin pathologists and that TCMS members "spread out" to discuss them with parent-teacher organizations, schools, and service clubs.

CHAPTER XII

PLEASANT DAYS, CONTINGENT CLOUDS

POLITICAL FIRE-storms about communism stirred the nation, which went to battle in South Korea so soon after World War II. Mobile Army Surgical Hospital (MASH) units would come into great prominence.

For the first time, Texas doctors did not volunteer in ample numbers and the obligation fell primarily on those deferred during the second world war. Some with previous service also were called back. The 1951 and 1952 Texas Medical Association directory listed the known members in the service from Travis County, citing Drs. Billy Frank Johnson, Sam N. Key, Jr., E. H. LaBosse, Walter K. Long, Vincent R. Murray, and David Wade. There would be many others. Dr. Lansing Thorne, called up for a second time, served nineteen months in Alaska with the territorial health department, where he was the only board-certified pediatrician.

Dr. Mathis W. Blackstock, who arrived in Austin in 1954, had been a surgeon in a Navy clinic for dependents in Kobe, Japan, from 1950 to 1951. He had graduated from

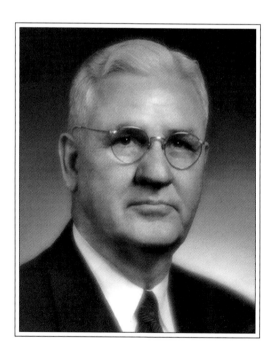

UTMB in 1948, served an internship in Houston, and completed a residency in Denver in 1951. His father, attorney Leo Guy Blackstock, a professor of business and military law at UT, had been chief of the prosecution division of the Supreme Command of the Allied Powers in Tokyo after World War II.

Austin's Dr. Gambrell, president of the Texas Medical Association from 1950-1951, called for doctors to meet their responsibilities in war. The United States instituted a physician draft and soon there were enough volunteers. Dr. Gambrell also received a letter from Army Surgeon-General R. W. Bliss thanking him for "the magnificent" job done in Texas by doctors volunteering their services for physical examinations of inductees and other needed tasks. In addition, Dr. Gambrell discussed the dominating topic of medical associations in this era—socialized medicine—declaring that no previous challenge compared to a paternal regimentation. He also complimented the TMA Woman's Auxiliary whose president was his wife, Patti McClung Gambrell.

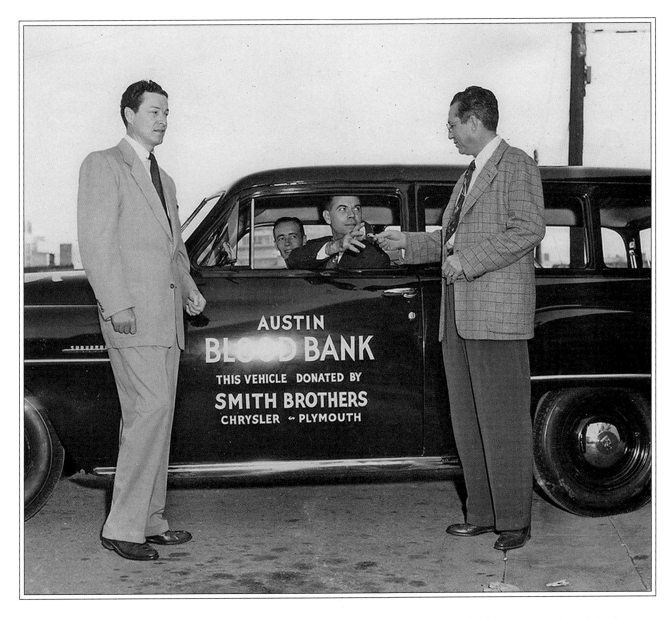

OPPOSITE PAGE: *Dr. William Gambrell was Texas Medical Association president in 1950-1951.* ABOVE: *Auto dealers Jay and Edwin Smith present the keys of the donated Blood Bank auto to Dr. R. O. Swearingen.*

The Travis County Medical Society developed a basic disaster plan covering mass casualty care. The *TCMS Journal* published details, including physical layouts for Brackenridge, Seton, St. David's, and Holy Cross hospitals, and the UT Health Center. When needed, all physicians were to report to assigned hospitals or locations.

September 24, 1951, was a special hallmark for Travis County medicine as the Austin Blood Bank opened its doors to donors at 1705 North Congress Avenue—or, as Dr. Charles Pelphrey recalled, "in the basement of Dr. Sam Todaro's building behind the state Capitol on Congress Avenue." County medical society members joined others to donate blood so that a sufficient volume could be built up for Austin and the surrounding area. Dr. C. H. "Hal" McCuistion chaired the blood donation committee, assisted by Dr. Wendell S. Sharpe. The administrator was Oliver Johnson and Dr. Sidney Bohls was director, with Dr. Pelphrey performing much of the daily work. Members had responded enthusiastically to financial pledges to enable a bank loan, and Dr. Raleigh Ross, TCMS president, sought guidance from Dr. E. Eric Muirhead, a professor at UT Southwestern Medical School (Southwestern Medical College had come under the UT umbrella in 1949). Dr. Muirhead, a highly regarded researcher on blood, plasma, shock, and hypertension, was a founder of the American Association of Blood Banks. Another valued service was initiated in 1951 when Austin physicians advanced $5,000 to establish a twenty-four-hour answering service, the Travis County Medical Exchange, which also helped people find a physician.

September 1952 saw the fruition of the Travis County Medical Society's 1948 initiative—the dedication of the new TMA building at 1801 North Lamar Boulevard. Facing Shoal Creek and Pease Park to the west, it was a modern 1950s structure designed for air conditioning with few windows. Among the speakers at the dedication were Texas Governor Allan Shivers and U.S. Senator Lyndon Baines Johnson. Unfortunately, Dr. Gambrell, who had been a spokesman for the new building, had died in July. Dr. Harold M. Williams of Austin, who succeeded Dr. Holman Taylor as TMA secretary and editor of the *Texas State Journal of Medicine*, oversaw the transfer of staff to Austin. After Dr. Williams resigned, Dr. Sam Key, Sr., was appointed briefly as secretary, succeeding himself by election. After an executive was employed to manage the association and a journalist to oversee the state journal, Austin physicians were named to the anonymous Journal Advisory Committee to review and select manuscripts for publication. Four years after the building dedication, Dr. Key died on September 17, 1956. In addition to his devoted work for the Texas Medical Association, he had been instrumental in starting a drive for a new St. David's Hospital building in 1945.

Physicians remembered Dr. George Decherd, who died in March 1951, and who had contributed his energy to the

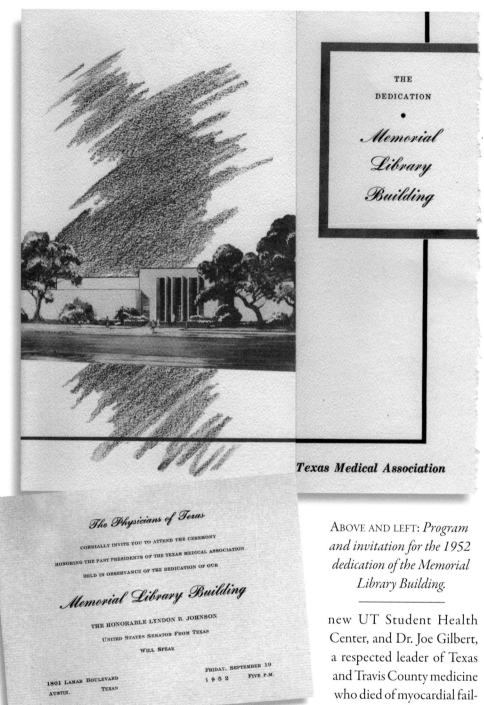

THE
DEDICATION
•
Memorial Library Building

Texas Medical Association

The Physicians of Texas
CORDIALLY INVITE YOU TO ATTEND THE CEREMONY
HONORING THE PAST PRESIDENTS OF THE TEXAS MEDICAL ASSOCIATION
HELD IN OBSERVANCE OF THE DEDICATION OF OUR
Memorial Library Building
THE HONORABLE LYNDON B. JOHNSON
UNITED STATES SENATOR FROM TEXAS
WILL SPEAK
1801 LAMAR BOULEVARD   FRIDAY, SEPTEMBER 19
AUSTIN,   TEXAS   1952   FIVE P.M.

ABOVE AND LEFT: *Program and invitation for the 1952 dedication of the Memorial Library Building.*

new UT Student Health Center, and Dr. Joe Gilbert, a respected leader of Texas and Travis County medicine who died of myocardial failure in October 1951.

When Dr. George Tipton completed his residency in 1949, he borrowed money for his first year of practice in Austin and his wife taught school. Surgeons then were doing house calls, for which he charged ten dollars. If he administered an injection, the fee was fourteen dollars. Surgical fees were modest, often only 150 dollars. Physicians typically covered most city hospitals, and Dr. Tipton's routine included twice-daily rounds, the first starting at 5:30 am. Patients typically were kept in the hospital for four to five days, although gall bladder patients remained for seven. Almost all patients with trauma or serious problems were transferred to Brackenridge Hospital. Certified by the American Board of Surgery in 1951, Dr. Tip-ton became chief of surgery and chief of staff at Seton and Brackenridge hospitals, and president of the Travis County Medical Society. As president also of the blood bank, he was the originator and chairman of the Disaster Medical Committee and the Travis County Civil Defense Medical Committee. Dr. Joe W. Bailey became his partner, with each physician having his own nurse but sharing a secretary.

With the goal of helping to assure consistently high standards of care, Dr. Tipton organized the first tissue audit committee in Austin at Brackenridge Hospital in January 1950. It "changed medicine in Austin," he recalled. A three-year process at Brackenridge led to heightened awareness among practitioners regarding their own abilities, resulting in a decline in faulty practices; an improvement in charts and more detailed case histories; and better ratios between pre- and postoperative diagnoses and postoperative and pathologic diagnoses. The American College of Surgeons' *Manual of Hospital Accreditation* in 1951 required such committees as did the Joint Commission on Accreditation of Hospitals (later the Joint Commission on Accreditation of Healthcare Organizations). In 1954, Dr. Tipton reported his work on the Brackenridge tissue audit committee in the *Bulletin of the American College of Surgeons*.

In 1950, Dr. William F. McLean opened a private obstetrics and gynecology practice in Austin. Born in Hereford, Texas, he was a Phi Beta Kappa at UT, where he worked his way through school as a laboratory technician. He graduated from UTMB in December 1942, took an

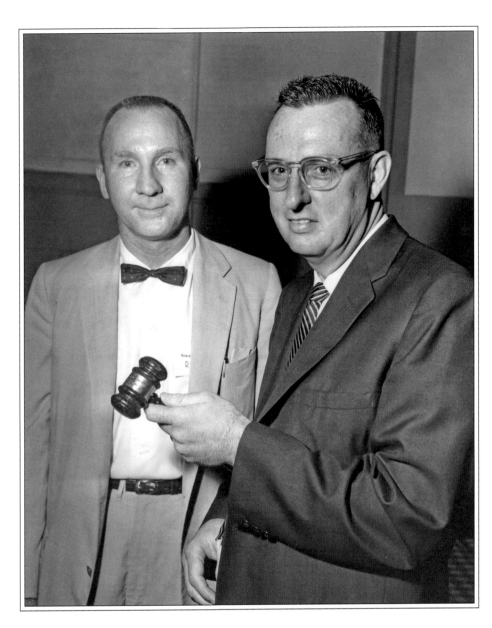

Drs. Raleigh Ross and George Tipton, Travis County Medical Society presidents, passing the gavel.

internship at the University of Iowa, and served in the Navy from 1943 to 1945. His residency in obstetrics-gynecology was from 1946 to 1949 at Parkland Hospital, Dallas, and he was chief resident from 1949 to 1950 at Watts Hospital in Durham, North Carolina. Dr. McLean established Gynics Associates in 1964.

Dr. Earl Lee Yeakel arrived in 1951 to join Dr. David O. Johnson as a partner in his anesthesiology group. An Oklahoma native and father of future federal judge Lee Yeakel, he was a graduate of the University of Oklahoma College of Medicine. He served an internship in Orange County, California, and was in the Army during World War II. Afterward, he took a fellowship in anesthesiology at the Mayo

Clinic and became a diplomate of the American Board of Anesthesiology.

Dr. Donald E. Pohl found no space when he visited Austin in 1951, but he returned from Minnesota the next year for the warmer climate and rented half a building at San Antonio and Fifteenth Streets. It took two years for him to begin earning enough to survive; fortunately, money earned earlier and additional work, including service at the UT Student Health Center, sustained the practice and his family. Like other Austin doctors, he taught and made rounds with interns and provided free clinic services at Brackenridge Hospital. The hospital's administrator, William King Brown, also asked him to make house calls for clinic patients for a dollar per person, and he began visiting seven or eight nursing-type homes per month, or as needed. After three years in the half-house, Dr. Pohl built an office with another physician at No. 1 Medical Arts Square—the first in the newest satellite area—and eleven years later moved to the new Medical Park Tower on West Thirty-eighth Street. A native of Council Bluffs, Iowa, Dr. Pohl graduated from the University of Iowa College of Medicine in 1944 and had begun a pathology residency but became interested in diagnostic medicine and followed that in residencies in Nebraska and Boston. He had been a captain in the Army Medical Corps for two years at the end of World War II and was certified in internal medicine in 1953.

Tuberculosis remained a great challenge. Besides crushing a phrenic nerve or performing thoracoplasty, air sometimes was pumped into the pleural cavity to allow the lung to collapse, or into the peritoneal cavity, thus pushing up the diaphragm to compress the lung. Every Wednesday or Thursday, Dr. Pohl recalled, about twenty patients arrived at the Brackenridge clinic to have their air pumped. Often, they brought about twenty friends, including a guitar player, and sat in the hall to wait. By the mid-1950s there were effective anti-tuberculosis drugs, like isoniazid, thus collapse therapies and lung resection became unnecessary except in cases of drug resistance.

Born in Rockland, Texas, Dr. F. Murphy Nelson graduated from UTMB in 1945. He served an internship at the U.S. Naval Hospital in Bethesda, Maryland, from 1945 to 1946, and a general surgical residency at John Sealy Hospital in Galveston, from 1952 to 1956. He became board-certified in surgery in 1957.

During the Korean Conflict, Dr. Clift Price was assigned to the Corpus Christi Naval Air Station on general family duty and also served on troop ships out of San Francisco to the Pacific, treating troops who had been exposed to sexually transmitted diseases in Japan and Korea and had to be treated on the return trip to the United States. Dr. Price left the Navy in 1953 and joined Drs. Coleman, Hanna, and Kelton at Children's Medical Center, the only pediatric group practice in Austin. Offered a guaranteed stipend of $900 a month, he was told he could keep patients that others referred to him if he chose. He typically made two or three house calls after five o'clock in the afternoon from the 1950s into the 1970s. In 1953, an office visit was seven dollars, and he cared for some patients without charge. A few families had health insurance, with rates from about forty-nine to fifty-nine dollars per year.

Dr. Joe C. Rude, a diplomate of the American Board of Radiology, moved to Austin in 1953 and became chief of radiology at Brackenridge Hospital. He was a consultant to Bergstrom Air Force Base, Austin State Hospital, and the Austin State School.

After a Veterans Administration residency in Dallas, Dr. John R. Rainey joined Drs. Bohls and Pelphrey in their pathology practice in 1952. In 1956, Drs. Pelphrey and Rainey purchased the private laboratory and it became known as the Clinical Pathology Laboratory. Dr. Thomas Gordon Price joined them in 1956 after a residency in Fort Worth. Later, Dr. Bennett Sewell, a 1957 graduate of Tulane University, board-certified in both anatomic and clinical pathology, would join them.

Although historically physicians had been chosen for the post, J. V. Irons, Sc.D., succeeded Dr. Bohls at the Texas Department of Health laboratories.

In 1953, both the Travis County Medical Society and the Texas Medical Association celebrated their centennial anniversaries. A gift marking the occasion came from Dr. Paul R. Stalnaker, son of Dr. John William Stalnaker, a Travis County physician who had served as an assistant surgeon in the Confederate Army during the Civil War. The elder Dr. Stalnaker had assisted in compiling *A Manual of Military Surgery*, an 1863 book of instruction on surgery and first aid. His son gave an autographed copy to the TMA Memorial Library.

Medical science was bubbling over again both from new discoveries and new applications. In 1953, James Watson and Francis Crick discovered the double helical structure of deoxyribonucleic acid (DNA) in 1953. Nationwide testing of Dr. Jonas Salk's killed virus vaccine for poliomyelitis began in April 1954 with mass inoculation of children. After it was licensed in April 1955, there were long lines at the city health department in Austin.

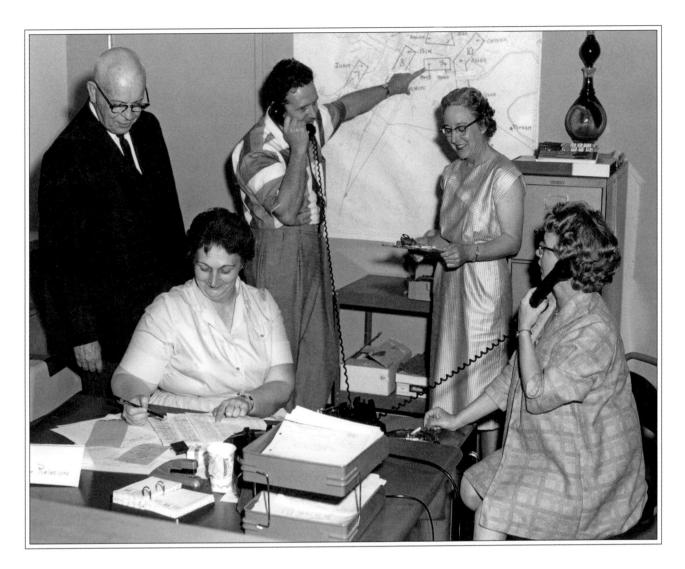

Travis County Medical Society sponsored a community-wide oral polio immunization program. Doctors Primer, Vickers, and Bain spot-check results in the Control Center.

By 1957, there would be an eighty-five percent decline in polio in the United States.

In 1954, Austin lost its first formally trained and board-certified pediatrician, Dr. Thomas D. McCrummen. Physicians and former patients remembered him as a fine, patient, and kindly gentleman.

Doctors' hard work was beginning to pay off and Drs. Griffin and Fox were able to move from their old house in 1954 and open a new clinic at 1010 West Nineteenth Street (later Martin Luther King Jr. Boulevard) designed by Austin architect Charles Granger. They now had room to open a physical therapy facility. They also saved bone that remained after clean amputations, wrapped it in sterile towels, and stored the aseptic package in closed, por-

celain containers in a downtown meat locker. During the 1950s and 1960s, they reused these hygienic fragments with no problems.

In 1949, Dr. J. Nelson Sanders had entered a two-year internship, including a year in general surgery, at the University of Michigan in Ann Arbor. After completing a urology residency at City Hospital, later John Gaston Hospital, in Memphis in August 1954, he moved to Austin to practice urology.

Dr. Thomas M. Runge, born in Mason, Texas, graduated from UTMB in 1947. He interned at Milwaukee County General Hospital and became a fellow in neurology and a fellow in medicine at the Hospital of the University of Pennsylvania. From 1950 to 1951, he was an instructor at the University of Pennsylvania School of Medicine. He served in the Navy for three years. He was board-certified in internal medicine in 1955, and from 1965 to 1966, he undertook a cardiology fellowship at St. Luke's Hospital and at Texas Children's Hospital in Houston.

His wife, Dr. Gretchen Herrmann Runge, born in Ann Arbor, Michigan, was the daughter of UTMB cardiology professor Dr. George R. Herrmann. She graduated from UTMB in 1947, interned at Milwaukee County General Hospital, and was a resident in pediatrics at the Hospital of the University of Pennsylvania from 1948 to 1950. Board-certified in pediatrics in 1956, she became a fellow in pediatric neurology at Baylor University College of Medicine, Houston, from 1965 to 1966. She was also medical director in pediatric neurology at the Austin Evaluation Center. The Runges' three children all became academic physicians.

One small Austin medical practice in the 1950s would grow far larger than the early participants imagined. Dr. Henry Renfert, Jr., a 1944 graduate of Cornell Medical College, spent the succeeding years at the University of Michigan Hospital in Ann Arbor. There, he served as an intern, an assistant resident, a resident. and as an instructor from 1944 to 1950. From 1951 to 1952, he was an assistant professor in internal medicine research and an associate instructor in industrial health. After serving as a lieutenant (jg) in the United States Navy from 1945 to 1946 and a lieutenant in the Naval Medical Corps from 1950 to 1951, he arrived in Austin in 1952 to practice internal medicine in the Capital National Bank Building.

In 1956, Dr. Virgil Lawlis, a 1950 UTMB graduate, joined Dr. Renfert and in 1957 the two physicians welcomed Dr. Leonard J. Sayers, a 1953 graduate of Northwestern University Medical School (subsequently the Northwestern University Feinberg School of Medicine). In 1958, Dr. Renfert moved to New York to serve

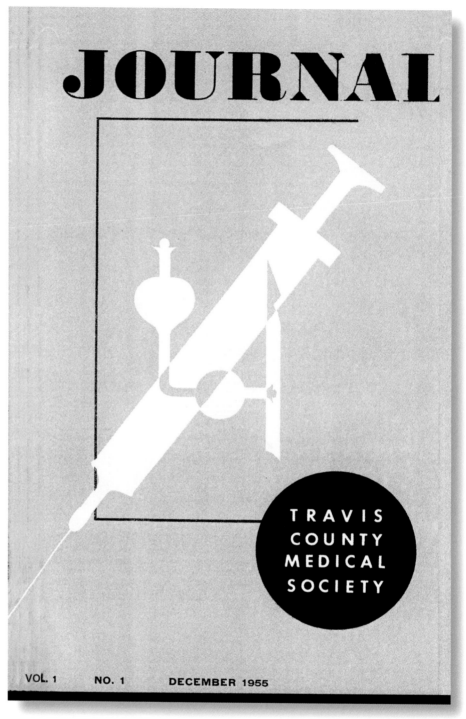

VOL. 1 NO. 1 DECEMBER 1955

The first issue of the TCMS Journal *was published in December 1955. TCMS President Dr. James Coleman and other leaders decided it was time to publish "a true journal or record of the proceedings of our society and the works of our doctors."*

two years as dean of students at Cornell Medical College. For a brief time, Drs. Lawlis and Sayers were the sole physicians in the practice, but shortly thereafter, Dr. Homer Goehrs joined them.

Dr. Virgil Lawlis had grown up on a dry land cotton farm in Sylvester, Texas, near Abilene, and graduated from McCaulley High School in Fisher County. He attended colleges now known as Texas Tech University in Lubbock and McMurry University in Abilene. After serving in the Navy for several months, he was accepted into the Navy's V12 training program at UT. Completing medical school at UTMB in 1950, he interned at King's Daughters Hospital in Temple, Texas. He served in the Air Force for two years, becoming a captain. While he was stationed at Reese Air Force Base in Lubbock, his wife, Dr. Marjorie Lawlis, was a general practitioner at Levelland, Texas. From 1953 to 1956, the Lawlises returned to UTMB, Galveston, where he was an internal medicine resident and she was a pediatric resident. From 1965 to 1966, he served a fellowship in gastroenterology at the University of Michigan.

Dr. Marjorie Lawlis, whom Dr. Virgil Lawlis had met in a UT laboratory, was born in Houston, the only child of a Certified Public Accountant father and a mathematics professor mother. She graduated from Milby High School in Houston, and after attending UT, received her M.D. degree from UTMB in 1950. She interned at King's Daughters Hospital in Temple, and, in 1956, completed a residency at John Sealy Hospital in Galveston. Certified by the American Board of Pediatrics in 1959, she was the infectious disease control officer and staff pediatrician at the Austin State School from 1956 to 1962. At the Austin State Hospital, she was a psychiatry resident from 1962 to 1965 and associate director of the children's psychiatric unit in 1966. She also was a resident in child psychiatry at Hawthorne Center, Northville, Michigan, from 1965 to 1966. When the Drs. Lawlis went to Michigan for advanced studies, they took their five children with them. Two of their sons later became physicians.

After the family returned to Austin, Dr. Virgil Lawlis was one of only two gastroenterologists in Austin for a time. Dr. Ted Edwards, the other, soon transferred into sports medicine. Dr. Charles Felger, who joined the Austin Diagnostic Clinic in 1968, also was a specialist in gastroenterology. While he was at Michigan, Dr. Lawlis studied endoscopy, including specifically the use of the gastroscope. At first, the instrument could only provide side views. Around 1950, the rigid sigmoidoscope, which reached the sigmoid, was used to detect colon cancer. Soon, however, endoscopy was greatly improved with fiber optic lighting and flexible scopes that provided views around corners. It also would be adapted to a variety of procedures in gastro-

enterology, including colonoscopy, which was developed later and which permitted examination of the large intestine. Improved, high resolution cameras also aided the advancement of endoscopy. The new technologies began allowing the use of endoscopy in numerous surgical and diagnostic procedures spanning specialties such as orthopedics; ear, nose, and throat; pulmonary; genitourinary; vascular; and other fields. Gynecologists previously had used colposcopy for the upper vagina and orthopedists began using modern arthrosocopy, based on the new technologies, for the knee in the late 1960s.

Discharged from the Navy in 1945, Homer Goehrs left for the University of Texas, where his roommate was Virgil Lawlis. After receiving his M.D. degree from Baylor University College of Medicine in Houston in 1950, Dr. Goehrs became an intern and assistant resident in surgery at Baltimore City Hospitals. He returned to the Navy as a lieutenant during the Korean Conflict. Serving on a heavy cruiser, he performed three appendectomies at sea. From 1954 to 1957, he was a fellow at the Mayo Clinic, including a year of rheumatology study with Philip Hench, the Nobel physician who was the first to use cortisone medically. Returning to Austin in 1957, he practiced briefly with Dr. Walter K. Long on Fifteenth Street before joining Drs. Lawlis and Sayers. He received his board certification in internal medicine in 1959.

Austin had no formal emergency medical system at that time and Dr. Virgil Lawlis and Dr. Goehrs loaded patients into their cars to take them to the hospital. A long transition period also would be necessary to encourage patients to go to a physician's office or clinic rather than to expect house calls. Often during a house call, doctors needed a blood count, an electrocardiogram, or other laboratory or diagnostic equipment. Matters like checking for anemia or internal bleeding simply could not be done adequately at home.

Dr. Leonard Sayers, born in Des Moines, Iowa, attended Iowa State University in Ames, Iowa, and graduated from Northwestern University School of Medicine in 1953. He interned in 1954, took an internal medicine residency from 1955 to 1956, and a fellowship in hematology in 1957, all at Cook County Hospital in Chicago. He moved to Austin in July 1957.

In 1958, the old Sigma Alpha Epsilon (SAE) fraternity house, across from Seton Hospital on Twenty-sixth Street, became vacant. Owned by Mr. W. O. Harper, proprietor of an Austin plumbing company, the house was rented and renovated by Drs. Lawlis, Sayers, and Goehrs. When Dr.

Renfert returned, the physicians formed a four-person group and bought the house. "Renfert, Lawlis, Sayers and Goehrs" then operated as an internal medicine group before coining the name, Austin Diagnostic Clinic. Dr. Walter K. Long briefly became a part of the group but joined the biomedical engineering department at UT, where he taught physiology for many years.

Dr. John P. "Pete" Vineyard, Jr., a 1955 graduate of UT Southwestern Medical School, Dallas, came to Austin in August 1961 at the request of Dr. Henry Renfert, joining him and Drs. Lawlis, Sayers, and Goehrs to practice in the old SAE house. As part of his internal medicine residency at Parkland Memorial Hospital, Dr. Vineyard had completed a two-year fellowship in infectious disease with Dr. Jay P. Sanford, the noted professor of medicine and chief of the infectious diseases service at UT Southwestern Medical School, Dallas.

In 1964, Dr. W. Donald Roberts returned to Austin after his internal medicine residency, and Dr. John Tyler, a board-certified cardiologist who had trained at Tulane University, joined the group at the SAE house. With no additional space on the first floor, Dr. Tyler was placed upstairs (a good stress test for the cardiac patients, the physicians recalled). Other physicians also soon joined the practice, including Dr. Terry Collier, a 1957 Baylor University College of Medicine graduate, who arrived in Austin in 1966. Dr. Robert "Bob" Anderson, Dr. Collier's roommate at Baylor, who had finished his training at UTMB, arrived in 1967. By now, the physicians knew they needed more space and began developing plans for a new location, settling on a Thirty-fourth Street site, where they moved after seven years at the old SAE house. In 1971, Dr. Vineyard left the group to set up a solo practice in internal medicine.

Dr. Charles E. Felger joined the Austin Diagnostic Clinic in 1968. Born in Victoria, Texas, he had graduated from Tulane University School of Medicine in 1961. After an internship and residency in internal medicine at Fort Sam Houston in San Antonio, the Army sent him to Stuttgart, Germany, as chief of the medicine service. He was president of the Travis County Medical Society in 1993 and was named its Physician of the Year in 1994. In 2004, he was named a top alumnus at Tulane University.

Among the active physicians in the 1950s and 1960s, Dr. Albert Terry was an early urologist in the city. Born in Nashville, Tennessee, in 1904, he was educated in the Dallas public schools and received his B.A. degree from the University of Texas. He attended Baylor University College of Medicine in Dallas and received his M.D. degree from Rush Medical College in Chicago, in 1931. He interned at Henry Ford Hospital in Detroit, and completed a residency there in 1934. He then undertook additional work in urology at the Cook County Postgraduate School (later the Cook County Graduate School of Medicine) in 1936 and was certified by the American Board of Urology in 1940. Briefly practicing general medicine and urology in Glasgow, Montana, he moved to Austin in 1936.

Austin gained the services of urologist Dr. B. Clary Bates, born in Lewisville, Texas. He earned his M.D. degree from UTMB in 1945, interned at the United States Naval Medical Center at Bethesda, Maryland, and served a residency at Wichita Falls Clinic and Hospital. He was also a lieutenant (jg) in the Naval Reserve from 1945 to 1947. Earning his board certification in urology in 1953, Dr. Bates would be praised for his diagnostic acumen.

In the mid-1950s, Dr. James Coleman, TCMS president, became concerned that "without adequate communication we may grow into a society of strangers." He and other leaders decided it was time to publish "a true journal or record of the proceedings of our society and the works of our doctors." The first issue was published in December 1955. Not designed as a literary medium or a place for scientific articles, the new journal was to provide "information that can serve as a basis for decision." A previous Travis County journal, although not owned by the society, was published from 1940 to 1943.

The Texas Medical Association opened membership to all races in 1955 by deleting the word "white" from the association's constitution. The new *TCMS Journal* in December 1955 reported that Dr. Carolyn J. Long of Austin, a black pediatrician, had been approved by the Board of Censors for society membership. A 1950 graduate of Meharry Medical College in Nashville, Tennessee, she served an internship and the first year of her pediatric residency at Homer G. Phillips Hospital in St. Louis. Her second year of residency was at Harlem Hospital, New York City, and she began her practice in Austin in 1954. Dr. Long died young in 1960 in Houston. Born in Waco, she had served on the staffs of Brackenridge and Holy Cross hospitals, and in conjunction with UT, had researched sickle cell anemia.

Dr. Robert N. Snider, looking for a new partner, invited Drs. Robert Ellzey and William L. DeGinder to talk with him in 1958. All three physicians became partners in the Austin Radiological Association, with quarters in a remodeled house at 2410 Rio Grande Street.

Dr. Ellzey graduated in 1950 from the University of Oklahoma and in 1954 from the University of Oklahoma School of Medicine. The Austin radiology group covered hospitals in Llano and Burnet one day a week with Dr. DeGinder, a 1947 UTMB graduate, piloting a Cessna 170 airplane. Dr. Thomas B. Fletcher, a 1983 graduate of UT Southwestern Medical School in Dallas, a radiologist specializing in vascular and interventional radiology, later joined the group, serving at Seton Medical Center. The partnership, which started in the late 1950s, would continue to grow and expand to satellite locations throughout Austin and the surrounding area.

Familiar names could be seen in Austin as descendents entered the medical profession. Dr. Frank H. Gregg, son of Dr. Francis Banner Gregg, became the fourth generation in his family to practice in Travis county. He was born in Austin, graduating with honors from UT Austin and in 1956 from UTMB with honors. He served an internship in Galveston and completed an ophthalmology residency at the State University of Iowa College of Medicine in Iowa City (later the Roy J. and Lucille A. Carver College of Medicine at the University of Iowa). After two years in the Air Force, he practiced in Austin for thirty years. In 1962, he was board certified in ophthalmology.

In 1957, Dr. Lee F. Scarborough, a psychiatrist, called on his colleagues for greater understanding of psychiatry. In a letter in the January *TCMS Journal*, he asked a common question, "How do I refer a patient to a psychiatrist?" He responded that the "psychiatrist is a physician who specializes. So, why not refer as you would to any physician? The answer is just that simple." He added, "Granted, there is

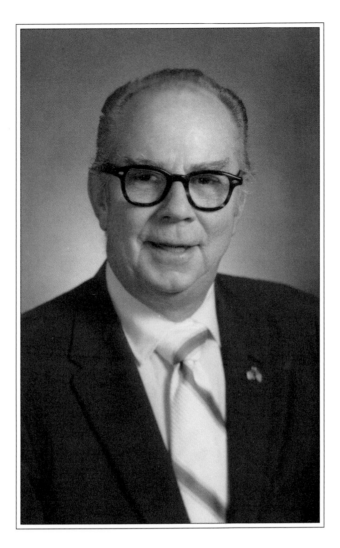

*Dr. C. H. "Hal" McCuistion, Travis County
Medical Society president, 1956.*

public misconception in the field of mental illness and mental health. There is resulting prejudice and erroneous judgment passed upon psychiatrists and their activities."

Born in Gould, Oklahoma, Dr. Scarborough graduated from Texas Military College in Terrell, Texas, in 1935 and from Baylor University College of Medicine in Dallas in 1939. He took a rotating internship in 1939 at Highland Sanitarium in Shreveport, Louisiana, and was a resident in neuropsychiatry at the Colorado Psychopathic Hospital in Denver from 1940 to 1941 and at the Galveston Psychiatric Hospital from 1946 to 1947. As an Army paratroop surgeon during World War II, he was wounded on D-Day in Europe in June 1944 while jumping into France. He later jumped into Holland, and from there he joined the beginning of the Battle of the Bulge, where he again was wounded. He retired as a captain.

The success of Travis County's blood bank in 1957 was recorded by Charles L. Collum, Jr., executive director of the blood bank and executive secretary of the Travis County Medical Society. It had seen an all-time high response with nearly 9,000 registrations and more than 8,000 accepted blood donors, with nearly 7,500 successful transfusions. He thanked those who had contributed services, including the Woman's Auxiliary, pathologists Drs. Pelphrey, Rainey, and Price, and also Dr. Charles Hardwicke for "his staunch support, his irrefutable logic in handling problems...." The 1957 year-end report of the Medical Service Bureau also revealed a successful year, with the Medical Exchange handling more than 165,000 calls from physicians and patients. A radio-communication plan to help improve the program was being considered.

A medical school for Austin was the major topic in the May 1958 issue of the *TCMS Journal*. The AMA's Council on Medical Education and Hospitals and the Association of American Medical Colleges believed that Austin offered a favorable milieu for a medical school. San Antonio, however, had been working longer to acquire a medical school, and in 1959, the Texas Legislature selected Bexar County for the South Texas Medical School. It would become the University of Texas Medical School at San Antonio, the third UT medical school.

Among doctors arriving in the late 1950s was Dr. W. Pruett Watkins who had begun practice in Luling, Texas, in 1940, assuming the practice of his father, Dr. John M. Watkins, above the Watkins General Store. He also practiced in Taylor before moving to Austin in 1958. Born in Luling, he attended UT Austin and UTMB, graduating in 1938, and interned at Jefferson Davis Hospital in Houston. During the Great Depression, he was in the Civilian Conservation Corps and in 1941 he joined UTMB's 127th General Hospital Unit, serving in England and France. He often volunteered his services, including at the People's Free Clinic in Austin, in Texas City during its 1947 disaster, and in Guatemala.

Dr. Francis McIntyre, a general practitioner who regularly wore his trademark bow tie, also opened his office on North Loop Boulevard in Austin in 1958. He had grown up in Wabash, Indiana, and attended Wabash College. During World War II, he was a navigator in the Army Air Corps, reenlisting after college and becoming an Air Force B-36 navigator. A graduate of UT Southwestern Medical School at Dallas, he had undertaken his internship at Brackenridge Hospital. From the beginning of his practice until he retired, he continued to make house calls.

Dr. V. C. Smart was born and grew up in ranching country in Spur, Texas, west of Lubbock—literally the end of a train route—where his father was a Ford automobile dealer. After graduating from high school in 1938, he attended Texas Technological College in Lubbock. In 1942, he joined the Navy as a Second Class Petty Officer and, after his discharge in 1945, he earned a degree in chemical engineering in 1947. His first job as an analytical chemist bored him, however, and he tried his father's business for a while before returning to school to study biological science. He was accepted into UTMB in 1952, graduating in 1956, and then interning at Brackenridge Hospital. With Dr. Charles E. Ferrin, he opened an office south of the Colorado River on South Lamar Boulevard. With only two other general practitioners south of the river, the two new partners immediately doubled the doctor population. An office visit cost five dollars and a house call seven to eight dollars. With health insurance rare, the partners assumed that fifteen to twenty percent of people could not pay. In 1980, Dr. Smart left his general practice to study allergy with another physician and, in 1981, joined Drs. Lobdell Exline and Harold Robinson in the practice of allergy.

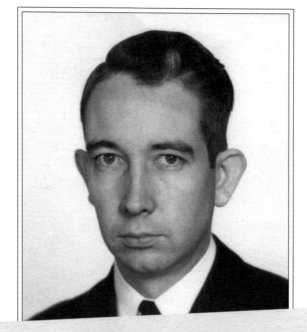

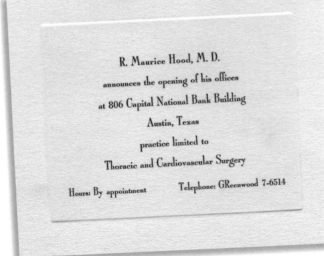

R. Maurice Hood, M. D.

announces the opening of his offices

at 806 Capital National Bank Building

Austin, Texas

practice limited to

Thoracic and Cardiovascular Surgery

Hours: By appointment   Telephone: GReenwood 7-6514

TOP: *Cardiovascular surgeon Maurice Hood established his practice in 1958.* ABOVE: *Medical ethics of the day dictated that announcements, signs, and advertisements should be understated and small.*

Born in Philadelphia, Dr. Albert F. Vickers had graduated from high school in Bensalem Township, Bucks County, Pennsylvania, in 1942. While studying to be an engineer, he entered the United States Army, shifting to the Army Specialized Training Program (ASTP). Changing his field to premedical education, he attended Princeton University under the original advanced ASTP, and before going on to medical school was assigned to Fort Dix, New Jersey, the entry point for troops being brought back from Africa and Europe. He served as an orthopedic technician, which, among other things, involved replacing casts hastily done on battlefields so troops could be sent to hospitals nearest their homes.

After the war, he completed his medical education at what is now called New York University School of Medicine, graduating in 1949. He served a rotating internship at Brooke Army Medical Center in San Antonio, followed by service at the Fourth Army Surgeon's Headquarters, before going to South Korea from 1951 to 1952 as an Army medical officer. At Brooke, he met his wife Virginia, a Texan who had been a flight nurse in the South Pacific during World War II. She had remained in the Army and was attending anesthesia school.

After leaving the Army, Dr. Vickers practiced in Giddings for six years before moving to Austin to practice family medicine in the late 1950s. He would be the 1968 president of the Travis County Medical Society. Virginia Vickers became a nurse-anesthetist at Holy Cross Hospital and worked with Austin anesthesiologists, primarily the Austin Anesthesiology Group. After the Allan Shivers Radiation Therapy Center, Austin's first cancer treatment center and a nonprofit outpatient facility, opened in 1973 next to Holy Cross Hospital, she often administered anesthesia to patients there. She earned the Certified Registered Nurse Anesthetist (CRNA) designation, which required extra training, and was one of the few CRNAs in Austin.

One of the early formally trained allergists in Austin was Dr. Theophilus S. Painter, Jr., an Austin native, who received his board certification in 1955. A 1947 UTMB graduate, he served his internship and residency and was a clinical instructor at the University of Michigan Hospital in Ann Arbor. From 1956 to 1958, he was a staff physician and chief of allergy at the Veterans Administration Hospital in Ann Arbor and instructor in allergy in the department of internal medicine at the University of Michigan Medical School. A captain in the U.S. Air Force from 1951 to 1953, he began his practice at the Capital National Bank Building in Austin.

In 1958, Austin welcomed cardiovascular surgeon Dr. R. Maurice Hood. Following the custom of new doctors, he set aside time to introduce himself to doctors in town and soon had all the work he could handle. This rite of passage for new doctors continued until the city and the number of doctors grew too large. Dr. Hood grew up in Lubbock, Texas, graduating from Lubbock High School in 1941 and attending Texas Technological College (later Texas Tech University) between 1941 and 1943. Accepted to Baylor University College of Medicine before the school moved to Houston in 1943, he instead entered the first class for the new Southwestern Medical College, graduating in 1946. He served an internship at Baylor University Hospital in Dallas, followed by a general surgical residency at the U.S. Naval Hospital in San Diego, California. He served as a staff surgeon at the U.S. Naval Hospital in Guam from 1949 to 1951. After serving a residency at the U.S. Naval Hospital in Oakland, California, from 1951 to 1952, he became a fellow in thoracic and cardiovascular surgery from 1952 to 1954 at the University of Michigan Medical School in Ann Arbor. He was board-certified in surgery and thoracic surgery.

Dr. John P. "Jack" Schneider opened his urology practice in 1958 in Austin, his home town. A Navy corpsman in World War II, he graduated from Tulane University School of Medicine in 1952. After an internship at Philadelphia General Hospital, he completed a four-year urology residency at the Mayo Clinic in 1957. Certified by the American Board of Urology, he would institute several changes in Austin. He recalled that he and Dr. James Reeves, a 1960 graduate of Baylor University College of Medicine, performed peritoneal dialysis using a large trocar needle in the abdomen. "It was tough doing that at night," he said, "and practicing urology in the daytime." He served as president of the Texas Urological Association and the Texas Association of Genitourinary Surgeons.

With Russia's Sputnik launched in 1957 and the U.S. National Aeronautics and Space Administration formed in 1958, a new world lay ahead. "Space Medicine, A New Science," a 1959 article from Randolph Air Force Base's Division of Space Medicine in San Antonio, told Texas doctors about a new medical field.

Austin physicians continued to donate time and expertise to training interns and residents at Brackenridge Hospital and to provide medical care for those needing it. Hospital emergency rooms were staffed primarily by interns or residents. There was a growing concern about health care costs for persons over sixty-five.

CHAPTER XIII

NEXT STOP: THE MOON

NUCLEAR BOMBS, CIVIL DEFENSE, and civil rights were major public issues. "Hippies," young people with long hair and colorful attire and their own ideas of society, populated Austin streets. President John F. Kennedy called for the United States to land a man on the moon by the end of the decade.

Doctors grew more alarmed about socialized medicine, and Dr. Nelson L. Schiller of Austin, a 1935 graduate of the University of Texas Medical Branch (UTMB), asked doctors to help "keep the priceless heritage of freedom" to practice the chosen work for which they had trained.

Medicine was vibrant in Austin. Dr. Francis Morris arrived in 1960 as Travis County's first plastic surgery specialist. Dr. R. Maurice Hood was beginning his extensive, year-long program to prepare for the county's first open-heart surgery. One essential facet was that Brackenridge Hospital, where the surgery was to be performed, had to establish an intensive care unit (ICU). The hospital also acquired a $10,000 heart-lung machine, donated by the Texas State Department of Health in 1961. The American Heart Association provided other equipment.

Until this decade, heart attack patients were treated in private rooms attended by private nurses. When Brackenridge set up the first intensive care unit in Austin in 1960, it also became possibly one of the first in the state to do so. Dr. Virgil Lawlis remembered that he, Dr. W. Donald Roberts, and Dr. Robert G. Farris served on the committee to instigate the ICU, wondering at the time if it really would be used. Their efforts, however, led to a watershed for criti-

cal care medicine in Austin. A nine-bed unit was constructed by the hospital maintenance department, and in 1965 it was enlarged to nineteen units. John Sealy Hospital in Galveston was just setting up its first ICU, and Dr. Robert Anderson, who had arrived in Austin from there, thought it was wonderful to have a nurse at each bed.

On August 31, 1961, Dr. Hood, leading a twelve-member surgical team, performed the first open heart surgery in Austin. The *Austin American-Statesman* wrote that Central Texans no longer had to travel to "Dallas or Houston for the most complicated type of heart surgery." Dr. Hood's team continued to work together and to train others.

At the Austin Diagnostic Clinic, Dr. Anderson performed the first invasive cardiology procedure using a coronary arteriogram in the later 1960s. An Austin native, he graduated in 1957 from Baylor University College of Medicine in Houston, and interned at the United States Naval Hospital inBethesda, Maryland. From 1964 to 1966, he undertook a residency at UTMB where he was a National Institutes of Health fellow in cardiology from 1966 to 1967. He served in the Navy from 1957 to 1961 and was board-certified in internal medicine in 1968.

In a 1960 issue of the *Texas State Journal of Medicine*, Dr. Robert L. Egan, chief of experimental diagnostic radiology at the University of Texas M. D. Anderson Hospital and Tumor Institute in Houston, emphasized the paramount "importance of roentgenograms of maximal detail" in mammography. He had begun using industrial-strength film for higher resolution, allowing earlier tumor identification. In 1961, Dr. Robert Ellzey began participating in

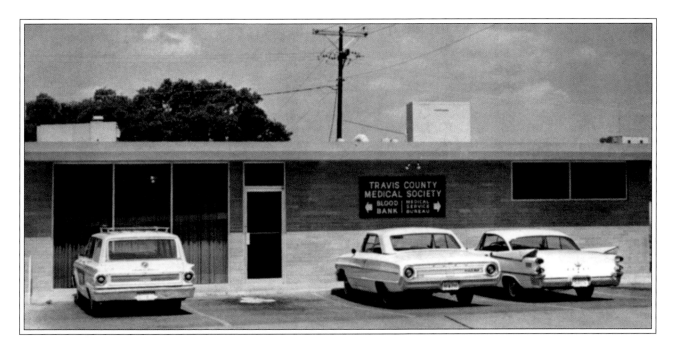

Travis County Medical Society and Blood Bank,
2908 Interstate 35, 1965.

Dr. Egan's Mammography Reproducibility Study done in conjunction with major teaching hospitals in twenty-two U.S. and Canadian cities. Spending a week with Dr. Egan in August 1961, he learned his method and how to modify his equipment for mammography. After medical school, Dr. Ellzey served a rotating internship at Denver General Hospital and General Rose Memorial Hospital, followed by a residency in radiology at the same hospital from 1955 to 1958. He was a diplomate of the American Board of Radiology. His military service included the Army and the Air Force Reserve. A founding board member of the Allan Shivers Radiation Therapy Cancer Center, he was active on TMA councils and was president of the Travis County Medical Society.

Dr. Joe C. Rude at Brackenridge Hospital is thought to have had the first automatic film processor in Austin. Howard Gatewood, the South Texas representative for Gilbert X-Ray and Surgical Company, recalled presenting a purchase request in the early 1960s to the Austin City Council. He also worked all night at Austin Radiological Association's old house on Rio Grande Street to install a processor. In offices, physicians were still hand-dipping x-rays, but these, too, would be replaced by automatic processors.

Dr. William A. Walker, a 1959 UTMB graduate, was chief radiologist at St. David's Hospital for forty-two years, from 1963 until 2005, while continuing with Capital Radiology Association (which became Capital Imaging). St.

David's, he would recall, in the latter 1960s obtained Austin's first image intensifier, which increased the intensity of an image about 5,000 to 6,000 times, and permitted the radiologist to discard the familiar red goggles that had been used in the fluoroscopy room. Other advances included the nuclear medicine camera in the late 1960s, and, when St. David's was not able to obtain a government certificate of need for a CT scanner in the late 1970s, his group purchased the equipment. For scanning, however, hospital patients had to be taken to Capital Imaging's site at 10 Medical Arts Square. Born in Beaumont, Dr. Walker had served an internship with three rotations at Charity Hospital in New Orleans and finished a radiology residency at UTMB. He was board-certified in radiology in 1964.

In June 1960, Dr. James M. Coleman died at age fifty-three while attending a postgraduate symposium on allergy in St. Louis. Dr. Coleman had compiled the history of early Travis County medicine, *Aesculapius on the Colorado; The Story of Medical Practice in Travis County to 1899.* Dr. Pruett Watkins, the editor of the *TCMS Journal,* wrote that too few readers realized that Dr. Coleman had contributed more to the journal than all others combined. "With his ever-present pipe and smiling face, he presented a picture of a relaxed, tolerant, wise man who is at once at ease with himself and his colleagues, as well as his fellow man...."

Dr. Grover L. Bynum arrived in Austin in 1960. A native of Henryetta, Oklahoma, he had graduated from Tulane University School of Medicine in 1953. After an internship in Denver, he spent three years as an Air Force flight surgeon before beginning his residency at the Mayo

Clinic. He joined Drs. Charles Darnall, Horace Cromer, and Francis M. Pearce, Jr., to form the Capital Medical Clinic with offices in the downtown Norwood Building, later renamed the Capital National Bank Building. Dr. Bynum became an advocate on many medical issues and served on the TMA Council on Socioeconomics, the State Legislative Task Force on Cancer, and the original board of the Texas Cancer Council. He was president of the Travis County Medical Society in 1973 and was named its Physician of the Year in 1997. In 2002, Tulane honored him as an outstanding alumnus.

Dr. Ben Cohen, thought to have been Austin's first neurologist, started a practice in 1960. Born in Williamstown, Pennsylvania, he graduated from Jefferson Medical College in Philadelphia. He served an internship at Williamsport General Hospital followed by residencies in psychiatry and neurology at Hines Veterans Administration Hospital in Chicago and Coatesville Veterans Administration Hospital in Pennsylvania.

In 1961, James Prentice of Austin, who was attending UT Southwestern Medical School at Dallas, served a summer externship in anesthesiology at St. David's Hospital. Then the newest and most modern hospital in Austin, St. David's had four operating rooms, with surgeries typically scheduled on weekdays from about 8:30 am to 3:30 pm. The future Dr. Prentice recalled that Dr. David O. Johnson and his anesthesiology partners made him feel part of the team from his first day and also gave him an appreciation for a hospital-based medical practice and the needs of the surgical patient and of the symbiotic relationship between surgeon and anesthesiologist. Dr. Johnson served as St. David's administrator for a time and "was everywhere."

Surgery volume in Austin was relatively small per capita with few emergency procedures. If a patient arrived in an emergency room, his or her physician was called to the hospital, regardless of the hour, to determine whether admittance was necessary. If surgery was indicated and the patient's physician was not a surgeon, he or she called on one. There were few Caesarean sections and vaginal deliveries were done under general anesthesia.

In January 1961, the Travis County Medical Society started its series of "Tell Me Doctor" television programs in conjunction with Austin's only commercial television station, KTBC. Austin physicians addressed an array of subjects—heart surgery, arthritis, allergies, and topics like blood and poisons. Similar programs were produced over the years, including a series entitled "Call the Doctor," in which patients could ask questions of doctors in the stu-

dio. Programs also appeared on public television station KLRN. The Travis County Medical Society sponsored its first Medical Career Day in November 1961 with 155 high school students participating and with physician-led tours at Brackenridge Hospital and the City-County Health Unit. At the Texas State Health Department, students saw exhibits of various services and laboratories.

Adele Zedler, wife of Dr. Garland G. Zedler, became president of the TMA Woman's Auxiliary in 1961. A graduate of the University of Wisconsin Law School, she practiced briefly in Madison, Wisconsin, and was admitted to practice in Texas in 1959. She also earned a private pilot's license.

On September 11, 1961, Hurricane Carla, a large Category Four storm, struck between Port O'Connor and Port Lavaca, affecting the entire Texas coast and parts of Mexico. Travis County, which was receiving evacuees, also was hit by high winds and rain. Physicians, nurses, and hospital personnel were placed on twenty-four-hour hold as were law enforcement officers, the Red Cross, and Civil Defense personnel. The massive evacuation of coastal residents reportedly saved countless lives. In the first hurricane to have live television coverage, much use was made of short-wave radios, "walkie-talkies," messenger units, and radio units of the Texas Department of Public Safety, sheriff's cars, and taxicab companies.

Travis County's existing flexible emergency plan, under Dr. George Tipton, was instituted. Approximately 1,800 people were sheltered in Austin and, as numbers increased, people were moved from schools into the City Coliseum and the Municipal Auditorium. First aid stations were set up, with medical society members making shelter rounds four to six times a day. Nurses were on continuous duty. Nineteen patients were moved to Brackenridge Hospital's emergency room for treatment, but only three were admitted to the hospital. Rest homes—as nursing homes often were called—provided care for the aged and infirm without charge. Respiratory disease was a problem. Facilities were available for making and refrigerating infants' formulas and, because many children had left home without shoes, the Red Cross provided footwear. Radios, television, live entertainment, and games provided diversion.

A sad event in 1962 led to major changes in the way football players and other athletes received fluids during workouts in the Texas heat. UT Longhorn football player Reggie Grob was taken to Brackenridge Hospital before the season's first game with the University of Oregon in 1962, suffering from heat stroke. Dr. W. Donald Roberts had been instrumental in encouraging Brackenridge Hospital to acquire kidney dialysis equipment, but physicians were not familiar with it. Dr. Jack Schneider and Dr. Roberts sought the help of Dr. Charles Baxter, then an assistant professor of surgery at UT Southwestern Medical School in Dallas, and they performed the dialysis. Reggie lived for seventeen days but his injuries were too great, and he had multiple organ collapse. A Southern Methodist University team member in Dallas also had died of heat exhaustion and two other UT players were taken to Brackenridge but recovered. Players thereafter were provided with ample water and innovations like Gatorade.

After learning about closed catheter drainage, Dr. Schneider purchased and introduced a disposable system to Austin hospitals. Previously, a rubber tube was inserted in the bladder with another tube running into a gallon bottle on the floor. Infections often were acquired almost immediately, he said, whereas the new system delayed the danger. When he began using fiber optics, he recalled the significantly brighter light, which provided a much clearer view through the cystoscope. Old instruments had tiny bulbs connected to a battery and, if they were not first covered with beeswax, they could short out when inserted into the bladder. Dr. James Reeves, he said, also used fiber optics while in the Navy in the mid-1960s. Among the first in Austin to use autologous banking of blood for patients before surgery—primarily because of concerns about hepatitis—Dr. Schneider also remembered introducing urology carts for Austin hospital floors after seeing an orthopedic cart on an elevator.

With no plans to stay in Austin, Dr. Joseph M. Abell, a native Houstonian, met Drs. Otto Brandt and James Graham in the lounge at Brackenridge Hospital. Dr. Graham proposed that he take the empty office adjacent to them in

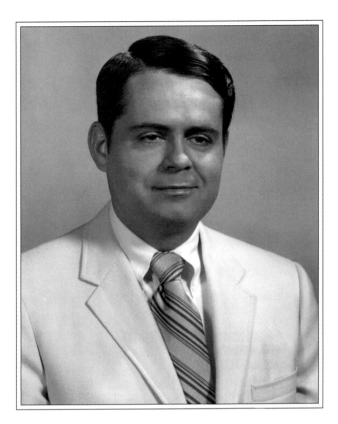

Dr. James Prentice served a summer externship in anesthesiology at St. David's Hospital in 1961.

a house renovated as a quadriplex. On August 1, 1962, Dr. Abell joined the aggregation of doctors around Fifteenth Street, locating at 1506a Guadalupe, in an office that had been occupied by obstetricians Drs. M. D. McCauley and William "Dutch" Hahn. Drs. Graham and Brandt helped by sending him patients. Dr. Abell also remembered learning from Drs. Frederick Lowry, Albert Tisdale, and Kermit Fox, three leading orthopedists.

Although major local and national crises would affect everyone, Austin retained a pleasant atmosphere. Dr. Abell was among a group of "running doctors," who met along Shoal Creek, including Drs. William "Bill" Barnes, Homer Goehrs, Theophilus (Theo) S. Painter, Clift Price, and Mr. John Kemp, executive director of TCMS. Afterward, they had breakfast at Harry Akin's *Night Hawk* restaurant on Guadalupe Street, where Mr. Akin sometimes joined them. He also ran with another group, the "early birds," on the UT track. Often, they also ended up at the *Night Hawk*. There were gatherings with neighborhood doctors like Drs. Jim Graham and Otto Brandt for breakfast and a chat at a corner drugstore, Renfro Drug Company No. 9, at the intersection of Guadalupe and Fifteenth Streets adjacent to their offices. The proprietor of Everette Kelly's Pharmacy across the street often spotted their arrival and joined them.

Born in Houston, Dr. Abell had graduated from St. Thomas High School there, attended Texas A&M, and earned his M.D. degree from Baylor University College of Medicine in Houston. He interned at Michigan Medical Center in Ann Arbor from 1957 to 1958, followed by a residency and appointments as a junior and senior clinical instructor, in the Department of Surgery, Section of Orthopaedics, at the University of Michigan Medical Center from 1958 to 1962. In 1965, he was certified by the American Board of Orthopaedic Surgery. Dr. Abell became active in community and medical organizations, and led many initiatives, including as TCMS president. He also held several leadership positions with TMA and was president of the TMA Foundation. He was an author and earned a B.A. degree with honors in 1991 from UT Austin.

Meanwhile, Drs Maurice Hood, Jack Schneider, and Francis Morris formed the Austin Surgical Specialties Clinic and invited Dr. Abell to join them in their project for a new building. Austin Specialties, Inc., opened at 3100 Red River in 1965. The structure was designed so each surgeon could take in one partner, but Dr. Hood's program grew rapidly and his group of cardiovascular specialists later moved to Medical Parkway.

In 1964, Caritas of Austin was founded by Monsignor Richard McCabe, chaplain at both Holy Cross and Seton hospitals. The organization would provide a broad range of assistance, from food to clinical care in its effort to fight poverty, hunger, and homelessness. Drs. Schneider and Abell had been among physicians in the St. Luke's Society who offered suggestions on the medical aspects of the charity program.

Another orthopedist beginning his practice in the 1960s was Dr. Philip M. Overton, who grew up in Austin, and whose attorney father had a long-time association with the Texas Medical Association. Born in Dallas, he graduated from UTMB in 1955, interned and served a residency at Parkland Memorial Hospital, followed by residencies at Baylor Medical Center and at Scottish Rite Crippled Children's Center, both in Dallas. From 1956 to 1958, he was a captain in the Army Medical Corps before returning to Austin to practice. He was certified in orthopedic surgery in 1965.

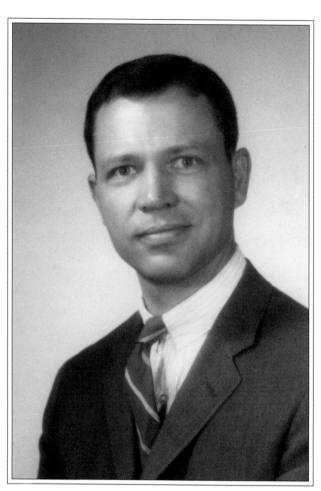

Dr. Joseph M. Abell, Jr., a Houston native, opened his Austin practice in 1962.

Dr. Will Watt, who set up his practice in 1916, died in February 1961 and was extolled by Charles Green, editor of the *Austin American-Statesman*, and by Dr. Charles M. Darnall, a colleague and friend who was one of Austin's early internal medicine specialists, having been board-certified in 1944. Dr. Watt had been in Rochester, Minnesota, undergoing treatment for lymphatic leukemia. Expressing his sentiment, Editor Green recalled his early years talking with Dr. Watt and Drs. John Calhoun Thomas, Joe and Horace Gilbert, and George Malcolm (Manny) Graham. "There were others and the town was not so lively then as it is now. We had time to gas...."

"Will E. Watt is dead," Dr. Darnall eulogized, "and Austin has lost her most colorful doctor as well as one of the most able that ever practiced medicine here or anywhere....Inside of Willie was a humanitarian quality that was frequently hidden by a rough exterior....He didn't want any one to think he was tender-hearted but actually he was. Many of the patients he treated were never sent a bill; they couldn't pay and he knew it. When one would try to pay him he might say, 'You don't owe me any money. The last rich patient I operated on paid for yours and his, too.' And that was probably true. Nevertheless the rich and the poor were equally devoted to him."

A native of Llano, Dr. Darnall had graduated from UTMB in 1930, interned at the Medical and Surgical Hospital in San Antonio, and had been a fellow at the Mayo Clinic. During World War II, he was a major in the Army Medical Corps.

In 1962, Dr. Ruth Bain became the first female president of the Travis County Medical Society. As her mother had assured her, she was opening doors, and even received praise from Dr. Raleigh Ross who let her know he hadn't been enthusiastic about women in medicine. Also in 1962, the Austin City Council reopened the Licensed Vocational Nursing School at Brackenridge Hospital to train more nurses, but in 1971 would close it to save money. Doctors would lament the loss, although other arrangements would be made.

Causing alarm in the early 1960s was the high incidence of phocomelia from the drug thalidomide. The synthetic drug, initially developed in 1953 by Ciba but discontinued, was picked up by a German company and marketed in 1957 as an anti-emetic during pregnancy. Its use was expanded to include treatment of insomnia. Accessible to U.S. travelers, including pregnant women, it was particularly destructive when used during the first trimester. The drug also was shown to cause polyneuritis. Stricter controls were instituted by the Food and Drug Administration in the early 1960s.

There was positive excitement about another development. After successful field trials, Albert Sabin's oral poliomyelitis vaccine, a live-attenuated virus, was licensed in 1962, replacing the Salk killed-virus vaccine. It was cheaper to produce, easier to administer, and was considered safer and more effective. Dr. Lansing S. Thorne wrote in the *TCMS Journal* that "Sabin vaccine has been in world-wide use since 1958 and has been given to millions of people. It apparently produces lasting immunity and, in addition, it produces intestinal resistance to infection (which the Salk vaccine does not). Thus, when an entire community is being vaccinated in a short time, there is a break in the chain of transmission of the polio virus and it quickly disappears from the population. A continuing program of vaccination of newborns should be rigidly followed." Initially administered in three separate doses added to a sugar cube, the vaccine later was made into a liquid. With pharmaceutical companies donating vaccine, Travis County Medical Society sponsored "Sabin Oral Sundays" to administer it to the public. Nurses and physicians volunteered time at sites around the county. Where there were 13,000 to 20,000 cases before the vaccines, there was a decline in 1960 to 2,525 cases of paralytic polio and by 1965 to 61 in the United States. By 1994, the western hemisphere was declared free of indigenous polio.

TCMS received more than $42,000 in contributions for the polio effort and with unused funds in 1963 established a foundation to support charitable, scientific, and educational medical programs. In its first five years, the new foundation contributed to a scholarship program for Bracken-

ridge Hospital School of Nursing and supported vaccination of children against diphtheria, pertussis, tetanus, polio, smallpox, and measles.

In addition to polio, pediatrician Dr. Clift Price recalled other suffering before effective vaccines were available. With pertussis, patients sometimes coughed themselves to death. Measles was rampant, and often when a mother acquired German measles during pregnancy, her child was born with brain and vision damage. Even in the late 1960s, there were outbreaks. Fortunately, Dr. Price rarely saw tuberculosis because of isoniazid. Streptomycin also was used but could cause deafness. "Thank God for antibiotics," he said. Because of them and the diphtheria-pertussis-tetanus toxoids (DPT) vaccine, he never saw patients with diphtheria.

In a 1960 state medical journal editorial, Dr. T. E. Dodd of Austin, chairman of the TMA Committee on Emergency Medical Service, called on physicians and county societies to review their preparedness programs. Noting that Red China planned to detonate an atomic device soon, he worried also about the dangers of Castro's Cuba. Crises came rapidly. In the fall of 1962, the country faced what could have been nuclear devastation during the Cuban Missile Crisis, and the government soon required all counties to prepare a civil defense plan in case of nuclear war. Fortunately, Travis County's disaster medical plan was in place. The Texas Medical Association basement and other locations became official Civil Defense shelter sites.

On November 22, 1963, as the American election season was in full swing, President John Kennedy was due in Austin after a stop in Dallas. Instead, Austinites learned shortly after noon that he had been assassinated and that Texas Governor John B. Connally had been wounded during a Dallas parade. Both were in Parkland Memorial Hospital, where physicians and staff worked feverishly to save them. Hours later, Dallas physicians dictated their reports, as they did again two days later after the alleged assassin, Lee Harvey Oswald, was gunned down. Travis County physicians played an important role in preserving the history of the medical and surgical treatment administered to President Kennedy, Governor Connally, and Lee Harvey Oswald at Parkland following their gunshot wounds. With the help of Dr. W. Pruett Watkins of Austin, chair of the Texas Medical Association's Journal Advisory Committee, the *Texas State Journal of Medicine* obtained what was believed to be the first publicly released dictation recorded by the Parkland physicians on their treatment of the three patients. The doctors' reports were rushed to Austin, and

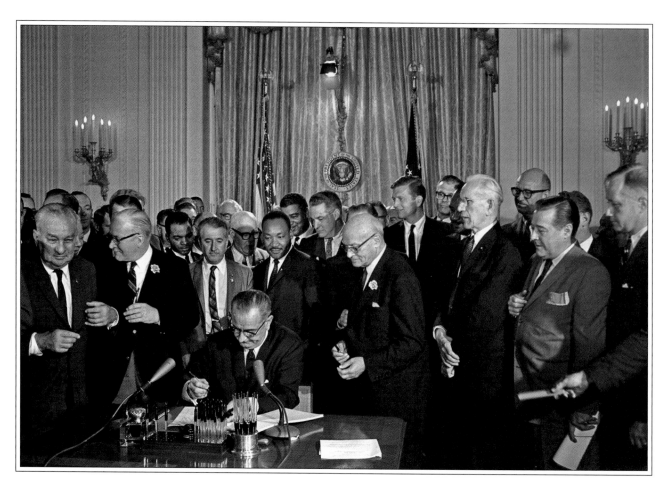

*President Lyndon Baines Johnson signing the
1964 Civil Rights Act.*

Travis County physicians, who made up the Journal Advisory Committee, decided to publish the accounts almost verbatim. Published in January 1964, the accounts would be quoted and referenced countless times. Dr. Charles Baxter, who had visited Austin a year earlier to help two Austin physicians in the use of kidney dialysis equipment, was among those reaching Parkland Hospital's trauma room where President Kennedy lay after he was shot.

Lyndon Baines Johnson was sworn in as president of the United States, and his ranch at Johnson City became the western White House. Austin physicians also looked after members of his family.

Dr. Glen Journeay would take an interesting route to practice dual roles as a family practitioner and college teacher. Born in Grange, Texas, in Jasper County, he graduated from high school in Angleton. He earned a B.A. degree in chemistry in 1945 and a B.S. degree in chemical engineering in 1947 from Rice University, where he was in the Naval ROTC's V12 program. He was on active duty with the Navy from 1943 to 1946. A 1952 Ph.D. graduate

in organic chemistry at the University of Texas, he became a research chemist at Dow Chemical Company at Freeport and spent five years in research at Monsanto Chemical Company in Texas City. Deciding to enter the medical field, he graduated in 1960 from UTMB and served an internship there in 1961. Besides teaching at St. Mary's School of Nursing in Galveston, he taught anatomy, physiology, and electrophysiology in the UT Biomedical Engineering Program. While he was in graduate school, Dr. John McKetta, the UT dean of engineering, had asked him if he could teach biomedical engineering, and he probably was the first person hired for the new cross-disciplinary area. He also taught environmental health and industrial toxicology in the UT Austin Civil Engineering department until 1999.

First practicing medicine in Texas City, Dr. Journeay moved to Austin in 1963 and set up his solo medical office in the Crestview Shopping Center on Woodrow Avenue, farther north than any physician in town. He remained there throughout his practice. Dr. Robert H. Zschappel filled in for Dr. Journeay when he could not be available. A native of Yoakum, Texas, Dr. Zschappel was a 1959 graduate of UTMB. He had interned at Philadelphia General Hospital in Philadelphia and served a residency in obstetrics and gynecology at UTMB. Dr. Teddy M. Sousares changed his field to psychiatry, and left the then more northerly site to work at the Austin State Hospital. In the young neighborhood where Dr. Journeay practiced , mothers often gave their children a check for the nurse to fill out and sent them on bikes to the office. Dr. Journeay also made house calls, even lugging around a cumbersome electrocardiographic machine. An author of technical and other articles, he also consulted with a number of state boards.

Dr. Robert L. Rock joined Dr. Hardy Thompson's ophthalmology practice on West Nineteenth Street (later Martin Luther King Jr. Boulevard) in 1963. In 1978, they moved to Burnet Road, developing a group practice later called Eye Physicians of Austin. Dr. Rock was a 1958 graduate of the University of Oklahoma College of Medicine in Oklahoma City and undertook his internship and residency in ophthalmology at UTMB hospitals, where he was chief resident. He also took a basic science course in ophthalmology at Illinois Eye and Ear Infirmary in Chicago and a post-residency fellowship in corneal and cataract surgery with Dr. Ramon Castroviejo at the New York Eye and Ear Infirmary in New York. Dr. Castroviejo had performed the first successful corneal transplant in the United States in 1941. A clinical professor of ophthalmology at UTMB, Dr. Rock is board certified in general ophthalmology and in cataract and intraocular lens (IOL) surgery. He maintained a special interest in volunteer service in third-world countries, and worked with Dr. Albert Schweitzer in Lamberene, Gabon, in West Equatorial Africa.

In May 1965, Dr. David Wade of Austin, a former president of TCMS, became the one hundredth president of the Texas Medical Association, the first psychiatrist to be chosen for the position in fifty years. In his first president's column, he observed that "History and tradition are never end products. They are but a foundation for the present generation to build upon. Our predecessors have left us a strong foundation....We can leave the generations to come an ever greater and more substantial foundation for their work."

A major national anti-smoking effort was launched in 1964 through the first *Report of the Advisory Committee to the Surgeon General on Smoking and Health*. The study found that cigarette smoking was the main cause of lung cancer in men and causally related to it in women; that it was the most important cause of chronic non-neoplastic bronchopulmonary disease in the U.S.; and that it could contribute to the development of cardiovascular disease and particularly to death from coronary heart disease. Health professionals were urged to do everything possible to dis-

courage cigarette smoking. Dr. William S. Brumage of Austin, who became chairman of the Texas Interagency Council on Smoking and Health, reported in 1971 that he was pleased with the progress of numerous Texas health-related societies, departments, and the Texas Parent-Teacher Association. The goal of the organizations was to produce a "smokeless generation."

Texas doctors supported the American Medical Association by participating in "Project Viet-Nam," sponsored by The People-to-People Health Foundation, Inc., with assistance by the Agency for International Development. Dr. Kurt Lekisch, then of Midland and later of Austin, was one of the volunteers helping the two hundred civilian South Vietnamese doctors.

More physicians were being drawn into the escalating war in Vietnam where laboratory quality was a problem at first but reached a high level of efficiency and quality in 1970, comparable to World War II. Wound severity was worse than in previous wars, but soldiers received better care more quickly. Experiences translated into civilian trauma management, emergency response systems, increased use of ancillary personnel, and the medical care team concept. Research into the pathophysiology of stress and of disabling cutaneous diseases also was a result. There were dramatic improvements in vascular surgery, advances in the hemodialysis unit in acute renal failure, and progress in knowledge of transplants when livers were destroyed by high-velocity missiles. Greater knowledge also was gained in the treatment of malaria.

Dr. Tracy Gordy, a 1961 UTMB graduate, served an internship at Wesley Medical Center in Wichita, Kansas, and completed his residency in psychiatry at the Austin State Hospital. He formed a Professional Association with Drs. Stuart S. Nemir, Jr., and Jim Clemons. He also served as president of the Central Texas Medical Foundation from 1977 to 1979, and for twenty-one years would teach in its psychiatric residency program. In 2001, he was named the Travis County Medical Society Physician of the Year.

Fluoridation of water was a controversial topic, with some opponents considering the intervention as socialized medicine or even a Communist plot. Others feared it might cause cancer, although public health advocates felt fluoride was safe in mild doses. In the capital, the Austin Dental Association sought fluoridation of city water to protect teeth from decay. Dr. Clift Price, who was involved in the six-year campaign, recalled that Mrs. Hallie Slaughter, wife of a grocery store owner, helped persuade the community to support the issue. Eventually, a nonbinding referendum called by the Austin city council passed by a few thousand votes.

Pediatrician Dr. Kaoru Dyo arrived in Austin in 1964. Born in El Paso, he had attended the Texas College of Mines, later the University of Texas at El Paso, and graduated from UTMB in 1954. He served an internship at Baylor Hospital in Dallas from 1954 to 1955. Originally a general practitioner in Harlingen, he had returned to UTMB for a pediatric residency, and was board-certified in 1966. When Americans of Japanese descent were placed in internment camps during World War II, he spent time in camps at Gila River, Arizona, and Crystal City, Texas. During the Korean Conflict, he served in the U.S. Army as a medic. Dr. Dyo was fluent in Japanese, Spanish, and English. One of his sons, Dr. Robert Dyo, also became a physician.

Austin was stunned again on August 1, 1966, as students around the University of Texas were heading to class or lunch in the noontime heat. Drs. Ruth Bain and C. B. Dildy, a 1935 graduate of Baylor University College of Medicine in Dallas, had an office at 504 West Seventeenth Street, not far from UT. Dr. Bain was calling in a prescription when her nurse interrupted her. "Something horrible is happening at the University. On the radio they're asking for doctors to volunteer." A cacophony of wails was heard as ambulances sped down Guadalupe Street. It was soon learned that Charles Whitman, a twenty-five-year-old UT student, posing as a delivery man and carrying guns, ammunition, and supplies, had climbed to the top of the UT tower, fatally wounding three victims on the way up. At 11:45 am, he began shooting across the great open expanse of the paved mall below the tower where students and visitors walked, hitting forty-nine people, fourteen fatally. Citizens and emergency personnel risked their lives to help the wounded and move the dead from the hot pavement of the mall to less open places. Whitman previously had killed his wife and his mother; he, too, was killed when Austin

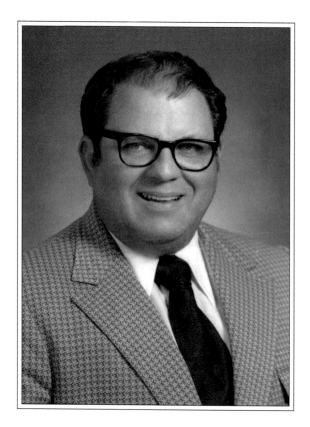

Psychiatrist Stuart S. Nemir, Jr.

policemen reached the top of the tower. The intern working in the emergency room as part of Brackenridge Hospital's medical education rotation asked for more help and the hospital disaster plan was activated. Funeral homes were providing ambulance services, and Hyltin Manor Funeral Home delivered the first victim to Brackenridge Hospital by 12:15 p.m.

Dr. Albert La Londe, chief of staff, heard about the situation on the radio and rushed to the hospital. He found a young lady shot through the chest almost at the midline. She died in the emergency room, probably of a massive lung hemorrhage. A young man in the Air Force Academy, who was visiting with his family and climbing the stairs to the tower, was struck in the head. The bullet pierced his scalp but did not penetrate the skull; arteriograms showed he had suffered only contusions, and no treatment was necessary. His younger brother, however, was killed and their mother, who suffered a spinal cord injury, was paralyzed permanently. Other victims bled to death on the hot pavement of the mall.

Dr. Bain had driven to Brackenridge Hospital, where her first task was to pronounce a victim dead. Radio stations warned listeners to avoid the campus area, and Dr. Jim Calhoon, a thoracic surgeon—as the authors of a Brackenridge history relay—had to drive a circuitous route from Seton Hospital, then on Twenty-sixth Street west of the campus, to Brackenridge Hospital on Fifteenth Street. That day, he was the only available Austin surgeon skilled in opening the chest during an emergency. He said he had never seen anything so devastating.

Dr. Joseph Abell looked out his office window near the University and gaped at the puffs of smoke from the observation deck of the UT tower. Only moments earlier, he had stopped by the University Barber Shop after coming from the hospital, but left because of a long line. From a rehearsal of Brackenridge's disaster plan, he knew to return to the hospital where nurses were effectively doing triage. He went directly to begin operating. Robert Heard, an Associated Press reporter whose arm was shattered by a bullet, did not want anything to affect his consciousness. With minimal anesthesia, the reporter underwent transfusion, debridement of his wound, and internal fixation of his humerus, and then began dictating his story. Dr. Abell had inserted a steel rod from his elbow to his shoulder and, with no time for measurement, had estimated the length. The rod turned out to be a perfect fit.

Of the thirty-nine victims brought to the hospital, twenty-seven survived, with twenty-one having been sent into surgery in the twelve operating rooms or to the cast room. Among other surgeons operating that day were Drs. Brian Forrister, Robert Dennison, William Moskovitz, Vernon Elledge, Bud Dryden, and Waldo Gonzalez. More than fifty doctors had reported to Brackenridge.

Dr. Robert W. Pape, medical education director, who oversaw the emergency room, became the hospital's resource for questions. Two police officers used two-way radios at the entrance to the Emergency Room to keep personnel in-

---

UT tower incident headlines The Austin American, *1966.*

formed of ambulances bearing patients. Also used was a Motorola Radio Page System, an auxiliary system for emergencies. Dr. F. Murphy Nelson, a former chief of surgery, recalled that the hospital's disaster plan had worked well and that the triage methods used were especially effective.

Learning of the tragedy about 12:15 pm, John Kemp, executive director of the blood bank called Dr. Douglas Terry, the medical director, and they estimated their needs. Mr. Kemp alerted radio stations to ask for donors from northeast Austin—out of the danger zone. "In five minutes," he said, "we had a traffic jam.... Two university students got out in the street and directed traffic. We had lines of people all around the building." He estimated that 500 people came to give blood; 125 pints were drawn, using all six drawing tables, from 12:25 pm until 10 pm. On a normal day, ten or twelve pints would have been drawn. After the tragedy, the blood bank established an emergency radio system to all local hospitals to facilitate a swifter disaster response.

Many physicians, having been in the military services, were familiar with field hospitals and trauma and were prepared for emergencies. Nevertheless, after the disaster, Dr. Abell recalled, physicians explored the status of Austin's emer-

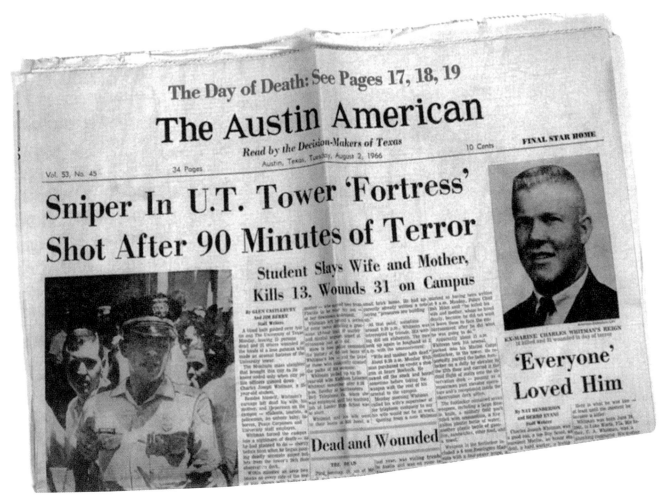

gency preparedness and the result was a better emergency medical services program.

Texas Governor John Connally also convened a nationwide panel of renowned scientists and physicians to investigate the matter. The governor, along with the chairman of the Board of Regents of the University of Texas, had called for a detailed investigation of "all the available medical and related psychiatric facts concerning" Mr. Whitman. The investigation was to determine the events and circumstances surrounding his actions on August 1, 1966; to examine any additional factual information indicated; to prepare material for "maximal utilization in evaluating the problem for our society"; and to offer recommendations on the detection and prevention of cir-

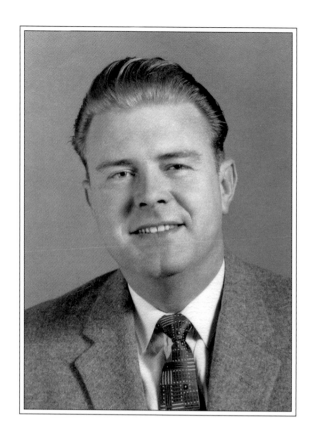

Dr. Robert W. Pape, Brackenridge director of education, oversaw the emergency room on the day of the UT tower shootings.

with clarity. It, however, made recommendations on mental health counseling and campus safety that could help all colleges and universities. Although its recommendation that Texas establish a statewide medical examiner's system was not followed, the advice helped spur further consideration of a medical examiner system then under study in Travis County. Both a new emergency medical system and the medical examiner system would become a reality in the 1970s.

Physicians continued to choose Austin for their practices. Dr. Joseph P. Quander, Jr., born in Washington D.C., grew up there and graduated from Dunbar High School. In 1957, he received his bachelor's degree from Yale University in New Haven, Connecticut, and in 1961 his M.D. degree from

cumstances that might lead to similar incidents. The findings of the panel were limited because the autopsy of Charles Whitman had been conducted about twenty-four hours after death; arterial and trocar embalming had been performed before the initial examination; many parts of the brain had been damaged by penetrating fragments of bone from multiple gunshot wounds and not all pieces of the brain were recovered; the brain had contusions and lacerations, and there was subarachnoid hemorrhage and cerebral edema. The brain further had been sectioned during autopsy. Two pieces of tumor reportedly were retrieved from the right temporo-occipital white matter by Dr. Coloman de Chenar, who had conducted the autopsy. The psychology study also could not be conclusive, but from the data available, the panel found no evidence that Mr. Whitman had a clinical neurologic abnormality or that the presence of an abnormality had interrupted pathways "leading to detectable neurologic signs." The panel, however, did recognize that abnormal aggressive behavior may be "a manifestation of organic brain disease." There also was no evidence of drugs. The task force concluded that the relationship between a brain tumor and Whitman's actions could not be established

Howard University College of Medicine in Washington, D.C. He interned at D.C. General Hospital and served his residency in obstetrics and gynecology in San Antonio through Bexar County and the UT Health Science Center at San Antonio, finishing in 1969. Between 1964 and 1966, he served in the Air Force. Becoming "Texanized," he wanted to remain in the Lone Star State.

Dr. Beadie E. Conner invited him to Austin to practice with him, disclosing that he had worked hard to obtain privileges for black physicians and feared that his efforts would be lost if no one came to succeed him. Although Dr. Quander, an obstetrician-gynecologist, did not join Dr. Conner's practice, he opened an office on East Nineteenth Street in 1969. He soon received a call from Dr. Paul Trickett, who wanted to hire a black physician for the UT Student Health Center, and he began working there half time while running his office practice. He served on staff at all hospitals, including Holy Cross, and received referrals from physicians throughout the community. In addition to TMA and TCMS memberships, he was president of the Lone Star State Medical Association and participated in an informal group of black physicians with Dr. Glen Johnson.

His wife, Arthuree, at times assisted in his practice.

Dr. Beverly Jewell Sutton, a 1957 graduate of the University of Michigan Medical School, became a resident in psychiatry in 1962 at Austin State Hospital. She earned certification from the American Board of Pediatrics and from the American Board of Psychiatry & Neurology, with a subspecialty in child psychiatry. Dr. Sutton established the first children's service in the state hospital system, serving as administrator until 1968. Following this, she developed the Child Psychiatry Training Program in 1971, serving as director until 1989, at which point she became director of the Austin State Hospital's residency program in psychiatry. She moved to Seton Shoal Creek in 2003.

Dr. Morris D. "Mac" McCauley discussed the new birth control pill in a 1967 *TCMS Journal* article. It had made the practice of obstetrics "considerably more pleasant and has brought better rapport between physician and patient than has been known for many years, simply because most of the pregnancies we see are desired and planned." He also added that the "dramatic reduction of the incomplete abortion in private practice is far too great to be contributed to anything but decreased fertility. The criminal abortion of married women is rapidly vanishing." Further, he said, "Last, but not least, the annual refill policy brings young women into our offices for annual pap studies they would not ordinarily have." In the previous year, his office had seen a significant number of high-stage Papanicolaou findings in young women between the ages of nineteen and twenty-five.

At Austin Diagnostic Clinic in 1964, the partners made a landmark decision—to hire only subspecialists—thus establishing subspecialty internal medicine in Central Texas. Patterned after the Diagnostic Clinic of Houston, considered the country's largest purely internal medicine group, the updated Austin Diagnostic Clinic became the second larg-

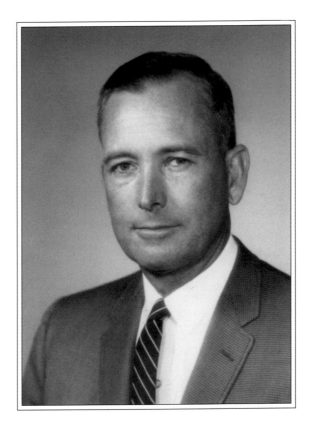

Dr. Thomas Runge, physician and professor in the Biomedical Engineering Department at the University of Texas at Austin, authored many publications and obtained more than 18 patents.

est in the country. In 1965, it occupied its new building on Thirty-fourth Street. In the 1980s, it would become a multispecialty clinic.

While retaining its existing location on Thirty-fourth Street, the Austin Diagnostic Clinic moved its main clinic to North Lamar Boulevard and Parmer Lane, and later established-clinics and centers for services in many other locations. By 1970, it had specialists in a variety of internal medicine fields and later added radiologists and neurologists. It acquired the city's first thyroid scanner and an isotopic brain scanner. Dr. Joseph A. Volpe, who had been an endocrinologist and had become a nuclear medicine specialist, joined the clinic in 1971. A 1962 graduate of Creighton University School of Medicine in Omaha, Nebraska, he was certified in internal medicine in 1968 and nuclear medicine in 1972. His internship and residency were served at Fitzsimons General Hospital in Denver, and he had served also as chief of the department of medicine at a U.S. hospital in Germany. A lieutenant colonel in the Medical Corps, he had been chief of the nuclear medicine clinic at William Beaumont Hospital in El Paso, after completing a nuclear medicine fellowship at Letterman General Hospital in San Francisco.

After returning from advanced cardiology training in Houston in 1967, Dr. Thomas Runge resumed his private practice and also became a professor in the UT Biomedical Engineering Department.

In 1967, Dr. H. S. "Hap" Arnold, a native Californian, arrived in Austin to practice thoracic medicine with Drs. Hood and Calhoon at Austin Surgical Specialties, then named Cardiothoracic and Vascular Associates. As a premedical student, Dr. Arnold had joined the Navy Reserve, which resulted in active duty in Vietnam, South Korea, and other foreign ports. In 1965 and 1966, he was a division surgeon on General Lewis W. Walt's staff. After graduating from

Northwestern University School of Medicine, he interned at Wesley Memorial Hospital in Chicago and undertook general surgery training at the U.S. Naval hospitals in Bethesda, Maryland, and in Oakland, California. He retired with twenty-two years of medical service in the Navy. From 1975 to 1988, he was a physician for the U.S. Olympic sailing team. He also was on the training faculty for Ethicon, a global medical device company, and became known for his work in video-assisted procedures (VATS). In 1993, he was Travis County Medical Society's Physician of the Year.

Dr. Tom Kirksey was born in Tientsin, China, and is the son and brother of physicians. He graduated from UTMB in 1959, took a flexible residency at Philadelphia General Hospital, and completed residencies in general and thoracic surgery at UTMB hospitals. Before arriving in Austin in 1969, he fulfilled his military obligation as part of the Surgical Research Unit at Brooke General Hospital in San Antonio and attained the rank of captain. There, he helped design the burn evacuation system for Vietnam. Dr. Kirksey joined the practice of Drs. Hood, Calhoon, and Arnold. He was certified by the American Board of Surgery in 1965 and the American Board of Thoracic Surgery in 1966. He also would serve as the 1984 TCMS president. Dr. Robert Tate of Sweetwater, Texas, joined the group in 1970. He earned his M.D. degree from UTMB, and took his general surgery residency at Brackenridge Hospital and his thoracic surgery residency at the University of Michigan Hospitals and Health Centers in Ann Arbor. He is a diplomate of the American Board of Surgery and American Board of Thoracic Surgery. He served two years as a general medical officer at Fort Leonard Wood in Missouri.

Austin otorhinolaryngologist Dr. Daniel B. Powell died unexpectedly in July 1968. He was the TCMS president, chairman of the *Texas Medicine* Journal Advisory Committee, and active in other TMA bodies and other local and state societies. A 1953 graduate of Tulane University School of Medicine, he interned at Baptist Hospital in Nashville, Tennessee, and was in general practice in Etowah, Tennessee. From 1954 to 1956, he served in the Army Medical Corps and in 1959 completed a UTMB residency in Galveston before moving to Austin.

Dr. Robert E. Askew, a native of Ferris, Texas, and a 1959 UTMB graduate, arrived in Austin in 1968. He had interned at the University of Michigan Hospital and completed a residency in general surgery there serving as chief resident and instructor. At Seton Hospital, he helped facilitate the tumor registry. The Travis County Medical Society selected him Physician of the Year in 1992 and in 1998

established the Robert E. Askew Endowment for Surgery. Active in many realms, Dr. Askew became a member of the steering committee for the Travis County Hospital District and chaired the advisory council for the UT School of Nursing. His son, Dr. Robert E. Askew, Jr., a 1986 graduate of UTMB, Galveston, later joined the practice.

Born in Marfa, Dr. Earl L. Grant attended Texas A&M and in 1959 graduated from UTMB. He joined the family practice group of Drs. Jerald R. "Jerry" Senter, E. V. Chauvin, and B. J. Smith. He later decided to return to school for specialty training in anesthesiology at Parkland Memorial Hospital in Dallas, where he worked with "one of the top anesthesiologists in the world," Dr. M. T. "Pepper" Jenkins, long-time chair of the anesthesiology department at UT Southwestern Medical School, who became his mentor and friend. Dr. Jenkins also was one of the physicians who cared for President Kennedy after his assassination in Dallas in 1963. Dr. Grant became the tenth member of the Austin Anesthesiology Group. He served on the TMA Board of Councilors and Board of Trustees, and would be named TCMS Physician of the Year for 1995. The Texas Society of Anesthesiologists also would honor him with its Distinguished Service Award in 2001.

Dr. Paul Burns, a 1963 graduate of Baylor College of Medicine, finished his residencies in otolaryngology and surgery in 1967, followed by a year of transitional or flexible training at Madigan Army Medical Center in Tacoma, Washington. After service in Vietnam, he arrived in Austin on July 1, 1970, a specialist in head and neck surgery. His partner was Dr. Ernest T. Butler, a 1962 graduate of Baylor College of Medicine, who had completed his residency in 1966. Dr. Butler would develop a means of soundproofing physicians' offices for hearing tests. Both physicians were certified by the American Board of Otolaryngology. In later years, Dr. Butler and his wife donated significant funds to the arts in Austin.

Dr. Stephen S. Clark, a 1968 graduate of UT Southwestern Medical School, Dallas, and 2000 president of TCMS, became a long-time general surgeon in Austin. He was born in Canistota, South Dakota. His residency in general surgery was at St. Paul Hospital in Dallas, and he received his board certification in surgery in 1974. His brother, Dr. Mark C. Clark, board-certified in internal medicine (pulmonology) and critical care medicine, is the husband of another board-certified internal medicine specialist, Dr. Margaret Kreisle Clark. She is the daughter of Dr. James E. Kreisle and granddaughter of Dr. Matthew F. Kreisle, Sr.

In 2004, like Dr. Sandy Esquivel, Austin orthopedic surgeon Dr. John A. Genung was inducted into the Univer-

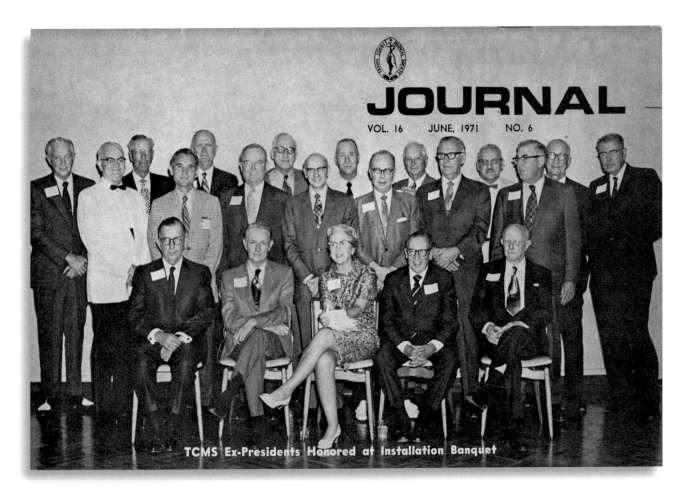

JOURNAL

VOL. 16   JUNE, 1971   NO. 6

TCMS Ex-Presidents Honored at Installation Banquet

Cover photograph of Travis County Medical Society presidents, TCMS Journal, *June 1971.*

sity of Texas Austin Men's Hall of Honor for his contributions as the Texas Longhorns' quarterback from 1960 to 1962. He led the team to an unbeaten season in 1962, and thus to the Southwest Conference title, engineering the last-minute drive against the University of Arkansas to win that game. A 1967 graduate of UT Southwestern Medical School at Dallas, he was a team doctor for the U.S. Naval Academy while in the military.

The day that Austin's first nephrologist, Dr. Jack W. Moncrief, arrived in 1969, a patient had been crushed by a car and was in kidney failure. He attempted peritoneal dialysis but with the patient having a rent diaphragm, he instead performed hemodialysis. Dr. Moncrief's arrival improved the life of Dr. Jack Schneider who remembered working day and night before then. Born in Beaumont, Dr. Moncrief graduated from Lamar University in 1959 and UTMB in 1962. He interned at Detroit Receiving Hospital in Detroit, Michigan, from 1962 to 1963, and served in the Air Force, where he was a captain. Joining a general medical office in Enid, Oklahoma, before returning to

UTMB for a three-year residency in internal medicine, he then became a fellow in nephrology at Georgetown University School of Medicine in Washington, DC.

Houston was the site of NASA's Mission Control and, as the nation watched on television on July 25, 1969, Astronaut Neil Armstrong and the crew from Apollo 11 landed on the moon's surface. The space program would foster much new technology and science for medical applications. In 1969, also, a new specialty—family practice—was initiated, requiring a residency training program. The venerable general practitioner, for the most part, became a family medical specialist. The federal government in 1965 had adopted Medicare and Medicaid amendments to the Social Security Act that led to sometimes complicated regulations and to predictions of physician shortages. World War II and Korean veterans also were aging and Vietnam soldiers were returning with wounds and disorders. The government thus offered incentives to expand medical education and add hospital beds and services. In little more than a decade, five new medical schools would open in Texas, and the curricula vitae of Travis County physicians soon would reflect graduation from the new schools.

CHAPTER XIV

FUTURE SHOCK

ALTHOUGH ALVIN TOFFLER'S *Future Shock* was a popular book, Austin remained a relaxing place to work in the early 1970s. Austin medicine in general, however, was about to experience a rapid sequence of significant changes.

Dr. Thomas B. Coopwood finished his hectic surgical residency in Houston and on June 30, 1970, pulled a trailer to Austin to join Dr. Raleigh Ross and Associates the next day. The old family friend paid his first month's income in advance. Dr. Coopwood was the namesake of his grandfather and father, both Lockhart physicians. An Army major during World War II, his father had been killed in Italy while serving with the Thirty-sixth Division. His grandfather and Dr. Ross's father, Dr. Alonzo A. Ross, had founded Lockhart Hospital. Graduating from Lockhart High School in 1956, the youngest Coopwood had received a degree under the University of Texas's Plan II program in 1959. After earning his M.D. degree from Baylor University College of Medicine in Houston in 1963, he was drafted into military service and served two years at Selfridge Air Force Base in Michigan, before returning to Houston.

New in the Austin landscape was Bailey Square Surgery Center. The ambulatory multispecialty surgery center opened in August 1973 at 1111 West Thirty-fourth Street, and was announced as the first "first free-standing out-patient unit" to open in Texas and as the largest such facility in the United States in square feet and in patient capacity. It was owned, financed, and operated by the Austin Doctors Building Corporation. Dr. Robert E. Askew was board chairman and members included Drs. Joe Bailey, G. R. Beiter (D.D.S.), Kaoru Dyo, C. Dale Parker, and W. Pruett Watkins. Dr. John C. Buckley was chairman of the medical advisory committee. Subsequently, the Park St. David ambulatory

surgery center, attached to St. David's Hospital, opened in the 1980s. Bailey Square later came under St. David's auspices. Dr. Grover Bynum, president of the Austin Doctors Building Corporation, guided the development of the medical district that included Bailey Square, the new Medical Park Tower, and the new Seton Medical Center.

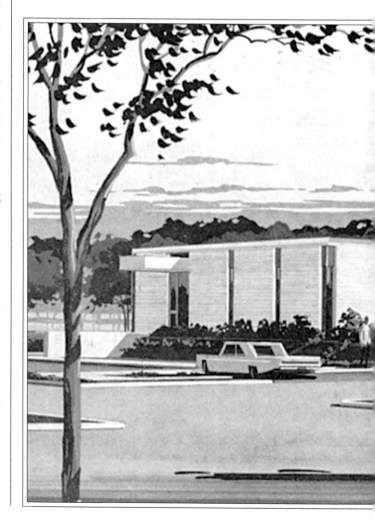

Tragedy struck on April 22, 1970, when Dr. Robert G. Farris, his wife and two daughters, and Dr. Edward Becker died in a private plane crash near the city's Mueller Airport. The doctors were associates of Drs. Albert A. La Londe and William R. Turpin in the Austin Neurosurgical Association. Dr. Becker, a Dallas native who had trained at the Mayo Clinic, had been in Austin for only a short time.

Dr. Farris had graduated from UT Southwestern Medical School at Dallas in 1949. He interned, served as assistant resident and resident in general surgery, and was junior and senior clinical instructor in neurosurgery at the University of Michigan's University Hospital in Ann Arbor from 1949 to 1954. He was a captain and chief of the neurosurgical service at the U.S. Army hospital in Tokyo, Japan, from 1954 to 1956. After completing his service at Brooke Army Medical Center in San Antonio, he moved to Austin. He was a diplomate of the American Board of Neurological Surgery.

After the deaths of Dr. Farris and Dr. Becker, Dr. Marvin R. Cressman, who was certified by the American Board of Neurological Surgery, joined Dr. La Londe in September 1970. Born at Pleasant Valley in Bucks County, Pennsylvania, his preliminary education was in Allentown, Pennsylvania, where he graduated from Muhlenberg College in 1955. He received his M.D. degree from Hahnemann Medical College (which in the late 1990s became Drexel University College of Medicine) in 1959. After medical school, he joined the Army and served his internship at Womack Army Hospital (later named Womack Army Medical Center) in Fort Bragg, North Carolina. He served his residency in neurosurgery at Walter Reed Army Medical Center in Washington, D.C., completing it in September 1965. Remaining in the Army for five years to fulfill obligations for his training, he served in South Korea, Tripler Army Medical Center, Hawaii, and Brooke Army Medical Center, San Antonio, where he came to know Austin neurosurgeons who met regularly with San Antonio colleagues.

In their neurosurgical specialty, Drs. La Londe and Cressman would experience a microcosm that reflected

An artist's rendition of the new TCMS and Blood Center Building, 4300 North Lamar, 1970.

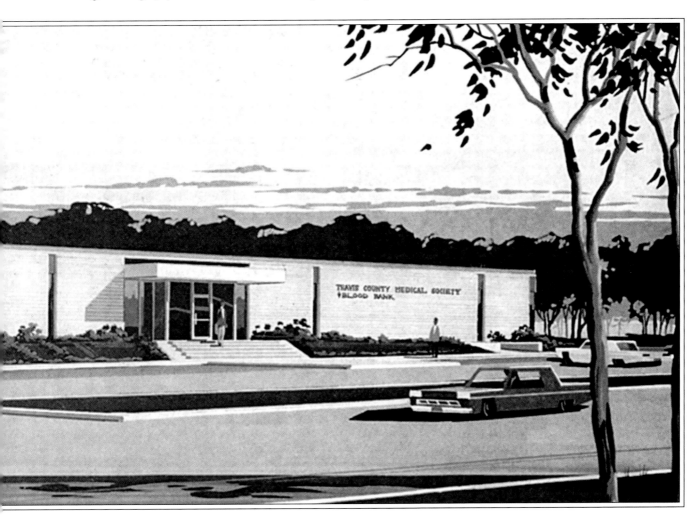

what was happening in the broader world of medicine as advancements in many other fields led to the to the refinement and enhancement of neurosurgery. The operating microscope, which Dr. Cressman first used in the Army in about 1966, had been introduced in Austin by Dr. Farris about the same time. "By the mid-1970s, the microscope was considered indispensable in most procedures in neurosurgery," he said. "Better ways became available to cope with cerebral edema in the 1960s, including steroids, diuretics, and hyperventilation. Anesthesiologists with more advanced training—and later those who were trained especially for neurosurgery—helped the neurosurgeon in the postoperative and post-head trauma patient with pulmonary problems. In the late 1970s, pulmonologists, who became intensivists, began managing the lungs and ventilation, and were a 'big boost.' In addition, infectious disease physicians arrived to care for problems such as pneumonia, meningitis, or other infections in a head-injury patient. With the explosion in the numbers and types of antibiotics, these specialists stayed attuned to the expanding array, and were especially important in the care of the patient. They also were helpful in the management of brain abscesses. Likewise, the arrival of emergency room specialists in the 1970s offered great support, helping early on with triaging and stabilizing acutely brain-injured patients."

Tomography, Dr. Jack Schneider believed, offered a significant advancement in imaging early in this decade. It could move over the body, focus on multiple levels, and provide images of thicker segments. The first in Austin, he believed, was in 1972 at the University of Texas Student Health Center.

Dr. Jack Moncrief had remained extremely busy since coming to Austin. With Margaret, who was his wife at the time and also a nurse, he set up a dialysis program at Brackenridge Hospital for patients with chronic problems, and for three years taught them to do dialysis at home on their own machines. In 1973, when Medicare payment became available, the first outpatient dialysis facility was established through his efforts at the Austin Diagnostic Clinic. He recalled it as the first non-university-affiliated outpatient facility in the state. He found particular satisfaction from his work in stimulating specialty care and in advancing the teaching program at Brackenridge, where he set up specialty clinics on hypertension, kidney, gastrointestinal disease, hematology, and cardiology. He established and obtained accreditation for the internal medicine teaching program and recalled that Drs. Thomas B. Coopwood and Thomas D. Kirksey did the same for the hospital's sur-

gery program, obtaining an affiliation with the University of Texas Medical Branch. He also developed a relationship with the UT biomedical engineering program, which continued for twenty-five years with numerous students receiving master's and doctorate degrees. Dr. Moncrief invented significant medical advances, receiving nine separate patents. He and Robert Popovich, Ph.D., a UT biomedical engineer, developed Continuous Ambulatory Peritoneal Dialysis, a procedure that freed patients from dialysis machines. At $8,500, the cost was significantly lower than a kidney dialysis machine, valued at the time at $25,000. The procedure remained a pivotal discovery in dialysis and the most frequently used method for ambulatory dialysis. Besides his UT affiliation, Dr. Moncrief was an adjunct professor at UTMB and at the State University of New York Downstate Medical Center. He left the Austin Diagnostic Clinic in the 1990s to establish the Moncrief Dialysis Center, later associated with DaVita, a national dialysis corporation.

This era saw a complicated evolution of federal health care planning laws, among which was the Health Maintenance Organization (HMO) Act of 1973. The Texas legislature passed its own HMO act in 1975. Austin had several big employers that were appealing to large HMOs. Travis County Medical Society had been working on a prepaid health insurance plan and in late 1975 established the Central Texas Health Plan as a separate non-profit corporation, an individual practice association (IPA). It was designed to provide the same benefits as an HMO while preserving aspects of a private medical practice. The plan would be implemented in the 1980s.

A new building for the Blood Bank, Travis County Medical Society, and the Medical Service Bureau was occupied at 4300 North Lamar Boulevard in October 1971. Austin Mayor Roy Butler formally dedicated the structure on November 21, with members of the Austin City Council participating in a ribbon-cutting ceremony. At an open house, donors who had given five and ten gallons of blood were honored. The blood bank now provided all blood components to the hospitals it served, filling 784 orders for various blood components in 1971. In February of that year, screening by immunoelectrophoresis had begun for the hepatitis-associated antigen. Twelve donors were identified as HAA-positive.

The first patient kidney transplant in Austin was performed at Brackenridge Hospital on October 13, 1970, and in 1971, the hospital became the first to open a separate twenty-six-bed cardiac care unit to monitor and treat patients with heart disease. In 1973, it opened the only separate pediatric intensive care unit in Central Texas and also in that year, a cardiac-arrest resuscitation team was formed for dispatching specialists anywhere in the hospital.

Dr. Gerald R. Baugh, a 1963 graduate of Johns Hopkins University School of Medicine in Baltimore, arrived in Austin in the early 1970s to join Dr. R. Maurice Hood's group of thoracic surgeons on Fortieth Street. He had taken his internship and surgical residency at Tulane University Charity Hospital in New Orleans and his thoracic surgical residency at the Medical College of Wisconsin in Milwaukee. He had lived in Austin since the age of two and had graduated from the University of Notre Dame in 1959. When he returned to practice, Dr. Hood and his colleagues already had performed open heart surgery. A bypass was performed perhaps every two weeks, but grew to once a week until three to five or more were being performed daily. Gradually, there were operations for double, triple, and then as many as five or six bypasses. After stents were patented in 1989 and became available for cardiac care, fewer single bypasses were necessary.

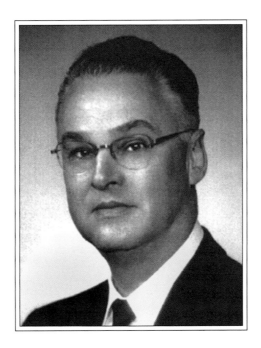

Dr. David Wade was appointed commissioner of the Texas Department of Mental Health and Mental Retardation in 1970.

Drs. Kermit Fox and Robert A. Dennison, Jr., had an experience of a lifetime in 1971 when they traveled to Wrightington, England, to learn from Dr. John Charnley (later Sir John Charnley) how to perform hip joint replacements. Observers and visiting "students" stood a few feet from the site of operation, separated by a glass panel that was part of the glass cubicle making up the operating room. The enclosure was supplied with specially filtered air, the medical team wore space-age suits, and the breath of individuals was vented away through attached tubes as the controlled environment was intended to minimize the possibility of any complicating infections, which were feared. The hip replacement procedure would be considered one of the greatest surgical advances of the twentieth century. After Dr. Fox returned to Austin, he implanted what was probably the first artificial hip in the capital.

In 1961, Drs. Fox and Griffin had moved into a building they constructed on East Thirty-second Street and, in 1963, Dr. Elwood "Woody" Eichler, Dr. Fox's nephew, joined the partnership. In 1968, Dr. Griffin left for a solo practice, and the name of the Fox and Eichler partnership was changed to The Austin Bone & Joint Clinic. In 1968, Dr. L. Don Greenway joined the group, and in 1970 the clinic incorporated and was designated a "Professional Association." Dr. Christopher S. "Kit" Chenault became the fourth member in 1971, followed by Dr. C. Bruce Malone in 1977. The office building was sold in 1989 to their neighbor, St. David's Hospital, as that institution expanded.

When internal medicine specialist Dr. Pete Vineyard decided to shift from group to solo practice, he rented space previously occupied by the late Dr. Leonard Paggi at 313 Medical Park Tower. He began his new practice on July 1, 1971. Born in Helena, Arkansas, where he received his preliminary schooling, he attended Sewanee, The University of the South, in Tennessee for three and one-half years. He earned his M.D. degree from the University of Texas Southwestern Medical School in Dallas in 1955. His general internal medicine residency, including a two-year fellowship with Dr. Jay Sanders in infectious disease, was at Parkland Memorial Hospital in Dallas, from 1958 to 1961. He also served two years as an Army captain in Fort Riley, Kansas, and Fort Stewart, Georgia.

In 1974, Dr. Vineyard invited Dr. Tom S. McHorse to come from Nashville, where he was completing a residency in gastroenterology. Dr. McHorse was a 1967 graduate of Baylor University College of Medicine in Houston and a board-certified internist and gastroenterologist. When he first arrived in Austin he spent about sixty percent of his time in general internal medicine and forty percent in gastroenterology, but the percentage of time would increase as the field became more and more important.

Dr. Nancy Thorne Foster, daughter of Dr. Clifford Thorne, completed her residency in internal medicine in 1986 and joined Dr. Vineyard. A side benefit, Dr. Vineyard said, was the desire of some women patients to see someone of their own gender. Dr. Foster was born in Austin, earned an M.D. degree from UTMB in 1983, and served a residency in internal medicine at the Eastern Virginia Medical Authority in Norfolk, Virginia, between 1983 and 1986. She was certified by the American Board of Internal Medicine. Dr. Foster's brother, Dr. George C. Thorne, Jr., a 1976 graduate of UT Medical School at San Antonio, became an ophthalmologist and joined Eye Physicians of Austin.

This era preceded the arrival of AIDS, and when the infectious disease specialists arrived in Austin, Dr. Vineyard concentrated on general internal medicine. Like other arriving doctors, he introduced himself to physicians in town; he also visited doctors in surrounding communities, like Taylor and San Marcos, and continued serving these communities as a consultant. Dr. A. Bryan Spires, an internal medicine specialist, had practiced at the Johns Clinic in Taylor but later entered administrative medicine, including serving as executive director of the Texas State Board of Medical Examiners. He remembered how he valued Dr. Vineyard's advice while he was in Taylor where he had some of the sickest of patients.

Since the 1950s, discussions had been leading toward a transformation that was about to affect internship and residency training in Austin and elsewhere. The Association of American Medical Colleges believed that graduate medical education should be the responsibility of academic medical centers and a 1966 AMA report addressed the discontinuity of medical education and accreditation from the undergraduate to the graduate years. In 1969, Dr. Robert Pape, Medical Education Director at Brackenridge Hospital, learned that forthcoming changes could cause the hospital's internship program to lose accreditation. In 1971, the AMA announced that, after 1975, internships had to be integrated as the first year of a residency training program. Six national organizations making up the Accreditation Council for Graduate Medical Education would establish the criteria. Freestanding programs not affiliated with medical schools would have difficulty meeting the new standards and could not depend solely on part-time faculty, which had been the historical basis of the Brackenridge Hospital program. Drs. Pape, Tom Kirksey, and A. Lobdell Exline, and Travis County Medical Society's executive director John Kemp had researched new options for graduate medical education and found a model county medical society program in Pensacola, Florida. The Travis County Medical Society refocused its existing non-profit foundation to form the Central Texas Medical Foundation (CTMF). Supported by Mayor Roy Butler of Austin, CTMF was chartered in 1972 to develop and operate a fully accredited, community-based graduate medical education program. Medical services were to be provided and emergency care was to be available around the clock at Brackenridge Hospital.

The final year of the old rotating internship at Brackenridge Hospital was from 1973 to 1974. From 1954 to 1974, Brackenridge had had ten to twelve interns each year. Their class photographs were found and preserved by Mary Micka for display at Brackenridge. When the new graduate medical education system began on July 1, 1975, it comprised four programs—family practice, internal medicine, pediatrics, and transitional.

A board of trustees made up of eleven physicians was appointed with Mr. Kemp as the CTMF executive and Ronald Goldstein providing administrative guidance. Dr. Pape became the first director of medical education and directed emergency room physicians in the 1970s. The Foundation also established its own medical clinic and each residency training program had a full-time director, an associate director, and other faculty. Mary Micka, for many years on the CTMF staff and who became Graduate Medical Education Program Manager for Austin Medical Education Programs, recalled the high degree of physician participation in the Brackenridge program.

Also in 1975, Dr. Earl B. Matthew became the first full-time director of medical services and education for CTMF. A graduate of UT Southwestern Medical School at Dallas, he had undertaken a residency and fellowships in Gainesville, Florida; Bethesda, Maryland; and the UT Health Science Center in San Antonio, where he was chief resident during his last six months. He earned a subspecialty certification in infectious diseases, and was a founding member and president of the Texas Infectious Disease Society.

Historically, relationships between osteopathic and allopathic physicians typically had been at arm's length although they had been governed by the same state medical board since 1907. In 1967, however, the Texas Medical Association agreed that "Doctors of Osteopathy who practice scientific medicine on an ethical basis are not cultists." In 1972, osteopaths became eligible for membership in TMA and county medical societies could accept applications.

In February 1972, Dr. Richard J. Alexander wrote in *Texas Medicine* about another development in Austin. A board-certified psychiatrist, he had graduated from UTMB in 1955. The counter-culture movement, he said, had brought many young people to Austin who were the age of most university students but were not enrolled. Often, they could not meet the city hospital's residency requirements for medical care.

Thus the People's Free Clinic was conceived, opening on April 7, 1970. Dr. Alexander reported that the impetus came from a registered nurse, Mrs. Georgia Whitaker. "She and her husband at that time, Dr. John J. Whitaker, an internist, were contacted informally by young people asking for treatment of various physical problems." With a small group of physicians and nurses, they found space in "the basement of the Congregational Church near the University area, put notices in the underground and campus newspapers announcing the opening, and on the first night saw 33 patients. The clinic subsequently expanded to a capacity of 80 to 100 patients each Tuesday night, with occasionally as many as 140 patients." Volunteers treated many problems, including venereal disease, and offered diagnostic services such as Papanicolaou smears. The Whitakers and Dr. Alexander handled administrative tasks until a full-time person could be hired. Renamed the People's Community Clinic, in 1972 it received a federal grant for women's health and family planning. In 1974, a city grant allowed it to broaden services to general medicine, and a county award covered prenatal care. Another clinic also opened at the Austin Boys' Club in South Austin.

Certified in internal medicine and oncology, Dr. Whitaker was the city's first oncologist in 1965. He graduated from Creighton University School of Medicine in Omaha, Nebraska, in 1958, undertook an internship at Mount Carmel Hospital in Detroit, Michigan, and a residency in internal medicine with a hematology subspecialty at the Mayo Clinic. In the Army, he was Chief of the Outpatient Department at Brooke General Hospital for two years, and then returned to the Mayo Clinic as an associate consultant in hematology and oncology. He also became a special consultant to the Oncology Drugs Advisory Committee of the U.S. Department of Health, Education and Welfare. In addition to his clinical research, he was a published author.

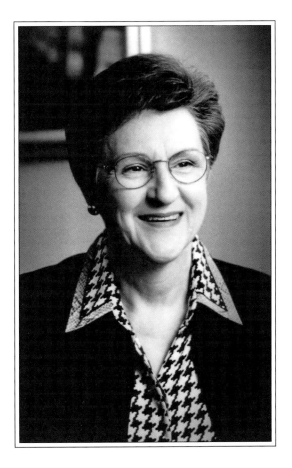

Pediatrician Dr. Karen Teel helped establish Children's Hospital of Austin in 1988.

Of mounting interest in the 1970s were end-of-life matters. Dr. Karen Teel offered her thoughts at a 1975 symposium, "Death and Dignity," sponsored by Baylor Law School. Published under the title, "The Physician's Dilemma; A Doctor's View: What the Law Should Be," in the *Baylor Law Review*, Dr. Teel's concepts included the idea of an ethics committee that is "readily accessible to those persons rendering medical care to patients...." The article is considered the first one known to suggest the formation of hospital ethics committees to consider individual cases.

A movement also was under way to care for mentally ill patients in communities rather than in state hospitals. In 1970, Dr. David Wade was appointed commissioner of the Texas Department of Mental Health and Mental Retardation, with a primary goal to develop community medical centers. Funds for local centers increased from less than five million to thirty million dollars during his tenure, and he left feeling that much had been done to advance the progress of community centers. Dr. Wade served the state in many other capacities, including as a member of the Texas Commission on Alcoholism; as assistant commissioner of the Department of Public Welfare; as consultant to the Texas Education Agency; and as director of health planning for Governor Preston Smith.

Dr. Clift Price had been in private practice for almost twenty-five years when he left his private pediatric practice to join the Texas State Department of Health. Several factors led to his choice, including the arrival in 1977 of what was to be called "managed care." A fourth of the medical practice at Children's Medical Center, where he practiced, had been lost when employees of the state and the University of Texas were enrolled in new insurance programs and assigned to other physicians. Some patients cried when informing Dr. Price that their insurance plan required them to see another doctor. At the health department, he learned to adapt to a bureaucracy, recalling that Dr. Robert Bernstein, Commissioner of Health, was very helpful in developing friendships in the public health community. Dr. Price also considered his era of medical practice a golden age when he did "not rush to see patients. There was an opportunity to get to know the family."

The road to Austin was not far for Dr. Linda Gilbert Prentice, pediatric endocrinologist, and her husband Dr. James A. Prentice, anesthesiologist, who grew up in the city. They had further insight into Austin medicine through Linda's father, Dr. Joe Thorne Gilbert. She graduated from UT in 1963 in zoology, after a prominent professor advised her against taking a premedical course because "women got married and had babies." While in San Francisco between 1964 and 1966, where she had a job as a chromosome technician, she worked for two female physicians who had families. She decided to apply to UTMB. After attending for one year and after her marriage in 1967, she transferred to Georgetown University School of Medicine in Washington, D.C., graduating in 1970. She took a residency in pediatrics at the Mayo Clinic from 1970 to 1973, and a fellowship in pediatric endocrinology from 1973 to 1976.

After returning to Austin in 1978 with her husband and family, she was in private practice in pediatric endocrinology for ten years and then served at the Brown Schools, Inc. In 1988, she moved to the State Health Department, expanding and overseeing a variety of programs, including newborn screening, and later worked in indigent care clinics. She would hold an academic position with Central Texas Medical Foundation from 1980 to 1985, and provide direct services and resident teaching beginning in 1995.

Dr. James Prentice attended Austin High School, entered UT Austin in 1955 as a premedical student, and re-

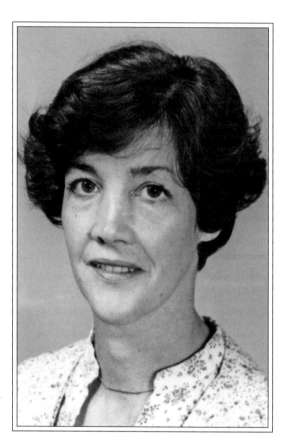

Dr. Linda Gilbert Prentice had a private practice in pediatric endocrinology and served at the Brown Schools and the State Health Department.

ceived a liberal arts degree in 1958. His M.D. degree was granted by UT Southwestern in 1962, followed by a general rotating internship at Hartford Hospital in Connecticut. Drafted into the Air Force, he served from 1963 to 1970. While stationed at Sheppard Air Force Base in Wichita Falls for two years, he decided on anesthesiology as a specialty, and undertook residencies at Bethesda, Maryland, from 1965 to 1967, and at Andrews Air Force Base in Washington, D.C., from 1967 to 1970. He then joined the anesthesia staff at Mayo Clinic in Rochester, Minnesota, where he was an assistant professor at the Mayo Medical School. He returned to Austin in 1978 and practiced with the Austin Anesthesiology Group until he retired in 2002. He was president of Travis County Medical Society in 1996.

As chief of pediatrics and later chief of staff at Brackenridge Hospital, Dr. Milton Talbot realized that changes were needed in children's hospitalization. Initially the children's area of Brackenridge Hospital was at the end of the sixth floor and a floating nurses' pool was used. Medication dosages for children weren't always known and there was no children's equipment. Dr. Talbot began talking about doing something. Dr. Karen Teel, chief of pediatrics, "a very conscientious physician," he said, spoke with hospital management. She was able to set up a pediatric intensive care unit on the sixth floor. Later the hospital remodeled space in the basement for a children's hospital. Hospital administrator Robert Spurck, Jr., helped pave the way with the city council, leading to construction of a separate hospital. Meanwhile, matters such as government requirements, including certificates of need, had to be addressed. Drs. Teel and Talbot sought a dedicated nursing staff with a separate administration, and eventually certified specialists were required to treat children. As the first chief of staff, Dr. Talbot wrote the hospital bylaws.

The first budget for Children's Hospital at Brackenridge was about $13 million, with groundbreaking in 1984. The hospital opened on February 14, 1988. Dr. Teel observed that the city had "always had an unusually sophisticated medical community. Even without a children's hospital, Austin has been blessed with a large number of qualified pediatricians."

Dr. Jacob Lindy Kay arrived in Austin in 1974 after a neonatal practice at Parkland Hospital and serving as a faculty member of UT Southwestern Medical School in Dallas. Born in Winona, near Tyler, he graduated from Baylor University, Waco, and from UT Southwestern Medical School in Dallas. During the Korean Conflict, he was an Army physician and served in Japan. In Austin, he established the Regional Neonatal Center at Seton Medical Center, the first facility for neonatal care in Central Texas, which opened in 1979. "We know now," he told the *Austin American-Statesman* in 1989, "that most premature infants can see, usually in the first week after birth." Dr. Kay also worked closely with various groups, including the Texas Medical Association, on legislative matters to help reduce neonatal deaths. Already, a study for the pediatric society had shown a significant reduction of neonatal deaths in Texas from 1960 to 1970.

Other pediatric specialists arrived in Austin. Dr. Abraham M. Besserman, a 1960 graduate of the Federal University of Rio de Janeiro, Brazil, and board-certified in surgery, practiced pediatric surgery in Austin. Dr. James Sharp, a 1963 UTMB graduate and a pediatric hematology/oncology specialist was certified in both fields, and established a clinic for children with cancer at Brackenridge Hospital. Dr. George L. Sharpe, a 1969 graduate of Dalhousie University Faculty of Medicine in Nova Scotia, was a specialist in neonatal and perinatal medicine and certified in both pediatric and neonatal-perinatal medicine. Children's x-rays were initiated. At first, there was not sufficient laboratory support for pediatrics and studies pertaining to pediatric endocrinology often had to be sent elsewhere.

Before the arrival of the pediatric surgeons, Dr. Lansing Thorne recalled, when a super complex surgery was required, the child was sent to medical centers in Dallas or Houston.

Shoal Creek Hospital, at 3501 Mills Avenue, offered 165 beds for acute medical and psychiatric care, and, in 1971, established a floor for rehabilitation medicine with a goal "to remove the disabled from forgotten beds in nursing homes or the back rooms of family homes" and also to provide patients with more independence and dignity. Dr.

Rodney J. Simonsen, a 1967 graduate of Johns Hopkins University School of Medicine and board-certified in physical medicine and rehabilitation, headed the program. By 1979, Shoal Creek Hospital had established the Central Texas Rehabilitation Center, the Renaissance Program to address addiction, a pain management program, and the Central Texas Arthritis Center.

Dr. J. Douglas Hudson, a leader in recruiting neurology specialties to Austin, graduated from UTMB in 1963, and completed a residency in neurology at the University of Iowa. He was the second neurologist in Austin and, in 1970, with Dr. Peter Werner, founded Austin Neurological Clinic and led the drive to bring Austin's first CT scanner, an EMI, to the city. Dr. Hudson's office reports that he also provided the city's first EEG laboratory with twenty-four-hour monitoring services, a neurochemistry laboratory, and one of the city's first neurovascular ultrasound laboratories. A founder in 1980 of what is considered one of the nation's first sleep laboratories, Dr. Hudson is certified by the American Board of Psychiatry & Neurology.

Dr. Stuart S. Nemir, Jr., in 1982 described the Renaissance chemical dependency program at Shoal Creek hospital as an "alternative treatment approach modeled after other successful treatment programs in Minnesota and Arizona." A graduate of Austin High School, the University of Texas, and UTMB, Dr. Nemir had served an internship in the Navy and had been an officer and flight surgeon. He practiced in Lubbock before moving to Austin in 1964, and was president of the Travis County Medical Society from 1983 to 1984. He also chaired the TMA Committee on Physician Health and Rehabilitation.

In the mid-1970s, the cost of professional liability insurance became a crisis. The Texas Legislature responded with laws to help relieve the problems, but they would rise to crisis level again.

Dr. S. H. "Bud" Dryden was elected to the Austin City Council in 1971 and served two terms. He supported bond issues that permitted a phased expansion of Brackenridge Hospital, neighborhood health clinics, and the fluoridation of Austin water. He also helped improve debt collection at Brackenridge, assured the establishment of its pediatric intensive care unit, and enhanced the hospital's inhalation therapy department. With others, he helped establish a new emergency medical system. Known for his care of the poor and patients living on the then-segregated east side of town, he relocated to East Twelfth Street after his office on Sabine Street, across from the old Brackenridge emergency room, was torn down.

In a 1972 *TCMS Journal* article, Dr. Maurice Hood wrote, "Traditionally the medical profession has taken little or no interest in medical care before hospitalization and that is not to their credit. This is an area where good medical care will often save many more lives than are saved in the emergency room." Existing funeral home ambulances were only vehicles, he noted, that moved a prone patient, attended by someone with limited training and equipment. He thus advocated modern ambulances equipped with cardiac equipment, intravenous units, endotracheal tubes, voice communication, and skilled medical attendants. His efforts and that of others would result in a modernized emergency medical system in Austin.

Dr. Hood had a special interest in firefighters and often monitored the Austin Fire Department's radio at home and in his car, showing up at incidents ahead of the firefighters. On his days off during the 1960s, he began teaching emergency techniques, including cardiopulmonary resuscitation, which supplemented the basic Red Cross training that firefighters received. In 1970, he was named honorary chief of the Austin Fire Department and given its outstanding service award in 1977. In 1978, Governor Preston Smith commended him for the teaching and organization of Austin's Emergency Medical Services (EMS) system. The city also honored him in 1976 as its Most Worthy Citizen, a "pioneer of open heart surgery and emergency care." The Austin firefighters, who nominated him, wrote, "There is no way for the people of Austin to know how many lives this man has saved." At heart, Dr. Hood remained a firefighter like his father, who had served Lubbock for forty-five years. In a 1992 speech to graduating cadets in the fire department, he offered practical thoughts and advice on learning tools, empathy, and courage versus foolhardy behavior. He also wrote a brief history of the Austin Fire Department. Noting the higher incidence of death from heart attacks in firefighters, he advised them that not all of the deaths were necessary. He cited inherited and preventable cardiovascular risk factors and suggested ways that firefighters could reduce their risks. He left Austin to hold faculty appointments as professor and chairman of the Department of Thoracic Surgery at Texas Tech University School of Medicine from 1972 to 1973, and then as Professor of Clinical Surgery at New York University School of Medicine. He also became a clinical professor of surgery at the UT Health Science Center at San Antonio, and held additional visiting professorships at various schools. He was a recipient of many honors in medicine and maintained a deep interest in teaching about the

"soul of medicine." A boundless writer, his topics spanned medical history, religion, and medical science, including thoracic and cardiovascular surgery, ethical decision-making in surgery, and medical evangelism.

As the EMS was being developed in the 1970s in Austin, the new specialty of emergency medicine also provided physician staffing at hospitals.

In 1976, Dr. Connie Yerwood became the first black physician to rise above a directorship in the State Department of Health. In addition to her forty-one years with the agency, she was active on many boards, committees, and commissions. She also had been president of the Lone Star State Medical, Dental and Pharmaceutical Association from 1955 to 1956. Dr. Clift Price succeeded her as chief of child and maternal health at the State Department of Health.

Dr. Mathis Blackstock joined the Rosewood-Zaragosa Clinic in the Austin public health system after twenty years in private practice and the 1974 retirement of his partner, Dr. Sigman Hayes. In 1978, Dr. Blackstock became associate director of the family practice residency program sponsored by the Central Texas Medical Foundation. His experiences had taught him that "the better exposure residents have to private practice, the better prepared they'll be." Upon his retirement in 1991, in recognition of his contributions to medical education and community health, the Central Texas Medical Foundation renamed its Family Health Center the Blackstock Family Health Center. He was named Physician of the Year by the Travis County Medical Society in 1991.

In 1975, Dr. Jim Kreisle, a highly respected Austin internist whom Dr. Virgil Lawlis called the best he had known, joined the Austin Diagnostic Clinic after twenty-six years in practice. A writer also, his published work included articles on the history of medicine in Travis County, poems, and a volume of letters to his parents from the front lines during the war. He remembered his father, Matthew Kreisle, Sr., as a pioneer internist who introduced electrocardiography to Austin. In 1990, the Travis County Medical Society selected him as the Physician of the Year. Two sons, James, Jr., and Bill, and one daughter, Margaret Clark, became physicians as did spouses of two of his children.

Amazing new imaging technology now offered a significant boost for the medical community and patients. A group of Austin neurologists and neurosurgeons funded a CT scanner, placing it at the Bailey Square Surgery Center. It was purchased at a cost of $450,000, recalled Dr. Robert M. Cain, a 1966 graduate of the Ohio State Col-

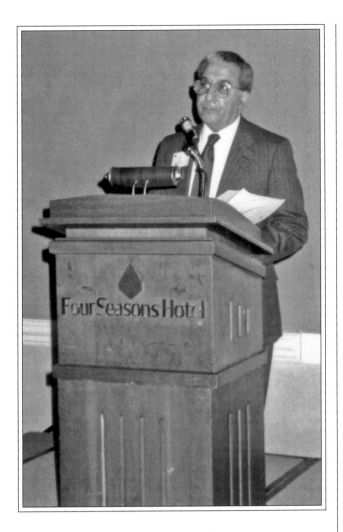

Dr. Hector Morales, 1998 president of the Travis County Medical Society.

lege of Medicine, who practiced neurology in Austin. He was among the group who purchased the EMI scanner in the mid-1970s. The CT or CAT scan (computerized tomography also known as computerized axial tomography) was developed by Godfrey N. Hounsfield at the Central Research Laboratories of EMI in London and produced cross-sectional images of the brain by scanning a beam of x-rays from numerous angles. Magnetic resonance imaging (MRI) would become available for humans in the 1980s.

Dr. Hector E. Morales arrived in Austin in 1977. He had earned a B.A. degree in 1953 and an M.D. degree in 1960 from the University of San Luis Potosí in Mexico. He interned at St. Clare's Hospital, New York City, from 1960 to 1961, followed by a residency at Washington Hospital Center in Washington, D.C., from 1961 to 1962. His studies took him to the University of Utrecht in Holland and then to a residency at Henry Ford Hospital in Detroit. He taught surgery and anatomy at the University of San

Luis Potosí for two years and practiced in Michigan and Illinois before joining Surgical Associates of Austin, leaving for a specialized practice in 2002. He chaired the Central Texas Medical Foundation from 1988 to 1997, later serving on the executive board of Austin Medical Education Programs. He became president of the Travis County Medical Society in 1998.

A recent state law had allowed Travis County to establish a medical examiner system, and, on July 1, 1977, the county inaugurated the system with a trained forensic medical specialist. The role of justices of the peace in overseeing inquest responsibilities was transferred to the medical examiner. Dr. Robert Van Zandt Bucklin of Los Angeles, an M.D. and J.D., who had started the Galveston examiner's office, became Travis County's first medical examiner. With an immediate business in postmortem examinations, his office also assumed responsibility for many counties. Because of the slow progress in obtaining proper facilities, however, Dr. Bucklin resigned in mid-1978. He was succeeded in August of that year by Dr. Roberto J. Bayardo who had worked as the chief deputy medical examiner for Harris County under Dr. Joseph Jachimczyk, who, in 1957, became the first formally trained medical examiner in Texas. Financial problems plagued the medical examiner's office but, in the 1980s, voters overwhelmingly approved a new morgue in a bond election. New facilities, however, would not be built until 1995. Working every day for fifteen years, Dr. Bayardo was the only medical examiner until Dr. Suzanna E. Dana joined him in 1993. By the mid-1990s, the office covered thirty-five counties. In 1995, Dr. Elizabeth Peacock joined the staff and served as deputy medical examiner.

Austin's first eye bank and eye laboratory in Central Texas was dedicated at Seton Hospital in 1976. St. David's Hospital announced in October 1972 that its radiology department had acquired a Pho-Gamma Scintillation Camera, providing images of internal organs. In 1979, Austin voters approved construction funds for another phase of Brackenridge Hospital's expanding programs and for razing the old red brick building, which was demolished in December 1984.

Besides endoscopy and fiber optics, medicine had seen nuclear-powered heart pacemakers, synthesis of the human growth hormone, and the first human baby conceived out of the body. Cardiac drugs made a significant difference in internal medicine. Surgery and neurosurgery, assisted by advances in many fields, saw major gains. Steroids also offered noteworthy results in specialties like dermatology.

CHAPTER XV

A NEW HEART

TRAVIS COUNTY IN THE 1980s suffered a boom followed by a severe downturn in the Texas oil industry, affecting everything from real estate to medical care. The trend toward managed health care caused consternation as services were denied.

By 1980, the World Health Organization had declared smallpox eradicated and children no longer had to be vaccinated against it in the United States. Still, the nation was confronting a new health issue—the autoimmune deficiency syndrome (AIDS). In 1983, the first death was reported in Austin and the Waterloo Counseling Center was established to help the ill. At one point, Austin's infectious disease specialists, who were few in number, were overloaded with work. Dr. Bruce Hurt wrote in the *TCMS Journal* that the medical profession knew little about "what is rapidly becoming one of the most frightening medical maladies to emerge within recent years...." Physicians were urged to report suspected cases. The People's Community Clinic expanded, providing leadership on HIV services. Although blood donations declined across the nation, the Central Texas Regional Blood Center in Austin set a record in 1985 because it established three programs to assure the safety of the supply—designated-donor, public education, and screening, including asking each prospective donor a set of forty-eight questions in advance of a blood donation. After the U.S. Food and Drug Administration licensed a new test for the antibody to the virus, the blood center immediately began using it.

In 1980, Dr. Norman Chenven, an Austin family practitioner, formed the Austin Regional Clinic (ARC). With pediatricians Drs. Thomas Zavaleta and Carol Faget, ARC entered into a partnership with PruCare, an experimental program of Prudential Insurance Company, to develop the first health plan and HMO in Austin.

In 1981, Austin physicians, often called upon to work with the Texas Legislature, were involved in the first "sunset" process for the Texas State Board of Medical Examiners. Although the process dealt with state agencies, by its nature it included the review of the state's Medical Practice Act with ramifications for all licensed physicians.

Dr. Willebrordus (Will) S. M. Van Wisse, a surgeon and graduate of the University of Leiden, the oldest university in the Netherlands, received the International Humanitarian of the Year award in 1982 from Sertoma. For three years, he had practiced medicine among Guatemala's poor, establishing five medical clinics in the mountains and a hospital, hiring a native Guatemalan physician to oversee the hospital. He arranged for at least one U.S. physician each year to work in the hospital and clinics and for a means of funding for young Guatemalans to study medicine, engineering, and other professions. In the mid-1970s, he founded the San Jose Clinic in South Austin.

Twenty years after serving as the first female president of the Travis County Medical Society, Dr. Ruth Bain became the second woman president of the Texas Medical Association in 1982. She would receive many other honors: the Texas Medical Association's Distinguished Service Award; the Travis County Medical Society's Gold-Headed Cane Award as the Physician of the Year in 1989; and in 1993, the University of Texas Medical Branch awarded her its Ashbel Smith Distinguished Alumnus

OPPOSITE PAGE: *In 1982, Dr. Ruth Bain became the second woman to serve as president of the Texas Medical Association.*

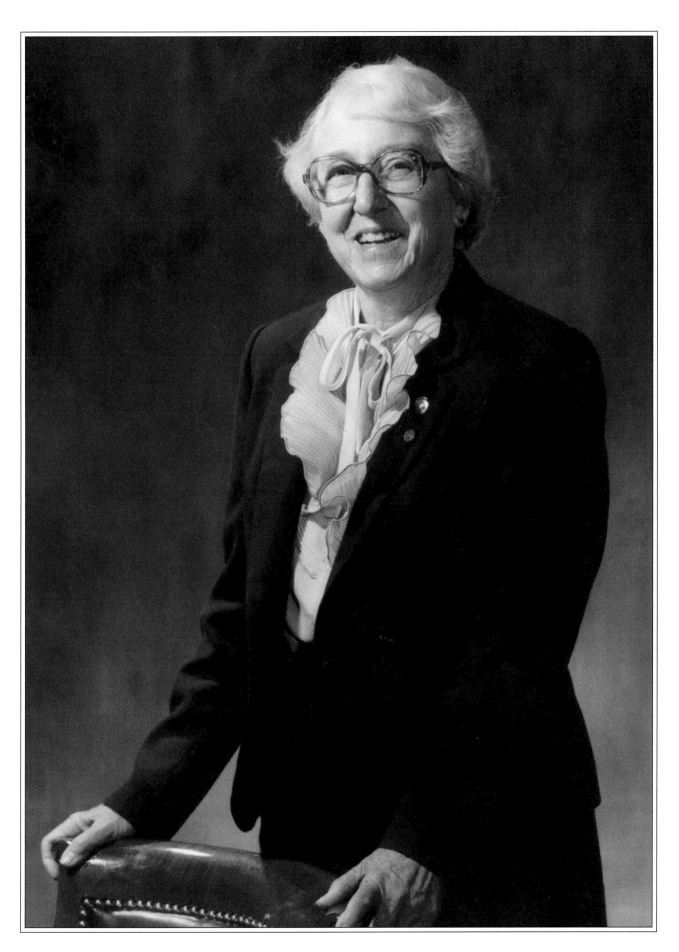

A NEW HEART   129

Award. Certified in 1977 by what would be the American Board of Family Medicine, she had served the CTMF Family Practice Residency in several capacities and in 1979 was appointed by the governor to the State Board of Medical Examiners.

The Central Texas Health Plan (CTHP) had been implemented in the early 1980s, and Dr. Bain served as medical director from 1985 to 1987 and as vice president of medical affairs from 1987 to 1990. Meanwhile, it became the PCA Health Plan of Texas. Dr. Bain later asked Dr. Lansing Thorne to join her as medical director. In June 1986, TCMS executive director John Kemp stated in a progress report that CTHP had proved "its popularity" in Austin, especially because it gave patients freedom of choice to select their own physicians. The plan, which worked well in Austin, Dr. Thorne remembered, later experienced financial concerns, partially because of problems in another state and perhaps, Dr. Bain believed, because it did not have a primary care "gatekeeper,"—although she did not particularly like the term.

In 1982, the Austin community said goodbye to Dr. Truman Morris, its first board-certified specialist in obstetrics and gynecology. His son-in-law, Dr. Douglas McIntyre, believed that he had delivered more than 10,000 babies. Austin obstetrician and gynecologist Dr. Marion Stahl remembered him as "very, very dedicated to our field and respected by all his fellow physicians." Dr. Morris had been the first chief of staff at St. David's Community Hospital.

Physicians had growing concerns about the corporate practice of medicine, and Dr. Milton Talbot, 1985 TCMS president, wrote that Texas statutes, the Texas Medical Association, and the American Medical Association stated that a corporation should not practice medicine. Dr. Talbot emphasized that "as physicians we feel" that a corporation "must not" practice medicine, observing that "A professional may be defined as one who holds the interest of his client or patient above his own personal or fiscal gain and above his social, political or personal advancement...." Acknowledging a corporation's ability to achieve efficiency, economies of purchasing, and other improvements, Dr. Talbot wondered whether a corporate philosophy "could allow medical care with the patient's welfare at the uppermost." He also recognized the likelihood of health care rationing.

Austin was being promoted as a "high tech" community. The computer had become integral to many realms of medicine, as had lasers, ultrasound, and miniaturization of equipment. There were increasing numbers of non-invasive diagnostic and surgical procedures and physicians were returning to school for training in new technologies, including laparoscopic, endoscopic, microscopic, and laser techniques. Radiologists had to know how to manage computed tomography scans and magnetic resonance imaging.

In 1980, Holy Cross Hospital established the first hospice program in Austin. On May 1, 1985, Austin's Star-Flight helicopter service began operating. The City of Austin and Travis County EMS and Brackenridge Hospital provided emergency care throughout a ten-county Central Texas region. Austin hospitals also continued to offer new programs and services, such as hyperbaric oxygen therapy at Brackenridge and development of an artificial ear at Seton in conjunction with Austin Otological Clinic.

At the time of Dr. Joe Thorne Gilbert's retirement in 1985, he and his father had served Travis County for eighty-five years. Also, on his seventy-eighth birthday, his family, friends, and patients had established the Joe Thorne Gilbert Lectureship in the Health Professions at the University of Texas, where he and his father had served the student health center since 1909. Dr. Gilbert's daughter, Dr. Linda Gilbert Prentice, was continuing the family medical tradition as would Dr. Laura Prentice Masters, daughter of Drs. James and Linda Gilbert Prentice, who graduated from UTMB in 2003.

After practicing for more than forty years, Dr. M. D. McCauley died in 1985 at the age of seventy-four. Dr. George Tipton praised him as a dynamic personality who championed excellence in medical care for Austin and was the conscience of the community.

In 1984, Dr. Jeffrey Youngkin, an obstetrician-gynecologist subspecializing in reproductive endocrinology and infertility with obstetrician-gynecologists Drs. Joe S. McIlhaney, Jr., Thomas Vaughn, and Harold Brumley, offered the first *in vitro* fertilization program at St. David's Hospital. Within a year, the first baby was born to parents from Bastrop. In 1987, a baby was born through gamete intrafallopian tube transfer (GIFT), a simpler and less costly approach. Dr. Youngkin believed he was the first Austin gynecologist to operate with a laparoscope. A Houston native, he graduated from Baylor College of Medicine in 1978 and completed a three-year residency in obstetrics and gynecology there in 1982.

The Travis County Medical Society established the Central Texas Bone Bank in 1985. Dr. Joseph M. Abell, a strong proponent of the bank, credited Drs. Atys DaSilva and Georgia and Carey Legett, along with TCMS administrator Edwin Smith as the four people most responsible for its success. Doctors earlier had instituted their own banks, storing bone in a frozen locker or freeze-drying it. The advanced new bank comprised skin, heart valves, and other materials for surgeries, including transplants. In 1985, the Central Texas Regional Tissue Bank was inaugurated and a retrieval program from cadavers was initiated. Dr. Edward S. Lewis, a board-certified orthopedic surgeon, performed the first tissue transplant in Central Texas at Seton Hospital using a donor tendon from the bank to repair a torn ligament, the most common and serious type of knee injury.

Cardiology and cardiovascular surgery continued to see major milestones. In March 1981, Dr. Robert W. Pederson performed the first angioplasty in the city at Brackenridge Hospital. A Corsicana native, he graduated from the UT Medical School at Houston in 1973. He served an internship and residency in internal medicine and was chief resident at the school's affiliated hospitals. He earned board certification in medicine in 1977, and from 1977 to 1979 was a fellow in cardiology at Vanderbilt University School of Medicine.

Dr. John D. "Chip" Oswalt joined Cardiothoracic and Vascular Surgeons of Austin in 1980. Originally from Fort Stockton, he was the son of Dr. C. E. Oswalt, a long-time leader in Texas medicine. A 1971 UTMB graduate, he served an internship at Brackenridge Hospital and in 1980 completed a residency at the University Health Science Center in San Antonio. Also the brother of physicians, Dr. Oswalt had intended to become a plastic surgeon until meeting many talented heart surgeons at Brackenridge Hospital. He is a diplomate of the American Board of Surgery and the American Board of Thoracic Surgery. At Seton Medical Center in 1986, Dr. Oswalt performed the first heart transplant in Austin and with Drs. David

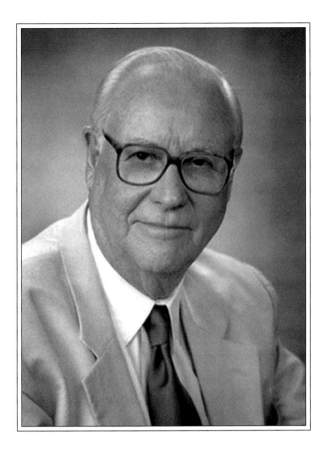

The Austin City Council honored Dr. Albert La Londe declaring Albert A. La Londe Day in 1985.

Morris and James Calhoon organized the transplant program. He also was the first physician in Texas to perform the Ross procedure, a durable aortic valve replacement devised by British cardio-thoracic surgeon Dr. Donald Ross. In 2000, Dr. Oswalt also established a nonprofit organization, HeartGift, to bring children to Austin from underdeveloped countries for heart surgery. In 1999, the Capital Area Division of the American Heart Association selected him as Austin's Cardiac Care Provider of the Year. Dr. Oswalt also taught the Ross procedure to others, utilizing the artistic capabilities of Dr. John Craig, a native Austinite and 1968 UTMB graduate. Initially an ophthalmologist, Dr. Craig developed dual careers in ophthalmology and medical illustration and later decided to devote full time to medical illustration. His work became internationally known.

The Texas Association of Neurological Surgeons named Dr. Albert La Londe its "neurological surgeon of the year" in 1984 and the Austin City Council honored him with Albert A. La Londe Day in 1985. The Travis County Medical Society named him Physician of the Year in 1996, and Seton Hospital recognized him for his "55 or more" years of service in December 2003.

In 1989, Dr. Earl B. Matthew of the Central Texas Medical Foundation obtained a grant from the American Foundation for AIDS Research for a seed grant to start a community-based clinical trials program. The HIV Study Group would be based at the Blackstock Family Health Center. Also in 1989, internist and rheumatologist Dr. Homer Goehrs became executive director of the Texas State Board of Medical Examiners.

Challenging health care issues remained: managed care; a maze of insurance plans; rising liability insurance premiums; hospital mergers; and mounting numbers of uninsured individuals seeking emergency care.

CHAPTER XVI

PUNCTUATING A CENTURY OF CHANGE

JOHN N. KEMP, A VETERAN of World War II and Korea, retired in 1990 as executive vice president of Travis County Medical Society. In 1965, when he arrived in Austin, the annual budgets of the society's four corporations totaled almost ten million dollars, and it had 304 members and a budget of $170,000. Mr. Kemp had overseen numerous programs, among them component fractionation of blood conversion from hermetically sealed bottles to plastic blood bags; tissue banking; construction of a new headquarters building; and a major enhancement of a graduate medical education program.

Thomas Young, former administrator of Brackenridge Hospital, succeeded Mr. Kemp, followed in 1994 by Marshall Cothran, formerly of the Dallas County Medical Society, who also had been in private business. The society and the blood center had been blessed with the voluntary activities of physicians and also had many dedicated staff.

Again, physicians were called to war, this time to Desert Storm. The *TCMS Journal* in 1991 cited six Austin physicians serving in the Persian Gulf. Other conflicts in this era, like the Bosnian war, also drew physicians into military service.

AIDS remained a challenge. Dr. Earl B. Matthew, director of medical services and education for the Central Texas Medical Foundation (CTMF) and chairman of the

TCMS Special Committee on AIDS policy, reported in 1990 that Austin had the highest per capita rate of human immunodeficiency virus in Texas. The need for physicians, he said, "could be staggering." A TCMS referral service comprised primary care physicians who agreed to accept a certain number of patients each year.

David Wright of Santa Monica, California, discouraged initially about medicine, had graduated with a degree in biology and joined Volunteers in Service to America (VISTA). In 1973, he was sent to Texas to set up a free clinic in South Austin, where Dr. Mathis Blackstock, "opened my eyes to the clinical side of medicine and showed me the influence a physician can have on a community." In 1980, Dr. Wright graduated from UTMB and returned to Austin for three years with Dr. Blackstock in the CTMF family practice residency program. After another absence serving as clinical director of the Mescalero Indian Health Service in New Mexico and as a teaching fellow at the Family Practice Faculty Development Center in Waco, he again returned to Austin as associate director and then director of the CTMF family practice residency program, serving until 1994. He "found an explosion in the numbers of dy-

---

OPPOSITE PAGE: *The new Texas Medical Association building under construction. TMA moved into the new structure at 401 West Fifteenth Street in 1991.*

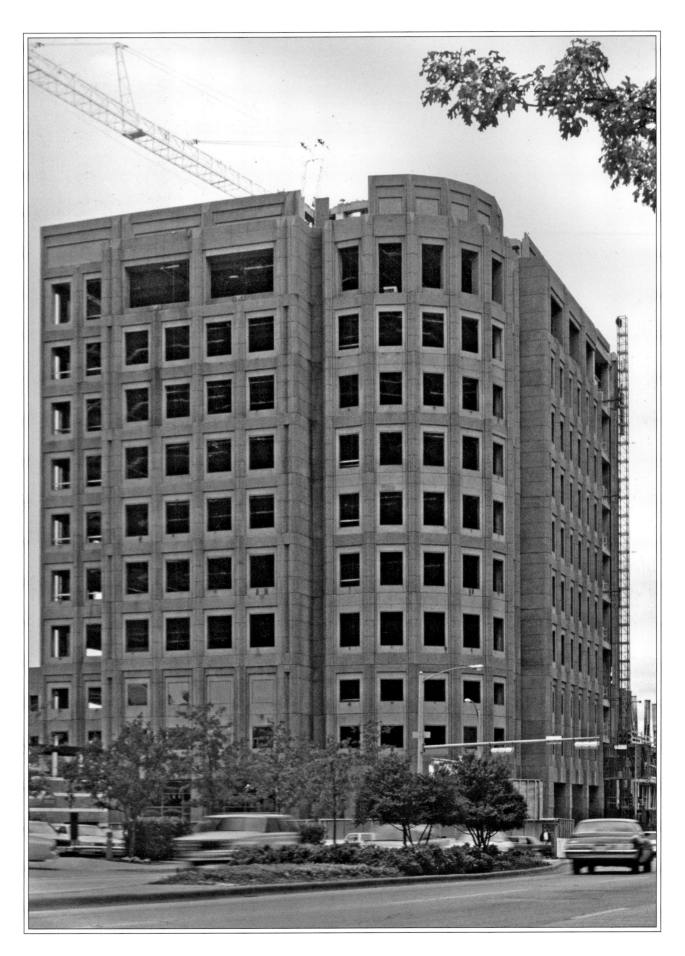

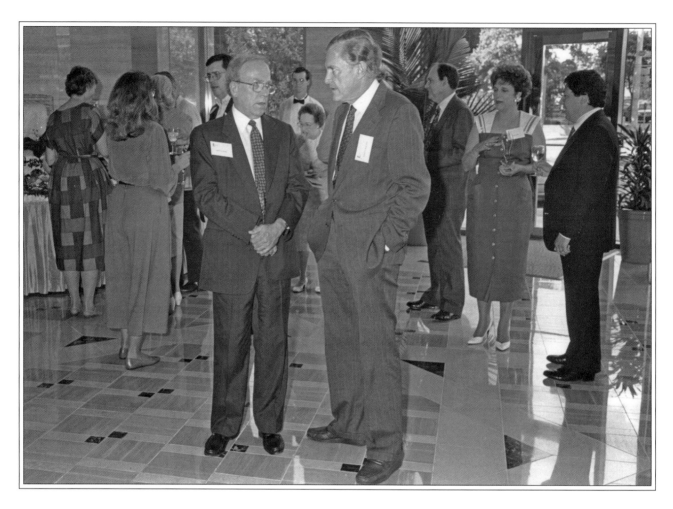

TMA Executive Vice President Robert Mickey (foreground, left) chats with Dr. Robert Rock at a reception at the newly completed Texas Medical Association building.

ing young men—my contemporaries," and would continue to see patients of all ages, including those with HIV.

The Texas Medical Association—which the Travis County Medical Society had led home to Austin in mid-century—had outgrown the building dedicated in 1952 on land donated by TCMS and had occupied three additional buildings across from the main building's side street, Martin Luther King Jr. Boulevard. In 1991, TMA moved into a new ten-story structure at 401 West Fifteenth Street near the state Capitol. The newest location also had sentimental value for Austin doctors. After World War II, many practitioners had remodeled old homes as offices in the area, and some, like Dr. Kermit Fox, had offices on the exact location where the new TMA building now stood.

In 1992, the Texas Osteopathic Medical Association moved its offices from Fort Worth to Austin, also locating near the Capitol at Fourteenth and Lavaca streets, a block from the TMA building.

Computerization was becoming integral to medicine. Simple browsers for the Internet would make it much easier to access global information. Web sites, including "drkoop.com," which originated in Austin, were devoted

to health information. Electronic mail became a routine method of communication.

Professional liability insurance again would reach crisis level in 1994, with reports that some physicians had abandoned high-risk specialties, such as obstetrics and emergency medicine.

Dr. Kurt Lekisch, who died in 1994, had graduated from the University of Bern-Switzerland in 1937. In 1992, at the new TMA building, he exhibited the history of tuberculosis through his private stamp and memorabilia collection. Dr. Paul C. Trickett, who had served at the UT Student Health Center, died in February 1994. He was a 1949 graduate of the Long Island College of Medicine.

In 1993, the Central Texas Medical Foundation was having difficulty keeping up with unfunded admissions at Brackenridge Hospital. Drs. Michael Mouw and Patrick Crocker called upon private physicians to help at the hospital and the trauma center. Dr. William J. Deaton, 1994

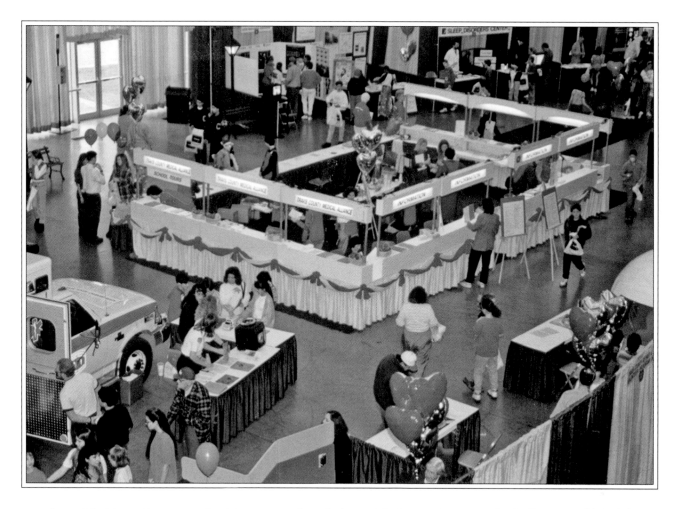

president of the Travis County Medical Society, attributed the problem to managed care plans having "no budget for indigent patients in their profit margins."

Dr. William G. Gamel, serving as TMA president, was involved in the 1993 "sunset" review of the State Board of Medical Examiners. A Lampasas native, Dr. Gamel majored in history at the University of Texas, graduated from UTMB in 1963, and completed an internship in internal medicine and a fellowship in gastroenterology at Parkland Memorial Hospital. The state board would be scrutinized again in 2005.

After the TMA Auxiliary changed its name to the TMA Alliance, the Travis County Medical Auxiliary became the Travis County Medical Alliance in 1992. It established a local HealthFest celebration to promote healthy lifestyles. Thousands of dollars were raised for programs such as the Children's Hospital, the Center for Battered Women, the Ronald McDonald House, the Mother's Milk Bank, the Volunteer Healthcare Clinic, and the Del Valle Children's Wellness Center. In 1997, the Alliance supported the "Baby Think It Over" program designed to help middle-school students better understand the responsibilities of parenting.

Among other creative endeavors were "Hard Hats for Little Heads," which promoted bicycle safety and included the distribution of free helmets to children. As it had in the past, the organization would continue to be a leader on health care issues, programs, and services.

In 1995, the City of Austin EMS Department, the Austin Fire Department, and the Travis County Emergency Services Department established a position for a full-time medical director over all services. In October 1995, Dr. Edward M. Racht, an emergency medicine specialist and board-certified in internal medicine, assumed the post. With the goal of providing a "seamless" patient care system, he had responsibility for all clinical aspects of out-of-hospital emergency care in the city and county. A 1984 graduate of Emory University School of Medicine, Dr. Racht would have medical oversight of approximately 1,700 providers in thirty-eight agencies.

On its twenty-fifth anniversary in 2006, the Austin Regional Clinic was cited as the largest multispecialty group practice in the metropolitan area, with thirteen locations in Austin, Round Rock, Cedar Park, and Pflugerville. It had discontinued its sole arrangement with Prudential, permitting patients to make choices among insurers.

Dr. Tom Coopwood, 1995 president of TCMS, talked about the changing medical environment, observing that the "issue is not about quality of care but how we can get more people into the system and decrease the cost. There has been a decided paradigm shift from a sick patient to a healthy one," he said.

Austin physician Dr. Thomas M. Runge, a founding member of the UT College of Engineering's Department of Biomedical Engineering, taught courses on cardiovascular dynamics, providing students with a medical-school-type experience in a hospital setting at Brackenridge Hospital. Also a professor in the Department of Surgery at UT Health Science Center at San Antonio, he conducted research on pulsatile flow blood pumps, especially for extracorporeal cardiac support and cardiopulmonary bypass. Spin-off results from his research included the process of pulsatile flow hemodialysis and the development of a whole blood substitute for use in cardiopulmonary bypass surgery and donor organ preservation. He obtained more than eighteen patents, including those on pulsatile cardiac assist devices and an aircraft lift, and authored numerous publications. His work involved a cross-disciplinary team at UT Austin and the UT Health Science Center in San Antonio. Drs. Runge and Patrick S. Pevoto had developed the pulsatile heart pump. Dr. Pevoto graduated from UTMB summa cum laude in 1979 with a B.S. degree in pharmacy and in 1983 received his M.D. degree from UTMB. He had been a registered pharmacist and became a board-certified obstetrician-gynecologist. In 2002, he earned an M.B.A. degree from UT Austin. He and his teammates, who had formed Private Concepts, Inc., at the UT McCombs School of Business, also won the Moot Corp®

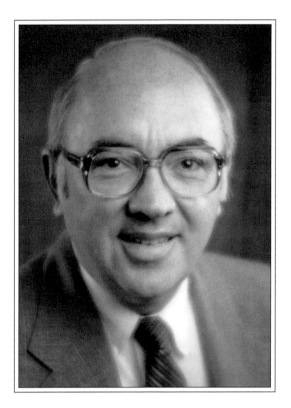

Dr. William Gamel was another Travis County physician who served as TMA president.

award in 2002, an international competition, for a take-home Pap smear test, the Pevlon Home Cervical Cancer Screen, which was patented and tested in clinical trials.

Also developing medical applications was ophthalmologist Dr. Stephen Dell, who held patents on several of his inventions. The brother of Michael Dell, the Austin founder of a global computer corporation known as Dell and a graduate of Baylor College of Medicine in 1988, he served his residency at Tulane University School of Medicine and was certified by the American Board of Ophthalmology. His research for the Food and Drug Administration resulted in approval of new laser treatments that modified the shape of the cornea by removing microscopic layers of tissue with incremental precision. In 2003, a new eye implant after cataract removal was approved by the FDA. It allowed a patient to focus on near or far objects. Dr. Dell implanted more than 200 of the lenses while participating in a three-year clinical trial.

In 1998, the Seton Network purchased the Central Texas Medical Foundation from Travis County Medical Society and Dr. Tom Kirksey became chairman of the board of trustees. In addition to his private practice, Dr. Kirksey had been clinical assistant professor of surgery at the UT Health Science Center at San Antonio and taught at UTMB. Degenerative disk disease forced him to retire after twenty-seven years as a thoracic and cardiovascular surgeon, and he returned to Brackenridge Hospital as part-time medical director. In 1995, he also was appointed to the Texas State Board of Medical Examiners for a six-year term and in 1999 was selected by TCMS as its Physician of the Year.

Individual groups historically had addressed specific diseases and their missions had evolved to meet a variety of needs. In the early twentieth century, the Texas Tuberculosis Association led the fight against tuberculosis and now, as the American Lung Association, worked to prevent lung disease and promote lung health. In mid-century, the Na-

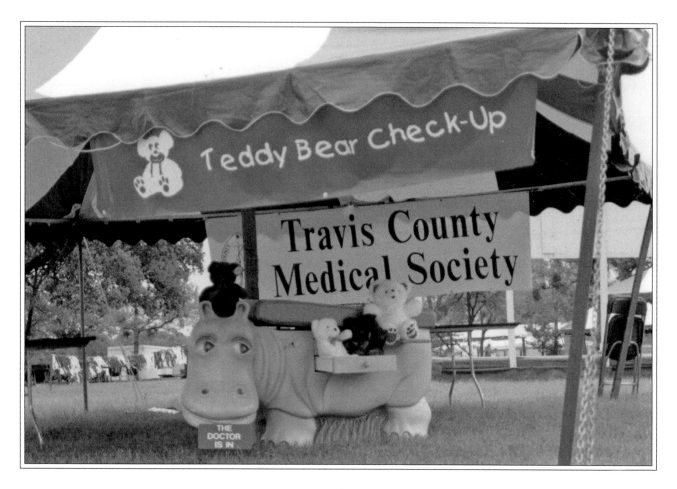

tional Foundation for Infantile Paralysis raised funds for polio solutions through its "march of dimes" and now, as the March of Dimes, focused its efforts on improvement of babies' health by addressing birth defects and premature births and infant mortality. Other state and local chapters of organizations also continued their long history as health care advocates, such as those of the American Heart Association, the American Cancer Society, the American Lung Association, and the American Diabetes Association.

Lance Armstrong, the seven-time winner of the Tour de France bicycle event, formed the Lance Armstrong Foundation in 1997 while undergoing treatment for testicular cancer. Its mission focused on survivorship and empowering people with cancer to live "strong," and provided grants to organizations. Its yellow wristband became an international phenomenon. In 1999, Michael and Susan Dell established a foundation with an emphasis on health and children, which, in 2004, offered one dollar for every two dollars raised, up to twenty-five million dollars in matching funds, for the construction of the Dell Children's Medical Center of Central Texas. The Dells also announced a gift of fifty million dollars in 2006 to help UT establish the Dell Pediatric Institute to look at critical health prob-

The Public Relations Committee has sponsored many programs, such as the Teddy Bear Check-Up, Call a Doctor, and Community Internship.

lems that impact healthy childhood development (including a focus on combating childhood obesity). Included also was funding for a new computer science building on the UT Austin campus.

Ethics in medicine once had seemed fairly clear, with principles codified for American physicians in the AMA's *Principles of Medical Ethics*. As medicine became more advanced, and developed artificial means to sustain life, bioethics issues grew more complex. The country's judicial system was hearing sensitive cases and Dr. Karen Teel's 1975 article on end-of-life issues was cited by the New Jersey Supreme Court in its opinion in the Karen Ann Quinlan case regarding the removal of artificial means of prolonging life in a comatose patient. Her commentary also had become the defining example in bioethics and legal textbooks. In 1999, the International Bioethics Institute in San Francisco presented its first Award of Distinction to Dr. Teel, recognizing her as a pioneer for proposing that hospital ethics committees be established to help institutions, family members, and physicians make ethical and humane choices near the end of life. A leader in developing the children's hospital in Austin, Dr. Teel, as the parent of a son born with abnormalities requiring years of surgery and treatment not available in Austin, well understood the problems that families faced. In 1995, she directed the founding of the Pediatric Physicians Alliance of Central Texas, serving as president through 1999. The Karen Teel Excellence Award was launched in 2003 to be given annually to the outstanding senior pediatric resident at Children's Hospital. Certified by the American Board of Pediatrics, Dr. Teel also served as an official examiner for the board.

In November 1994, Dr. Raleigh Ross died in Austin. In 1980, the surgical unit at Brackenridge Hospital had been named for him in recognition of his dedicated work with interns and surgical residents. Dr. Ross had served as president of the Texas Surgi-

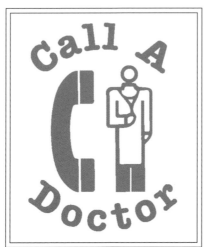

cal Society and for ten years on the Board of Texas State Hospitals and Special Schools, including three as chairman. In honor of his father, a Lockhart physician for more than sixty years, Dr. Ross provided for the Alonzo Alverly Ross Professorship in General Surgery at UTMB in 1975. It was designated a Centennial Chair in 1991.

Dr. George Edmund Bennack, Brackenridge Hospital's first intern (1931-1932), died in 1995 at age ninety-four in Raymondville.

In 1995, Dr. Tracy Gordy, who had had been editor of the *TCMS Journal* since 1984, providing many cover photos, completed his service. He also was active in other publishing circles,

---

Call a Doctor is a joint venture between KVUE-24 and the Travis County Medical Society. Volunteer physicians like Drs. Tom McHorse and William Halden staff phone banks, answering anonymous questions from people in the viewing area.

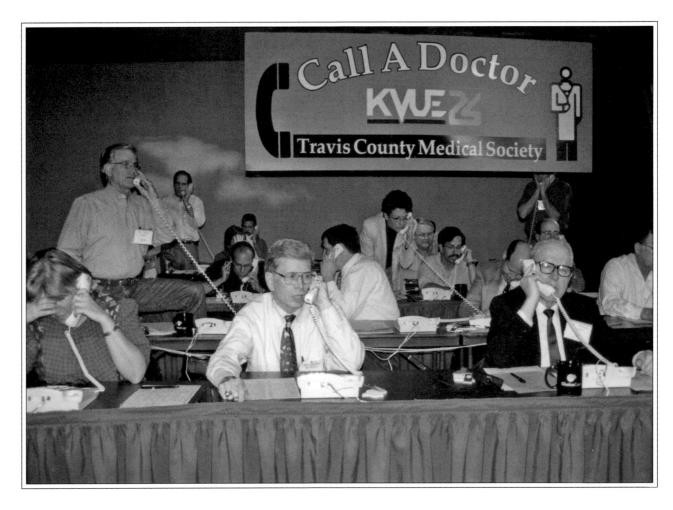

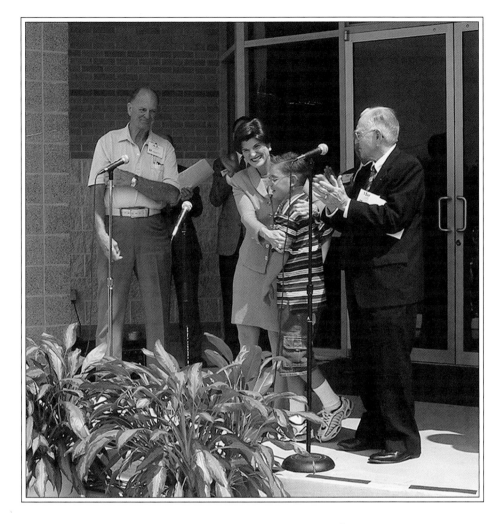

Luci Baines Johnson (above, center) spoke at the 1999 dedication of the Blood and Tissue Center's new facility expansion.

also held its groundbreaking in 1997 in Central Park at Thirty-eighth Street and North Lamar Boulevard.

At that time, Austin had the highest concentration of managed care in the state, a 1996 TMA study showed, with nearly sixty percent of the capital's population enrolled in a Health Maintenance Organization or a Preferred Provider Organization. "Austin Regional Clinic (ARC), one of the oldest and strongest physician-led groups in Austin, shepherded managed care into Austin and was the first physician group in the area to accept capitated contracts," the report stated.

In 1998, the Travis County Medical Society sold its nonprofit Central Texas Medical Foundation to the Seton network, and in 2000, CTMF became Austin Medical Education Programs.

including as a reviewer for *The New England Journal of Medicine*. In 1999, he became chairman of the AMA's Current Procedural Terminology panel. He was certified in psychiatry and geriatrics by the American Board of Psychiatry & Neurology.

Two major hospital systems emerged from existing hospitals in the 1990s. In October 1995, the City of Austin leased the assets of Brackenridge Hospital and Children's Hospital of Austin to the Seton Healthcare Network. Under the terms of the long-term contract, Seton would manage the institutions. In 1996, St. David's Hospital merged with the Columbia/HCA Health Care Corporation.

In the late 1990s, the Christopher House reopened in Austin. Previously an AIDS specialty hospital, it had been acquired by Hospice Austin, one of the country's oldest and largest nonprofit hospice programs, as the first inpatient hospice for Central Texas. The Heart Hospital of Austin

The Blood Center and Tissue Bank became the Central Texas Regional Blood and Tissue Center in 1999 and held dedication ceremonies at its enlarged facility. Participants included Dr. E. Randy Eckert, vice president of the center's board, and Luci Baines Johnson, daughter of former President Lyndon Johnson. She had donated blood to the center for twenty-seven years. Dr. Joe Abell and his wife Mary chaired the capital campaign, which raised nearly three million dollars to build the new blood center. Dr. Abell recounted its history and purposes, noting that the Travis County Medical Society remained unique in owning and running a blood and tissue bank. In 1999, the Center also participated in a stem cell research project to determine if stem cells in bone marrow transplantation would enhance treatment for leukemia and breast cancer.

Physicians, even the most optimistic, occasionally felt there was a shadow on freedoms once enjoyed by the profession. Managed care, the professional liability insurance crisis, and myriad regulations from agencies contributed to the changing medical climate.

CHAPTER XVII

CHAOS AND SERENDIPITY

THE MILLENNIUM PASSED without chaos or meltdown of the world's computer systems but on September 11, 2001, the nation was shocked when a long-planned attack on U.S. soil by al Qaeda, an Islamic extremist group, caused nearly 3,000 deaths. The country responded immediately. Local, state, and federal governments intensified efforts to address future terrorism. The Texas Medical Association established a Bioterrorism Task Force, which produced a tool kit on physician protocols and patient information on biological agents.

Long before 9/11, the Travis County Medical Society had mechanisms for effective and efficient communication to physicians in community emergencies, and, as early as the 1980s, disaster notification drills had been conducted yearly through the Medical Exchange. When emergency situations occurred in later years, more targeted communication approaches became possible because of improved computerization and the widespread use of cell phones. Text messages could be sent via cell phones or pagers to preassigned tiers of physician responders according to the nature, level, or location of the disaster. In the case of an extreme community-wide crisis, a single message could be sent to physicians advising them to go to their assigned emergency locations. The medical society also remained prepared to communicate by backup means, such as ham radio, should electronic or computer systems be affected.

Physicians again were serving in war zones. In 2001, American troops were sent to Afghanistan and, in 2003, to Iraq. Ever more specialized skills now could be applied to the care and treatment of soldiers on the battlefield. Early in the Iraq war, the last unit of the Korean-type mobile hospital, MASH, was decommissioned. The replacements, dubbed Combat Support Hospitals (CaSH), expanded on the earlier models, adding

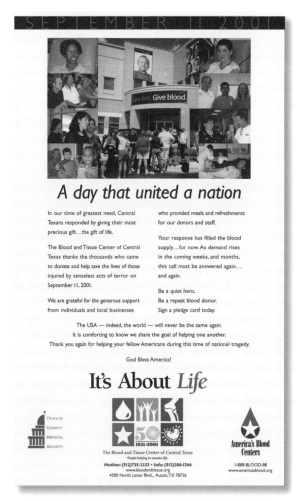

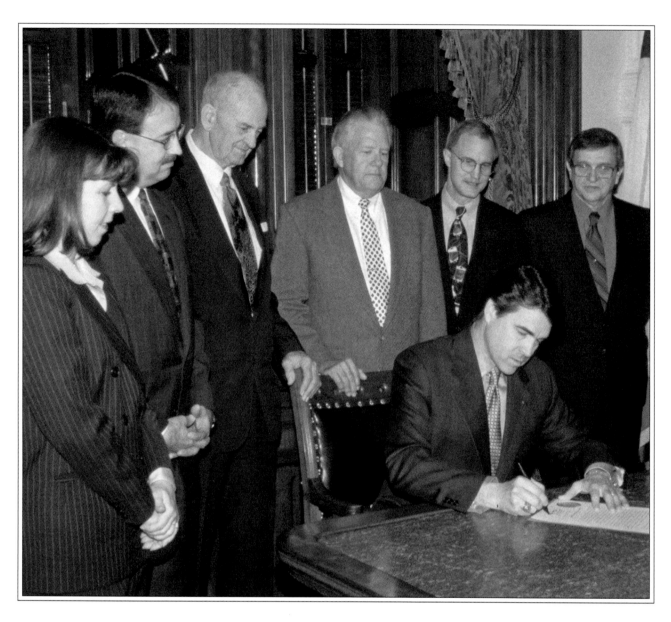

ABOVE: *Governor Rick Perry signs Blood Donor Month proclamation, 2001.* OPPOSITE PAGE: *"A day that united a nation." Thousands of people waited in line to donate blood on behalf of those injured on 9/11.*

features such as a deployable radiology unit and support for telemedicine. The wars in Afghanistan and Iraq would bring unique types of injuries, particularly traumatic brain injuries from improvised explosive devices (IEDs), and the need for long-term rehabilitation for physical injuries and post-traumatic stress disorder. The wars also would demonstrate remarkable medical advances and skills on the battlefield.

Among physicians serving early in the Iraq war were two Austin ophthalmologists-to-be who were in Kuwait when the war began in March 2003. Lt. Col. Sean Blaydon, who

had been director of ophthalmic, plastic, orbital, and reconstructive surgery and director of the ocular trauma service at Brooke Army Medical Center in San Antonio, was Commander of the 286th Eye Surgical Team. Major Shari DeMartelaere served with him. She remained with the Forty-seventh Combat Hospital in Kuwait but Lt. Colonel Blaydon and others on his team were redeployed to the twenty-eighth Combat Support Hospital in Baghdad on July 4, 2003, where he served for a year. Dr DeMartelaere joined Texas Oculoplastic Consultants in Austin in 2004. A graduate of the University of Minnesota Medical School, she completed her residency in ophthalmology at the University of Colorado and became a board-certified ophthalmologist. Dr. Blaydon also became an associate at Texas Oculoplastic Consultants. A native of the U.S. Virgin Islands and schooled in England, he had received his M.D.

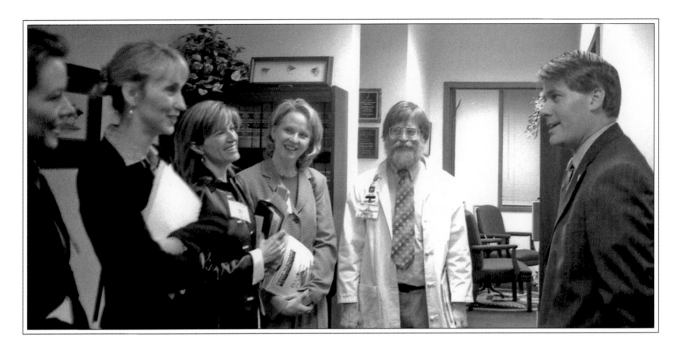

First Tuesday is a grassroots movement for tort reform. Travis County Medical Society and Alliance members with Rep. Todd Baxter.

degree from Tulane University School of Medicine in 1989, had served an ophthalmology residency at Walter Reed Army Medical Center in Washington, D.C., and a two-year fellowship in ophthalmic plastic surgery at Texas Oculo-plastic Consultants.

Dr. Bud Dryden, Austin's Most Worthy Citizen in 2001 when he was honored for his work for the poor, died in 2002. Travis County also said goodbye in this decade to many other senior physicians who had been leaders since the post-World War II era. Among them were Drs. James E. Kreisle, David O. Johnson, Oliver Suehs, Charles B. Dildy, Robert B. Morrison, Rexford Carter, David Wade, Thomas M. Runge, Sam N. Key, Jr., Morris Polsky, Stuart Nemir, Margaret Sedberry, Pruett Watkins, William F. McLean, Kaoru Dyo, John Buchanan, Glenn Capps, William "Bill" Hart, William "Dutch" Hahn, George Sharpe, Frank Gregg (a fourth-generation Travis County physician), Elmer C. Baum (who had represented osteopathic physicians and served on the Texas State Board of Medical Examiners), Martin Legett, Robert "Bob" Anderson, and Sam W. Wilborn. Among the list also was John Kemp, Travis County Medical Society's long-time executive and Roy J. Cates, his predecessor, who was the society's executive from 1959 until Mr. Kemp arrived in 1965.

In 2003, nearly two years ahead of schedule, the international collaborative effort on the Human Genome Project, comprising the mapping of the genome, was completed.

The Texas Medical Association and the Travis County Medical Society held yearlong sesquicentennial celebrations. In 1853, Travis County physicians had made history when they brought Texas doctors to Austin to form a state association. Two district societies also had been formed, one of which was Travis Medical Society, a predecessor to TCMS.

In 2003, the Texas Legislature passed tort reforms to improve the medical care climate and address the professional liability crisis. Voters ratified the changes in a constitutional amendment. Among many assisting in the effort was Dr. William Gamel, a past TMA president and the chief executive officer of the Texas Medical Foundation's Health Quality Institute. TCMS named him Physician of the Year in 2003.

Travis County leaders remained well represented in the American and Texas medical associations. Dr. Joseph P. Annis was elected in June 2006 to the AMA Board of Trustees, the first TCMS doctor to serve on that body. He was a 1969 graduate of the Medical College of Wisconsin and board certified in anesthesiology. Dr. C. Bruce Malone, III, became chair of the TMA Board of Trustees in May 2006. A 1969 graduate of Duke University School of Medicine, he had earned board certification in orthopedic surgery, and specialized in orthopedic surgery and sports medicine.

Physicians also held key roles in other state and national medical organizations. In 2003, Dr. Thomas D. Kirksey, a former member of the Texas State Board of Medical Examiners, became the chief elected officer of the Federation of State Medical Boards and in 2001, Dr. Donald W. Patrick, who held degrees as a doctor of medicine and a doctor of jurisprudence, became executive director of the Texas State Board of Medical Examiners. Effective September 1, 2005, the Texas Legislature changed the name of the venerable board formed in 1907 to simply the "Texas Medical Board."

In 1981, Dr. Charles B. Mullins had become executive vice chancellor for Health Affairs for the University of Texas System, a position he held until 2001. In 1996, he was named the holder of the newly established J. Fred Schoellkopf, Jr., Chair in Cardiology at UT Southwestern Medical School in Dallas. Dr. Mullins received his undergraduate degree from the University of North Texas and his M.D. degree from UT Southwestern Medical School, where he had been a tenured faculty member since 1971.

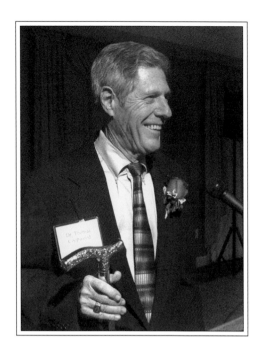

Dr. Tom Coopwood was among the initial appointees to the Travis County Healthcare District board of managers.

As the needs of members and the community changed, the Travis County Medical Society had adapted. Traditional monthly meetings had evolved into special annual occasions and more frequent focused gatherings. Particularly since the 1970s, hospitals and specialty medical societies largely had assumed the mantle of continuing education, but the society served a neutral role in a variety of realms that spanned individual institutions. For instance, Dr. Tom Coopwood had chaired a committee to study and address the risks of wrong site, wrong procedure, and wrong person surgery errors, bringing in representatives from Austin area hospitals and outpatient facilities. The effort resulted in a uniform set of risk-reducing guidelines to be incorporated by each area institution into its operating policies and procedures. Although it had sold its notable graduate medical education program, TCMS continued to oversee the Blood and Tissue Center of Central Texas and to expand the call center services provided by its subsidiary, the Medical Service Bureau.

As president of TCMS a few years earlier, Dr. Joe Abell had initiated the Physicians' Forum for retired physicians after his "good friends Drs. Homer Goehrs and Earl Grant" inspired the concept. "Until then, retired physicians just

seemed to fade," he said. Now, they attended regular Forum meetings, which featured talks on timely subjects.

In 2002, the Travis County Medical Society established Project Access, a coordinated system of physicians and institutions to help provide diagnostic services and medication for patients without funds. Dr. Tom S. McHorse became the first chairman and, in 2005, was named TCMS Physician of the Year.

The need for charity care had grown rapidly and Dr. McHorse, also a former TCMS president and former Seton trustee, called for a regional solution to the many unmet charity needs. "If we can make primary care services available in a non-emergency setting, and if we manage the whole medical process rather than isolated events," he said, "we can prevent small problems from becoming crises."

Until 2004, Austin had been the largest Texas city without a hospital district. In that year, however, county residents voted to establish a district by a significant margin, thus enlarging the tax revenue base of public health care facilities to all county residents. The goals were more efficient management, tax fairness, better delivery of health care, and reduction of overcrowded emergency departments. A board of managers was appointed to oversee Brackenridge Hospital; Children's Hospital of Austin; and Austin Women's Hospital (a general hospital offering women's health services on a separate floor of Brackenridge Hospital and operated by UT Medical Branch, Galveston). Among the initial appointees to the Travis County Healthcare District board of managers were Dr. Thomas B. Coopwood, Sr., Dr. Donald Patrick, and Thomas N. Young, who was a former Brackenridge hospital administrator, a former TCMS chief executive officer, and a former Austin Regional Clinic administrator.

In 2004, Dr. Robert Askew was co-chair of the steering committee of the Indigent Care Collaboration, an alliance of health care safety net providers. He also was director of the Seton Development Fund, on the board of directors for the Shivers Cancer Foundation, director of the UTMB

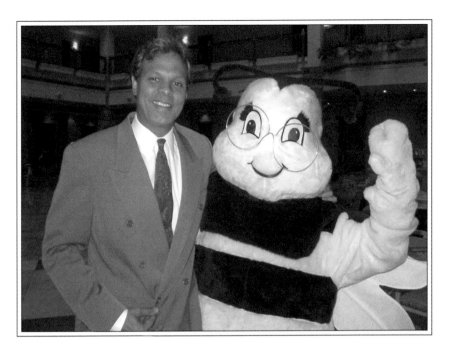

Texas Commissioner of Health Eduardo Sanchez with Be Wise mascot. The Texas Medical Association Foundation program promotes immunization.

development board, and member of the board of trustees of the Central Texas Institute for Research and Education in Medicine and Biotechnology.

In September 2004, the Texas Legislature consolidated the state health department and other agencies to form the Department of State Health Services. Dr. Eduardo Sanchez, Commissioner of Health at the time, had begun an Austin medical practice in 1992. A board-certified family practitioner, he also had served as chief medical officer for the Austin-Travis County Health and Human Services Department from 1994 to 1998. He was a Corpus Christi native, a 1988 graduate of UT Southwestern Medical School at Dallas, and held a master's degree in public health.

A symbol of modern trends was evident in August 2005 when a majority stake of Clinical Pathology Laboratories, Inc. (CPL), was bought by an Australian company. CPL was said to have been the largest privately owned medical laboratory company in the country, with operations in Texas and five other states. In 1989, CPL's chief executive Dr. Robert Conner and its president David Schultz had expanded on the pathology practice launched in 1948 by Dr. Sidney Bohls, who had soon brought in Drs. Charles T. Pelphrey and John Rainey.

Specialization continued to evolve. Doctors and clinics focused not only on an organ, but on specific areas and functions. Hospital-based specialties had fostered new terms like hospitalists. Cornerstone Healthcare Group provided long-term acute care in hospitals like St. David's and in free-standing settings. Rehabilitation units dealt with aftercare for burns, Parkinson's disease, and other illnesses. Outpatient dialysis care was offered.

Dr. Christopher Chenault, 2004 president of the Travis County Medical Society and an orthopedic surgeon specializing in hand surgery, marveled at the changes he had seen. As he left his office to replace a knee seriously damaged by arthritis, he passed radiographic equipment that developed film in ninety seconds and multiple computer terminals at nurses' desks that offered instant access to laboratory results. His patient was anesthetized with an epidural anesthesia, a continuous process monitored and measured by a computerized machine. A similar device provided and monitored the intravenous solution. During surgery, the new knee was secured with a plastic polymer that hardened in fifteen minutes and would hold the knee in place for at least twenty-five years. When he entered medicine in the early 1960s, a patient's only option had been a wheelchair. A 1964 graduate of Baylor College of Medicine, Dr. Chenault had interned at the University of California at Los Angeles (UCLA) School of Medicine, serving at Harbor General Hospital (the County of Los Angeles-Harbor-UCLA Medical Center). His orthopedic residency was with what became the University of Iowa Hospitals and Clinics in Iowa City, Iowa.

In the late summer and early fall of 2005, two hurricanes, Katrina and Rita, struck the Gulf Coast, causing enough destruction for the World Meteorological Organization to retire their names. After Katrina made its second landfall at Buras, Louisiana, on August 29, large numbers of people across the mid-Gulf Coast were affected. Many waited for rescue from water-logged conditions without food, water, medical treatment, or medicines. Volunteers and emergency responders traveled to the Greater New Orleans area to help and Austin received scores of evacuees. An efficient emergency system was in place with representatives of key organizations and government agencies customarily meeting monthly as the Interagency Disaster Council. The Travis County Medical Society had been represented on the council by its chief operating officer, Belinda Clare, for more than fifteen years and the relationships that were formed over that time helped during the crisis. The society also was experienced in notifying physicians and spouses and when the time came Ms. Clare requested volunteers by e-mail. More than 400 Travis County physicians plus countless nurses, emergency medical technicians, mental health, pharmaceutical, and other health professionals arrived to help over 4,000 evacuees. With them also were Marshall Cothran, the chief executive officer of TCMS, and Ms. Clare, both of whom spent the Labor Day weekend helping organize the massive rescue effort.

The operation was run from the City of Austin's Emergency Operations Center (EOC). In addition to the county medical society, participants included the American Red Cross; Brackenridge, Seton, and St. David's hospitals; the UT School of Nursing; and numerous volunteers.

On Saturday, September 3, and Sunday, September 4, hourly waves of airplanes brought evacuees to Austin-Bergstrom International Airport. A medical team met them to do triage and then sent them by bus to the Austin Convention Center for more extensive evaluation. Individuals needing urgent care were sent to Brackenridge Hospital and others were transported to the Palmer Events Center, where a medical center had been set up. The constantly changing situation called for ever-shifting responses. Many people were separated from families, and volunteers helped them via computers and cell phones. Most individuals just needed to be clean. Many needed prescriptions for their normal medications and others required chemotherapy. Patients with chronic diseases had to be treated and some needed nursing home and psychiatric care.

A medical microcosm quickly formed. At the Palmer Events Center, rows of cots made a hospital ward; a full pharmacy of free drugs was provided by CVS Pharmacy; and a clinic was ready to treat those not sent to the hospital. Fire and EMS personnel were prepared to help. Mr. Cothran said he had "never seen a more effective collaborative effort."

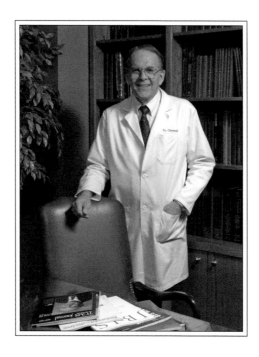

President Christopher S. Chenault on the cover of the TCMS Journal, *January/February 2004.*

Two volunteers found themselves at the helm. Dr. Ann Messer was a board-certified family physician and a 1979 graduate of Rush Medical College in Chicago. Dr. Peggy Russell, board certified in internal medicine and geriatric medicine, was a 1979 graduate of the University of North Texas Health Science Center's Texas College of Osteopathic Medicine.

Meanwhile, Brackenridge Hospital invoked the updated disaster plan developed after September 11, 2001. An emergency services area was set up in a parking garage beneath the helipad, reported Dr. Patrick J. Crocker, medical director for the hospital's Department of Emergency Medicine. Most patients had chest pains and skin and foot infections. One had a possible hypertensive hemorrhage and another dysrhythmia. Only six were admitted and others were returned to the convention center. The hospital also saw patients with acute diarrhea, hypertension, and diabetes. Dr. Crocker, a graduate of the Des Moines University College of Osteopathic Medicine in Des Moines, Iowa, is a board-certified emergency medicine specialist.

Dr. Guadalupe "Pete" Zamora, the 2005 Travis County Medical Society president, writing in the *TCMS Journal*, was awed at the kindness and generosity of Central Texans. The Blood Center also was overwhelmed with donors. Numerous citizens, including physicians working the 24-hour triage centers in 12-hour shifts, emergency medical technicians, nurses, and medical staff made "a huge contribution to the lives of those devastated people."

The medical community experienced a special serendipity—the great joy of practicing freely and helping those in need. A registered nurse, Carolyn Curry de Cordova—certified also as a hospice and palliative nurse—reported on her work with special-needs' patients. She was impressed with the response of the Travis County Medical Society. "Dr. Racht and Dr. Messer were in the eye of the storm so to speak," she said. "They were calm and efficient. Not only were they asked to practice medicine that was a cross between field hospital triage in a war zone, general medicine, and palliative care, they were also expected to make deci-

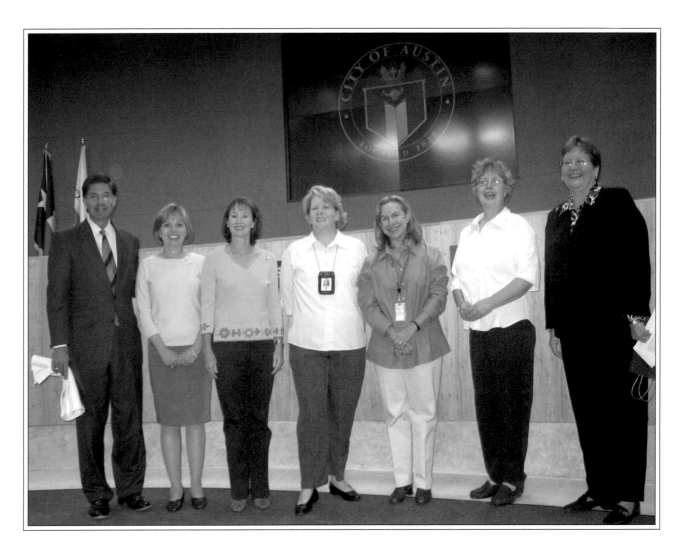

sions in a situation where major decisions were changed regularly...."

On September 24, 2006, a second hurricane, Rita, sent evacuees to Austin, but most did not require serious medical attention.

Austin now had two major hospital systems—Seton Family of Hospitals and St. David's HealthCare Partnership. The Austin/Travis County Emergency Medical Services System was integrated with the networks and the independent Heart Hospital. Seton's Brackenridge Hospital had a Level II Trauma Center. Also integrated were Children's Hospital, two hyperbaric medicine centers, and a number of specialty hospitals. The Austin Interagency Disaster Council was meeting monthly with the EMS System representatives.

In June 2007, the 200-million-dollar Dell Children's Medical Center of Central Texas, which could expand to 300 beds, opened at 4900 Mueller Boulevard. On June 30, the official opening date, patients were moved from Children's Hospital of Austin on Fifteenth Street to the new

Mayor Will Wynn recognized representatives of community groups that responded to the victims of Hurricane Katrina. Immediately to the right of Mayor Wynn above are Belinda Clare, COO, Travis County Medical Society and Patty Loose, President, Travis County Medical Alliance.

medical center. Three times larger than the former children's hospital, with nearly a half million square feet, the new Center received critical acclaim for its "breathtaking and innovative" design. It also was recognized for its "environmental and artistic feast for the senses: a three-acre multilevel healing garden with labyrinth, human sundial, and reflecting pond and bridge; a four-story waterfall; five self-contained ecosystems, each corresponding to a distinct area of the 46-county service area; and a collection of healing art, sculpture and photography unmatched in a clinical facility anywhere." The new medical center is providing much greater capacity for services such as the pediatric intensive care unit, the emergency department, a comprehensive trauma program, and plastic and reconstructive surgery. It also offers many new services and its presence has fostered medically related construction. A new facility with thirty rooms is being constructed by Ronald McDonald House Charities of Austin and Central Texas. The existing thirteen-room facility on Fifteenth Street will be kept for downtown hospitals. By establishing a healthy environment for the healing of its patients and implementing an environmentally conscious commitment to the region, the Dell Children's Medical Center of Central Texas also is considered an exemplary "green" facility and is on track to earn the platinum status from the Leadership in Energy & Environmental Design (LEED) and the U. S. Green Building Council.

The former Children's Hospital of Austin became the home of a new clinical academic center. Although Austin has become a significant center for medical research and medical education, it does not yet have its own medical school. In 1881, Texans had voted to place the University of Texas in Austin and the university's medical department in Galveston. Later, UT also established medical schools in Dallas, San Antonio, and Houston. Meanwhile, efforts have been under way to establish an academic health campus in Austin. From an internship established by Brackenridge Hospital in 1931, Austin has steadily built a major graduate medical education program. Through the foresight of the Travis County Medical Society, which had fostered the Central Texas Medical Foundation in the 1970s, an accredited training program has continued to expand. UTMB and UT have established joint M.D./ Ph.D. programs in neuroscience, bioengineering, and molecular biology. The Seton Family of Hospitals and the University of Texas Medical Branch also have signed a thirty-year agreement on graduate medical education. In the effort to further advance medical and health education in Austin, a coalition of organizations named the Central Texas Institute (CTI) has been formed, with Dr. James C. Guckian, executive director of the UT Medical Branch-Austin Outreach effort, serving as president. Member organizations of CTI include the University of Texas at Austin; the University of Texas Medical Branch at Galveston; the University of Texas Health Science Center at Houston School of Public Health; the University of Texas Health Science Center at San Antonio; Seton Family of Hospitals; St. David's HealthCare Partnership; Central Texas Veterans Healthcare System; and the Greater Austin Chamber of Commerce. In 2005, Dr. Guckian wrote about the advantages of an academic health center in a *TCMS Journal* article, pointing out that a new medical campus would take advantage of Austin's great neuroscience strengths; academically oriented clinicians and practitioners; UT faculty and investigators; and the resources of Austin and Central Texas institutions. CTI's website contains a statement explaining its goals, observing that "Inasmuch as resources may not be presently available to create a new medical school in Austin, CTI believes the most efficient, fastest, least expensive, and least complicated path to achieving the goal of having a preeminent research intensive academic health center in Austin is to establish a geographically separate clinical campus of the UT Medical Branch in Austin."

The capital area is also drawing other academically related medical institutions. Temple's Scott and White has grown into a large multispecialty and teaching hospital for Texas A&M, has set up nearby clinics, and is developing the University Medical Campus in adjacent Williamson County.

A statistical snapshot of Travis County Medical Society members in 2007 showed 2,800 members and growing, representing ninety-five of the one-hundred different specialty designations from which they could select. The most senior member until her death on September 5, 2007, was Dr. Marie Tisdale, who would have turned 98 four days later. In 1944, during World War II, she had been so proud—and relieved—when she was accepted as a member of the Travis County Medical Society. Dr. George Tipton was the oldest living former president. The beloved figure of early Texas, the general practitioner, was rare. From being the majority of doctors in mid-twentieth century, only around thirty remained and some had limited their focus. Austin's Chamber of Commerce showed that thousands more individuals also served in the health care professions.

The Blood and Tissue Center of Central Texas remains the exclusive provider of therapeutic blood products to more than thirty health care facilities in ten Texas counties. The Center also collects blood from volunteer donors at its donor centers in Austin and Round Rock and at on-site mobile blood drives hosted by community organizations, schools, churches, and employers throughout the region. The Tissue Services division, established in 1985, provides a full range of human allograft tissue products for orthopedic, neurological, cardiac, and burn surgeries.

Austin still touts its quality of life, including its inviting pool fed by underground springs and its "crystal-clear" lake.

This short history sketches only a few of those who have contributed to Travis County's history. Once again, new doctors have moved into town. They will make their own history. Time has shown, after all, that much work remains for the "medicos"—with perhaps a little serendipity over the next hill.

PROFILES IN TRAVIS COUNTY MEDICINE

THE HISTORY OF MEDICINE IN TRAVIS COUNTY stretches back over 150 years and provides a fascinating picture of the staggering changes that have taken place since the first doctor made his rounds on horseback in the early 1800s. It shows how hard physicians in Texas have worked to establish the sound practice of medicine through establishing a stable government, health and sanitary laws, the regulation of medicine, and tougher standards in medical education. On the following pages can be found a representative sampling of those men and women who are carrying on the legacy of providing quality medical care in Travis County. These profiles offer a glimpse of how the communities within the county continue to be shaped by its men and women of medicine. Whether they practice alone or as part of a group, whether they are just starting out in their practice or nearing the end of their public service, their commitment to their patients, to science, and to the public ensures that the heritage of healing in Travis County and beyond will be carried on well into the future. Though the niches they have carved out for themselves in the medical world are rich and varied, these physicians all bring to their profession a sense of dedication in treating their patients. This sense of integrity and responsibility often pours out into other parts of their lives and the people, organizations, businesses, and communities to which they contribute are the stronger for it. We give our thanks to these dedicated and talented physicians for sharing their stories.

This turn-of-the-century photograph of Austin shows Congress Avenue, looking towards the Texas State Capitol.

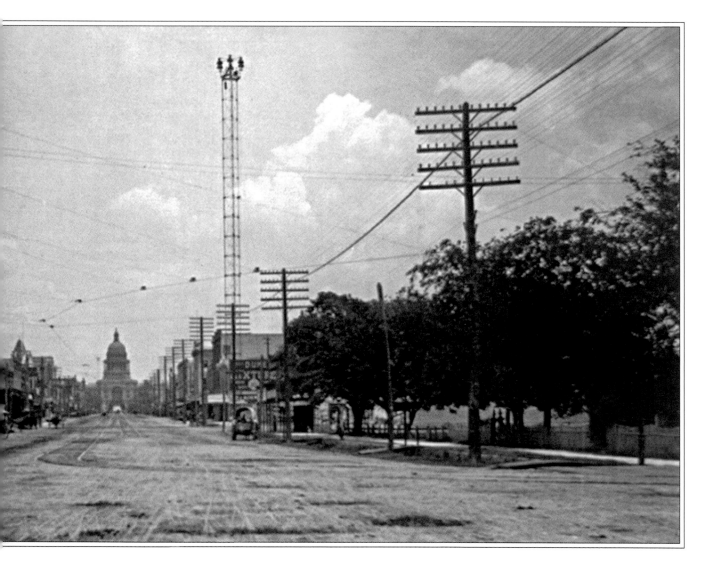

TRAVIS COUNTY MEDICAL SOCIETY

THE YEAR 2003 MARKED THE 150TH ANNIVERSARY OF THE Travis County Medical Society (TCMS), a professional organization of licensed physicians and a component society of the Texas Medical Association. With more than 2,700 members, representing 90 percent of eligible physicians in the greater Austin area, TCMS is one of the five largest county medical societies in Texas. Throughout its history, it has facilitated the joining together of physicians to share medical knowledge and to raise the standard of medical care. The Society has a history of addressing matters of importance to the profession and to the community it serves, including assistance in enacting and enforcing medical practice and public health laws as well as providing information to the public on important medical issues.

Travis County Medical Society was chartered in 1853, when Texas had been a state for only eight years and construction of the State Capitol had just begun. At its second meeting on October 22, 1853, the Texas Medical Association recognized two district medical societies: Bexar Medical Society, organized one month prior, and Travis Medi-

cal Society, officially organized that very day. Since that time, Travis County physicians have worked in partnership to address issues of public health, ethics, training, standards, and medical services.

One such example was the movement by TCMS to develop a community blood bank for Austin. A committee of five physicians undertook creation and financing of the project and in 1951, the Travis County Medical Society Blood Bank, a non-profit community blood bank governed and operated by the Medical Society, opened its doors. Known today as The Blood and Tissue Center of Central Texas, it is the exclusive blood supplier for more than 30 health care facilities in ten Central Texas counties, and provides tissue procurement services for 60 hospitals in central, east, and south Texas. The Blood and Tissue Center is the only such facility in the country still integrated with its found-

BELOW: *Deep in the Heart of Texas Medicine.* OPPOSITE PAGE: *TCMS and Project Access staff celebrating the Medical Society's sesquicentennial.*

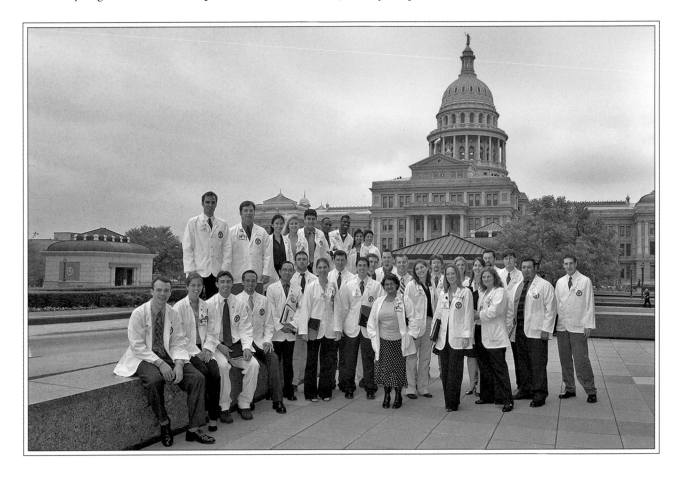

ing medical society. "Historically, Travis County physicians see a community need, and they collectively respond and take a leadership role in addressing it. This pattern has been the hallmark of the TCMS at least since the mid-twentiety century, and is what has driven the evolution of its unique organizational structure," says Marshall Cothran, TCMS Executive Vice President and CEO.

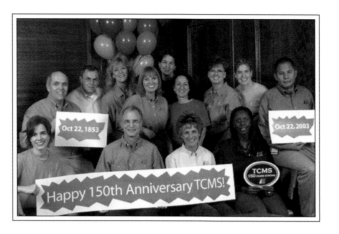

Since its inception, TCMS has strived to meet physicians' practical needs as well. In 1955, it took over operation of the Medical Exchange, and in 1957, incorporated this wholly owned subsidiary of TCMS as the Medical Service Bureau. In times past, it has provided such varied services as printing, computer consulting, cellular phone and pager sales, and patient account collection. As physician needs have changed with time, so have the services offered. One of only a few medical society-owned call centers in the country, the Medical Exchange is a high tech medical call center, processing 1.5 million transactions per year. Operators take emergency and non-emergency calls from patients, physicians, and hospitals and relay these to physicians as requested. In addition, the Medical Service Bureau provides medical records management, patient lab results reporting, virtual staffing, and other medical office services through Patient Plus. With more than 1,000 physician subscribers, the Exchange is open 24 hours a day, 7 days a week, 365 days a year.

Created in the 1960s as a subsidiary of TCMS, the Travis County Medical Society Foundation (TCMSF) has undertaken a mission of charitable, educational, and scientific endeavors. It began providing nursing scholarships at Brackenridge Hospital in 1965, and made measles inoculations available to 25,000 needy children in 1967.

In May 1972, TCMSF established another non-profit corporation, the Central Texas Medical Foundation, the objectives of which were the promotion, development, and encouragement of medical education and the distribution of medical health services and care to the people of Central Texas. In 1998, after more than 25 years of development and operations, TCMSF sold the residency programs to the Seton Family of Hospitals which operated them for eight years before transferring their sponsorship to the University of Texas Medical Branch (UTMB) in 2006 and

2007. Today, the full-time faculty, adjunct volunteer faculty, and residents of UTMB-Austin programs continue to provide medical services to anyone seeking treatment at the city-owned Brackenridge Hospital.

In an effort to provide medical information to the community, in the 1980s, TCMSF purchased telemedicine tapes and provided access to them to the public by phone. In 1991, it joined with the TCMS Alliance, a philanthropic organization of physicians' spouses, to endow a chair at the University of Texas School of Nursing, and in 2001, TCMSF sponsored the Medical Society's Symposium on Weapons of Mass Destruction.

"The Society's activist history has included the creation of many other programs, some of finite duration, that addressed particular needs of a particular time and others that are ongoing today. These have included, among others, the Central Texas Health Plan, Credentials Verification Office, Continuing Medical Education Consortium, the Austin-area common credentialing form, and the multi-facility physician identification and access badge project," says Cothran.

Project Access is yet another example of Travis County physicians stepping forward to meet a need. Project Access is a coordinated system of volunteer physician care, hospital care, diagnostic services, and medication assistance for low-income, uninsured county residents. Its ultimate goal is to deliver more care to the target population, in more appropriate settings, and for less overall cost to the system than before. Initial funding for Project Access infrastructure, staff, and acute medications was provided by grants from the Indigent Care Collaboration, TCMSF, the RGK Foundation, and the Travis County Healthcare District. In its first four years of service, Project Access physicians and partners donated $5.2 million of free care to eligible patients.

The physicians of Travis County have a long tradition of service to the profession and to the community. They have given back through volunteerism and philanthropy; they have held elected and appointed offices on school boards, city councils, state boards, and commissions; and they have served in the trenches and at all levels of leadership in organized medicine for more than 150 years.

—Barbara James

THE BLOOD AND TISSUE CENTER
OF CENTRAL TEXAS

THIS YEAR, MORE THAN 60,000 whole blood and apheresis donations were collected by The Blood Center of Central Texas at its mobile blood drives and fixed site donor centers. These donations are tested extensively to assure suitability for transfusion and processed into life saving components—red blood cells, plasma, and platelets—which go to help over 120,000 patients annually. The Center is the exclusive blood supplier for more than 30 health care facilities in ten Central Texas counties and also works with the Marrow Donor Program of Central and South Texas to increase the number of Central Texans on the National Marrow Donor Registry. The Tissue Center was established in 1985. Today, it provides tissue donor family services and performs surgical tissue recovery in communities throughout Central and South Texas. It also distributes a full range of human allograft tissue products for orthopedic, neurological, cardiovascular, and burn surgeries.

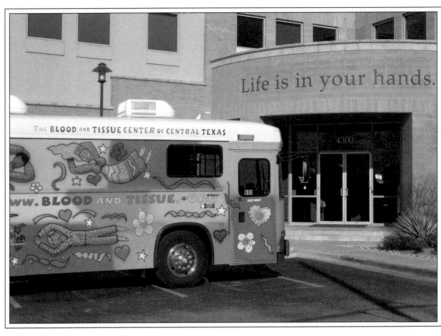

Chartered by the Travis County Medical Society (TCMS) on April 10, 1951 and opened on September 24, 1951 at 1705 North Congress Avenue, the Center was one of the first community blood banks in the nation established and operated by a medical society.

In 1947, TCMS appointed a blood bank committee made up of Drs. Sidney W. Bohls, Happy Scott, John F. Thomas, Revace O. Swearingen, and Emerson K. Blewett, with Dr. Bohls as chairman. Dr. Bohls's selection as chairman was no accident. Appointed director of laboratories for the Texas Health Department in 1928, the pathologist instituted the processing of blood plasma for civilian emergency use during World War II. The committee asked the TCMS Board to obtain the signatures of 100 members willing to pledge $200 apiece so that the blood bank could obtain a loan from one of the local banks. The response was enthusiastic and the Travis County Medical Society

Opened in 1951, the Center was one of the first community blood banks in the nation established and operated by a medical society. The Tissue Center was established in 1985.

Blood Bank, which later was named The Blood and Tissue Center of Central Texas, was chartered, thanks to the commitment of these physicians.

The history of the Center is rich with support both by and for the community. The University of Texas' pledge drive in December 1951 set a goal of 5,000 pints to benefit U.S. soldiers in Korea. The Austin Police Department presented an "Outstanding Service" award for services rendered by the Blood Bank staff during the University of Texas Tower incident on August 1, 1966. Donors immediately came to the Blood Bank following notification of the shootings and the facility stayed open late into the night. Such has been the response of this community and its Blood Center to many local and national tragedies over the last 50 plus years.

The name and location of the Blood Bank has changed several times over the years as The Blood and Tissue Center of Central Texas evolved to serve a much larger population and hospital base as a full-service, fully accredited, regional blood and tissue center.

ADULT CARE OF AUSTIN

THE FIRST THING YOU WILL NOTICE upon entering Adult Care of Austin is a "greeter"—someone to personally welcome each patient and give that person whatever is needed, whether it's a snack, something to drink, or just a friendly face with whom to talk. When you are in the waiting room, you feel as if you are in your living room—a warm, welcoming atmosphere. When you are in some of the exam rooms, you'll see pictures of Dr. Sonstein's patients adorning the walls. Each room has a distinct personality: one displays artifacts from Dr. Sonstein's mission trips while others have themes such as the University of Texas-Aggie rivalry. The hallway is lined with pictures of staff members and their families.

Because a large portion of Dr. Sonstein's practice is older people, his practice is specially equipped to serve the senior community. Dr. Sonstein likes dealing with the whole person concentrating on the physical and emotional well-being by practicing continuity of care. To insure that continuity, Dr. Sonstein has nurse practitioners who make house calls, assisted living, and nursing home visits, a physical therapist, an audiologist and speech pathologist, and a social worker, all available to serve his patients' individual needs. Dr. Sonstein and his partners are considered "traditionalists"—they take care of their patients both in the office, and at the hospital where they round twice a day.

Almost yearly, Dr. Sonstein can be found in the impoverished villages of Central America. For one week a year, Dr. Sonstein, his wife and part of his staff, at their own expense, treat and care for needy patients.

Dr. Sonstein has been in practice in Austin since 1978 and several of his staff members have been with him for over 20 years. He arrived in Texas via the National Health Ser-

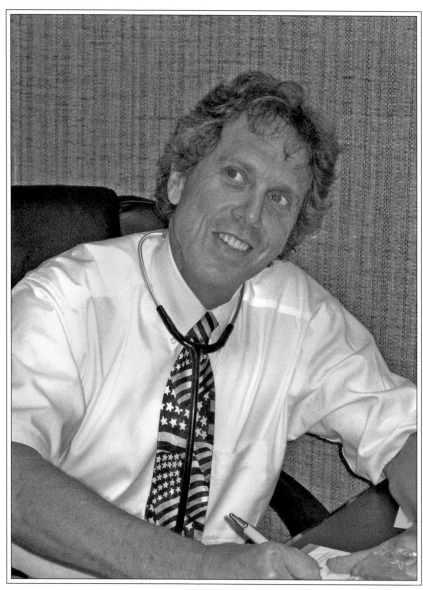

Allen Sonstein, M.D. of Adult Care of Austin.

vice Corp where he served two years in Waelder, Texas, a rural, medically underserved area. For those who remember the TV show *Northern Exposure*, this was him but in Texas rather than Alaska. Dr. Sonstein is an advocate for the patient and strongly believes in excellent care. He also believes in partnership, empathy, respect, and support for his patients. The mission statement of Adult Care of Austin best summarizes his belief: *"The best possible continuous, comprehensive, and personal care delivered with the kindness, understanding, respect, and dignity that you deserve."*

ALLERGY & ASTHMA CONSULTANTS

A NATIVE AUSTINITE AND a doctor for over 50 years, Dr. Theo Painter has more than just watched the changes in medicine and Austin's landscape; he has been a contributor, as the first allergist in Central Texas certified by the American Board of Allergy and Immunology, a founder of Texas Allergy Society, and president of Austin Doctors Building Corporation (ADBC). He also started the first charity allergy clinic at Brackenridge Hospital and was a bank director for many years.

Soon after Pearl Harbor, Painter's medical training quickly transformed into year-round medical school in a navy training program, where he graduated at the age of 22. He then did general practice in Columbus, Texas for three months

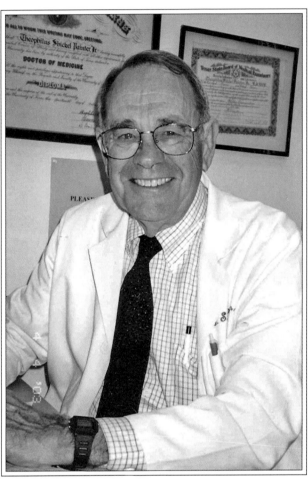

Theo S. Painter, Jr., M.D.

while he waited to begin a rotating internship and internal medicine residency at the University of Michigan and to be certified by the American Board of Internal Medicine. He then served with the Air Force in California and helped manage allergy patients. After practicing internal medicine for two and a half years in San Antonio, he returned to a fellowship in Allergy Medicine at the University of Michigan. In 1958, Dr. Painter returned to Austin to establish his allergy practice.

During the 1960s, he joined with eight physicians to pool together money to build new office space. They formed ADBC, which eventually involved 65 shareholders—all physicians and dentists except for one business manager, Mr. M. K. Hage—and changed Austin at 38th and Lamar. They acquired 190 separate lots of land in central Austin, built Medical Park Tower and Bailey Square

Office Building, arranged the construction of Shoal Creek Hospital, and sold 15 acres to Seton (at cost) for building Seton Medical Center. Dr. Painter served as president of ADBC during its decade-long era of construction. "I enjoyed being involved in major business decisions. It was an interesting time," admits Dr. Painter. Drs. Joseph Bailey, Pruett Watkins, Robert Ellzey, George Shia (DDS), William Turpin, and Stuart Nemir, among others, also played prominent roles. Mr. Hage provided business sense and imagination.

On the top floor of the Bailey Square Building, the doctors' corporation built the first outpatient surgical center in Texas, beginning the trend to reduce the cost of some surgical procedures by as much as two-thirds. This facility gained national attention for its planning and management, and as a result, Mr. Hage and Dr. Painter traveled to Kuwait to discuss building such a facility there.

The corporation expanded its mission to develop a regional medical center. Also, before dissolving, the corporation donated and dedicated Seiders Park and prepared it for the city as part of Austin's hike-and-bike trail.

Today, Dr. Painter practices in offices two blocks from where he was raised. Outside his office window, he can see the results of his leadership. "I can hardly believe what was here when we started, gravel roads and small homes, and now all these medical buildings." His favorite satisfaction, though, still comes from being a doctor, giving medical care to people—some restricted all their lives due to allergies or asthma—so they can lead normal, healthy lives.

AUSTIN FAMILY MEDICINE ASSOCIATES

"I ENJOY KEEPING MY PATIENTS HEALTHY AND GUIDING them to improved health through close attention to sound preventive health practices," says David Sneed, D.O., whose practice certainly focuses on wellness and treatment of a variety of illnesses commonly seen in family medicine such as diabetes, heart disease, hypertension, and depression. Dr. Sneed first opened his medical practice in Austin in 1985. "There have been many changes in Austin and medical practice in those years," he says, noting that many of his patients have been his patient for many years and that that aspect of family medicine makes it a personally rewarding profession.

Dr. Sneed has served on the South Austin Hospital board of trustees and as its chairman. "Austin has a great medical community that everyone can be proud of," he says. He wants to thank all the consultants throughout Austin that have helped him and his patients over the past 22 years. He looks forward to the future in Austin and anticipates continuing to practice for many years, but also looks forward to adding new physicians to his practice.

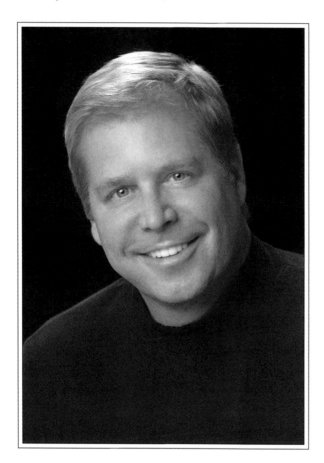

David Sneed, D.O.

A longtime interest in dermatology led Dr. Sneed to incorporate a wide range of non-invasive cosmetic dermatology procedures into his practice when he created Aesthetica MedSpa, one of the first Medspa clinics in Austin. "Our office is set up to take care of ninety percent of the medical needs that a person might have and the addition of our cosmetic services through Aesthetica MedSpa has expanded our potential patient care even further. Advances in light and laser technology, as well as new injectable treatments such as Botox Cosmetic," and various tissue fillers have revolutionized cosmetic dermatology," he says.

Dr. Sneed has achieved state and national recognition for his esthetic practice and has achieved some of the highest levels of recognition for Botox Cosmetic™ injections and the use of Restylane™ for tissue rejuvenation. Additionally, he has become a leader in the placement of Contour Threadlifts. The threadlift is a non-invasive procedure that provides an option for those patients that desire a skin lifting procedure, but either do not want or do not need a full surgical facelift. Patients from across the state and even other countries come to Austin for his help with these cosmetic procedures.

One of the aspects of medicine that initially attracted Dr. Sneed to a medical career is the variety and continual change that takes place in the practice of medicine. "Even with all the frustrations of health insurance issues, I can honestly say that I look forward continually to seeing my patients and helping them achieve better health through what we do in our clinic," says Dr. Sneed. He notes that patients still surprise him in a variety of ways and the challenge of today's medical environment still intrigues him. "Where else can you impact the lives of people so directly?" he asks. "Both aspects of my practice are evolving, family medicine will see many more changes before I hang up my stethoscope and some of the most rapid advances are being made in the field of cosmetic dermatology right now," he concludes.

Dr. Sneed's office offers a wide variety of solutions for both medical and cosmetic dermatology issues and he is passionate about the care his patients receive, embracing the changing treatments and technologies that improve their health and well-being.

ANNE L. ALEXANDER, M.D.

AFTER BEING GENTLY NUDGED IN THE direction of medicine by an encouraging high school biology teacher and inspired by Dr. Grover Bynum, her parents' longtime internist, Dr. Alexander committed herself to medical school. Before then, she gained some experience in the business world, which included assisting Dr. Donald Ward in running a clinic at the People's Community Clinic in Austin. Now, with her business know-how, specialized medical training, and "a lot of help" from her family in Austin, she has achieved success as a solo practitioner in primary care.

"Because it's a small office, I can be more responsive to my patients, which helps increase patient compliance. They also have more access to me at the hospital because I'm part of a five-doctor call group," says Dr. Alexander. "Having my own practice also

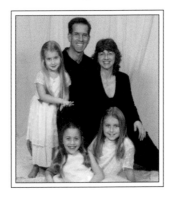

Clockwise from top left, Miriam Rose Kessler, David J. Kessler, M.D., Anne L. Alexander, M.D., Rachel Kessler and Danielle Kessler.

means more control over my personal life."

In 1990 she graduated from medical school at University of Texas Southwestern Medical Center at Dallas, where she next completed her residency program in primary care and internal medicine. She stayed in Dallas as a faculty member for three years, and then worked for Scott & White Clinic in Temple, both teaching and providing patient care. After eagerly returning to Austin with her husband, a cardiac electrophysiologist and now father of her three children, she opened her practice in February 2003. "Never the same day twice," she says. Dr. Alexander provides comprehensive care that includes the diagnosis, treatment, and management of everything from heart failure and diabetes to routine female visits, skin examinations, and blood work.

LOUIS W. APOSTOLAKIS, M.D.

DURING HIS TRAINING AT MEDICAL school in his home state of Ohio, Dr. Louis Apostolakis was inspired by an excellent teacher in Otolaryngology to pursue his first specialty, Otolaryngology. During his residency at the Otolaryngology-Head and Neck Surgery Department at the University of Iowa School of Medicine, the next pivotal teacher in his life appeared, this time a facial plastic surgeon.

While working on his fellowship with renowned plastic surgeon Dr. E. Gaylon McCullough in Alabama, the head nurse there, who was a Texan, often encouraged Dr. Apostolakis to consider Texas in his search for a home for his family and future practice. "My wife said she never wanted to see snow again and everyone said that Austin was the best city in Texas, so we decided to visit,"

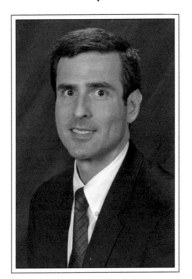

remembers Dr. Apostolakis. "We thought it was beautiful."

Once he had moved to Austin, taken out a business loan, and opened shop, Austin's economy was diving from its original tech-driven peak, but the city still seemed inviting. The competitive nature of the plastic surgery business was tempered with congeniality, and patients were drawn to "Dr. A.," a doctor they felt they could "really talk to." "I have a lot of fun with my patients," admits Dr. Apostolakis. "It's nice to do surgery on people who are looking forward to it, instead of dreading it."

In 2007, six years after arriving in Austin, Dr. Apostolakis finds the city recuperating economically, his business growing steadily, and the time when he can broaden his horizons and get more involved with his community approaching quickly.

ASSOCIATES IN GENERAL SURGERY

THESE THREE GENERAL SURGEONS FROM DIFFERENT CULtural backgrounds all agree: Austin is a great place to live and to practice medicine, its educated population engendering an advanced and invigorated medical environment. The doctors also share an attraction to the hands-on, technical work that is among the most diverse of the medical specialties.

Founder Dr. Jean-Pierre Forage first worked in Austin as part of Houston's St. Joseph trauma unit. After his time at Brackenridge Hospital and after considering locations across the country, he decided to settle in the livable and friendly *third coast*, and set up his solo practice in Austin in August 1983. Since 1989, Dr. Forage has been using the minimally invasive techniques of laparoscopic surgery,

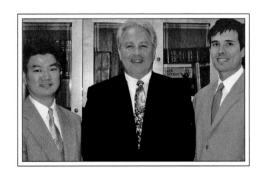

From left to right, H. Christopher Shin, M.D., Jean-Pierre Forage, M.D., and Alex Esquivel, M.D.

which he learned from inventor Eddie Reddick, to which he added his own developed techniques.

By 2000, the growing practice made room for another doctor, Dr. Christopher Shin, a hard-working, "bread-and-butter" general surgeon who had migrated to the U.S. from South Korea at the age of ten. Dr. Shin left his private practice in Corpus Christi to move to Austin. "It was a great opportunity in a great city."

The next year, Dr. Esquivel, who was practicing in Omaha at the time, learned that the team was "ready for another partner." The doctor, who came to the United States from Mexico City, also at the age of ten, was ready to move his new family to Austin. Since then, he has become well-known in the city for his laparoscopic surgery. Together, the three now serve their patients in their North, South, and Central offices.

AUSTIN ALLERGY ASSOCIATES

IT SHOULD COME AS NO SURPRISE that among the busiest of doctors in Travis County are allergists and Austin Allergy Associates is no exception. Drs. P. Dennis Dyer and T. Ray Vaughan say there are only two months of the year, August and November, when their practice isn't swamped with people in need of allergy relief.

Of course, asthma is one respiratory affliction that never takes time off. Both doctors treated asthma patients early in their careers. "My number one admission (to the hospital) was asthma," says Dr. Dyer of the beginning stages of his long career. Both doctors agree that a break in helping asthmatics came in the early 1980s when the medical profession recognized asthma as an inflammatory disease rather than one of airway constriction. Dr. Vaughan says

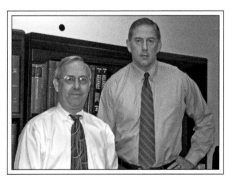

T. Ray Vaughan, M.D. (left) and P. Dennis Dyer, M.D. of Austin Allergy Associates.

through treatment they are able to make many of their patients feel "asthma free," "a gratifying, positive part of being an allergist," he adds.

One of the most satisfying cases for the practice was a young boy whose mother had restricted his activity for fear of an asthma attack. When the child came to the practice, Dr. Dyer changed his medication to a steroid spray, did peak flow monitoring, and instituted an asthma action plan to treat the boy at home. This change turned the child's life around, freeing him to participate in sports and play outdoors with his friends. The doctors share a past as both educators and military physicians. They also envision a future of helping central Texans breathe more easily in one of the country's most allergic climates.

AUSTIN ASSOCIATION OF PLASTIC SURGEONS

IT'S RARE TO FIND A GROUP OF PHYSICIANS WHO WORK AS closely together as the Austin plastic surgeons. This group of doctors doesn't appear to compete with one another. In fact, they work as a cohesive team, referring patients to the plastic surgeon they feel will best serve the patient's needs. Their reach stretches far beyond cosmetics, restoring function to burn and assault victims, and helping children with birth defects and other deformities.

The rich history of Travis county plastic surgery can be traced to one man. Dr. Francis Morris is known as the father of plastic surgery in Austin. It was 1960, and plastic surgery was an uncharted specialty in central Texas. That's when Dr. Morris first came to town and began performing miracles on grateful patients. "I was well received by the medical community in Austin which consisted of between 75 and 80 physicians," said Dr. Morris. He specialized in caring for those with burns and deformities. He also helped patients who were injured, restoring hands to working order.

Following Dr. Morris, was William Barnes Jr., M.D. Dr. Barnes set up practice in Austin in July 1964. Like his colleague Dr. Morris, Dr. Barnes studied plastic surgery at Duke University. Although he initially treated cases of trauma and burns, in 1973 he turned his practice toward cosmetic procedures, including more than ten thousand breast augmentations. In addition to his plastic surgery practice, Dr. Barnes is an accomplished artist in bronze, scrimshaw, and photography.

It was several years later that Austin got its third plastic surgeon when Dr. Patrick Beckham set up practice here in 1971. Dr. Beckham is recognized by his colleagues for several achievements. He was president of the Texas Society of Plastic Surgeons from 1979 to 1980, and was the first physician to have a hand fellowship. He is a member of the American Society of Hand Surgeons. Dr. Beckham is well known for his work with children suffering from cleft lips and palettes and is one of the founders of Austin Smiles, a non-profit organization providing reconstructive plastic surgery to children from Austin to Latin America. The Austin Smiles team generously provides surgery to children in need, regardless of their familys' ability to pay. Most of the surgeries performed are to repair cleft lips and palates which help to restore speech and breathing functions to children and give them healthy, normal lives.

Shortly after Dr. Beckham's arrival in Austin, plastic surgeon Dr. Richard Parker joined the central Texas medi-

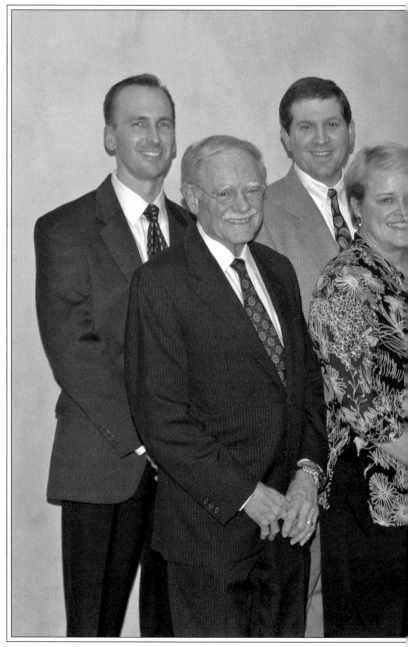

cal community. Like Dr. Beckham, he is also one of the founding partners of Austin Smiles. Dr. Parker is known for a lot of firsts in Austin: He began the very first outpatient surgical center here, he started the cleft lip and palate team, and he started breast cancer reconstruction surgery in Austin. Another plastic surgeon to come to Aus-

tin in the early 1970s was Dr. Victor LiPalaez. Like Drs. Beckham and Parker, Dr. LiPalaez was instrumental in setting up Austin Smiles. Although he has been in practice for a long time, Dr. LiPalaez still takes emergency calls. He is also known to service the poor and underinsured. In addition, Dr. LiPalaez is able to serve the Spanish-speaking population of central Texas, as he is completely fluent in the language.

James Fox, M.D., who came to Austin around the same time as Drs. Beckham, Parker, and LiPalaez, is another of the founding partners of Austin Smiles. He is a general plastic surgeon who is known for his work with cleft lips and palates. He is a past president of the Texas Society of Plastic Surgeons and is one of the few plastic surgeons in central Texas known to assist in gender re-identification surgeries. Another founder of Austin Smiles is Dr. Robert Clement, whose plastic surgery practice is dedicated to breast reconstruction and who was voted one of the best plastic surgeons in America by his peers an impressive seven times. The results were published in *The Best Doctors in America*. Other plastic surgeons to join the Austin community in the 1970s were Drs. William Davis and Robert Ersek. Dr. Davis performed the first thumb transplant in Austin. Dr. Ersek is considered the most published plastic surgeon in Austin. He has developed his own breast implant and is known worldwide for his Lipoplasty University.

The 1980s brought eight new plastic surgeons to Austin, including its first female plastic surgeon, and several who went on to become president of the Texas Society of Plastic Surgeons. Dr. Karin Montero is not only the first female plastic surgeon in Austin, she is among the few who are bilingual. Dr. Montero is a contributor to Austin Smiles, making journeys to Latin America to help

Members of the Austin Association of Plastic Surgeons, back row, left to right: Kelly Tjelmeland, M.D., Steven Holzman, M.D., James Cullington, M.D., Sanjay Sharma, M.D., and Dustin Reid, M.D.; front row, left to right: Patrick Beckham, M.D., Karin Montero, M.D., Ashley Gordon, M.D., and Ned Snyder, IV, M.D.

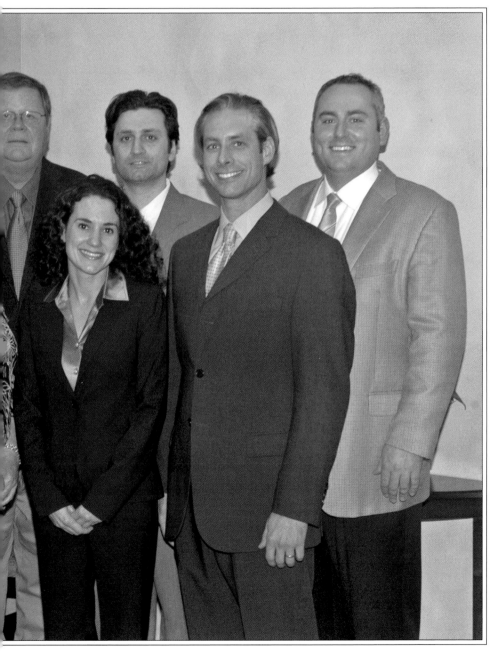

poor children with birth defects. Dr. N. D. Moscoe is also one of the founders of Austin Smiles. He has his own surgical center, but is also affiliated with all of Austin's major hospitals, giving patients a choice when it comes to their care. Drs. Alfred Wilder and David Wishnew also both came to Austin in the 1980s. Dr. Wilder is a founding member of Austin Smiles and travels the world repairing cleft lips and palates. *Austin Monthly* magazine has recognized Dr. Wilder as "one of the best plastic surgeons in Austin." He is quickly becoming known for his treatment of formerly obese patients and is able to remove excess skin giving patients a much improved overall look. In addition to a multidimensional plastic surgery practice, he also performs traumatic reconstructive surgery.

Other plastic surgeons who came to Austin in the 1980s include Drs. James Cullington, Umesh Gadaria, William Gorman, and David Turner. Dr. Turner is a past president of the Texas Society of Plastic Surgeons and specializes in breast reconstruction and cosmetic surgery. He is also on the cleft palate team and donates his time to the Austin Smiles Organization. Like Dr. Turner, Dr. James Cullington is a past president of the Texas Society of Plastic Surgeons. Dr. Cullington's organizational skills are well documented. He is responsible for creating the Austin Society of Plastic Surgery. He also established the emergency call schedule to serve Austin's indigent community, a practice he has maintained for more than 20 years. In addition to those roles, Dr. Cullington also established the Brackenridge Hospital Wound Management Clinic and he is among the founders of Austin Smiles. In the operating room, he is best known for his microsurgery and flaps, which he performs for cancer and trauma patients.

Dr. Umesh Gadaria, along with his wife, Patty, runs the Advanced Skin Care and Laser Surgery center. In addition to anti-aging skin care techniques, Dr. Gadaria also performs general plastic surgery. Dr. Gadaria has contributed his time to the Austin Smiles organization. Dr. William Gorman has been practicing medicine since 1983. The bulk of his practice is aesthetic surgery but also performs cancer reconstruction. Dr. Gorman has been a contributor to Austin Smiles.

By the 1990s, word was circulating about the cohesive, friendly atmosphere enjoyed by Austin plastic surgeons and several other physicians joined this dynamic group. Among them is Texas native, Dr. Jeffrey Hall. Dr. Hall has served as chief of Plastic Surgery at Seton Medical Network, and is a past president of the Austin Plastic Surgery Society. Like many of Austin's plastic surgeons, Dr. Hall participates in the Austin Smiles organization, traveling to countries the world over to help disadvantaged children. Dr. Steven Holzman specializes in several types of cosmetic surgery, including an extensive number of dermatological procedures. He has served as president of the Austin Society of Plastic Surgeons. Partnered with Dr. Holzman is Dr. David Mosier, a past president of the Austin Society of Plastic Surgery. At the Plastic Surgery Center of Austin, Dr. Mosier does a great deal of cosmetic surgery on the face and breast, as well as other parts of the body.

Dr. Timothy McGee serves the Round Rock area. His practice is multidisciplined, but specializes in reconstructive and cosmetic surgery. Dr. Troy Thompson has opened a general plastic surgery center in Round Rock. Dr. Martin Schaeferle, III, joined Dr. Ersek at the Personique practice. He served the United States as a naval doctor in both South Korea and Vietnam and is a recipient of the Naval Achievement Medal. Following his military service, he practiced plastic surgery in Washington state before coming to Austin. Dr. Deidre Rhoad, whose practice includes traumatic reconstruction along with cosmetic surgery, is the second female plastic surgeon in the Austin area.

Five physicians joined the Austin community of plastic surgeons between 2000 and 2005. These include: Dr. Sanjay Sharma, a hand specialist; Dr. Kelly Tjelmeland, who operates his own surgical center for trauma and cosmetic surgery; Dr. James Robison, IV, who has a full-service plastic surgery practice; Dr. Sergio Maggi, who has delved into brachioplasty reconstruction and who is the founder and served as director of the Austin Plastic Surgery Center; and Dr. Robert Caridi who serves the Austin community with a wide range of cosmetic plastic surgery services. He and his family have been featured on the ABC network television show *Good Morning America*. Dr. Patrick Kelley has been in the Austin area since July 2005 and is the chief of craniofacial and reconstructive plastic surgery at the new Dell Children's Medical Center of Central Texas.

The following physicians have also joined the Austin plastic surgery community: Dr. Scott Haydon, who has set up a full cosmetic and reconstructive practice servicing a surgery center in West Austin and who has partnered with the newest member (as of this writing), Dr. Ashley Gordon; Dr. Dustin Reid who opened a general plastic surgery center in Central Austin; and Dr. Ned Snyder, a fully trained plastic surgeon who has partnered with his wife, Dr. Renee Snyder, a dermatologist. Together, the Snyders are running a cosmetic and dermatology practice and are quickly becoming an asset to the Austin community.

AUSTIN NEUROLOGICAL CLINIC/SLEEP MEDICINE CONSULTANTS

Dr. J. Douglas Hudson graduated from The University of Texas Medical Branch in Galveston. Following his residency in Neurology at the University of Iowa he came to Austin as the second neurologist in town. Since then, Dr. Hudson has dedicated himself to pioneering the community's neurological services. Joined by Dr. Peter Werner, Dr. Hudson founded the Austin Neurological Clinic in 1970, and three years later introduced Austin's first CT scanner. Dr. Hudson also provided the city's first MRI, EEG lab with 24-hour monitoring services, neurochemistry lab, and one of Austin's first neurovascular ultrasound labs. In 1980, he co-founded one of the nation's first sleep labs.

Dr. Hudson has enriched the field of Neurology in a broader capacity and is the reputed local "father of neurology." In 1972, he aided the formation of the Austin Neurological Society and also served as president of the Texas Neurological Society. Dr. Hudson helped recruit Austin's first physical medicine and rehabilitation physician, neuroradiologist, pediatric neurologist, and the first neuropsychologist to establish a private practice with neurologists. He is board certified in Neurology and Neuro-rehabilitation.

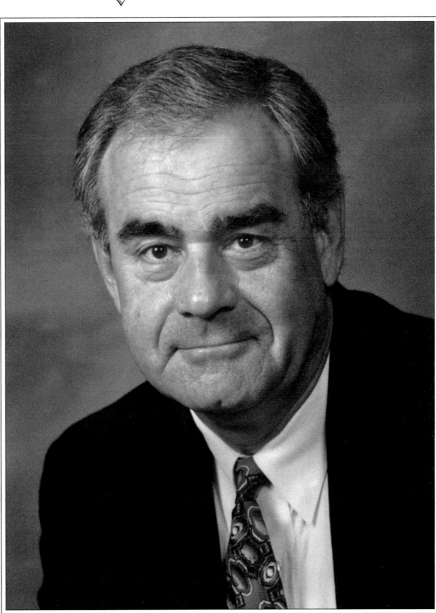

Dr. J. Douglas Hudson, the "father of Neurology" in Austin.

In recent years, Dr. Hudson has refocused his attention to sleep medicine. His passion to explore sleep and its effect on serious health conditions led him to become the first board certified sleep medicine doctor in Travis County and a renowned leader on the subject of sleep. Dr. Hudson founded Sleep Medicine Consultants in 2001. In addition to his private practice, hospital, and community work, he is currently the medical director of several area sleep labs. As an international speaker on sleep disorders, a principal investigator in sleep and neurology-related drug research, and a well-respected practitioner, Dr. Hudson continues to treat patients and educate health care professionals and the public on sleep and other neurological concerns.

AUSTIN BONE AND JOINT CLINIC, P.A.

AFTER WORLD WAR II, FORMER CLASSMATES DR. KERMIT Fox and Dr. Lawrence Griffin met at the Campbell Clinic in Tennessee. In 1948 they moved to Austin and established the foundation for the Austin Bone and Joint Clinic, the oldest orthopedic clinic in Austin.

Since then, the fledgling specialty of orthopedic surgery has developed to include highly sophisticated treatments for the musculoskeletal system. The clinic did the first total hip replacement in Austin in 1971 and the first total knee replacement in 1972. Today, they continue to expand the variety of procedures they perform and have developed a reputation for their work in all aspects of orthopedic surgery.

Following in the founders' footsteps, the clinic's physicians maintain a culture of tolerance and information-sharing within the group and share it with their greater commu-

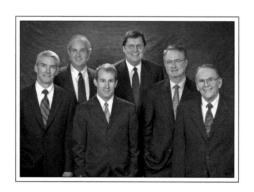

nity. All of the doctors at the Clinic have served as instructors for residents from Austin and San Antonio and have served on countless committees in the community hospitals, as well as the Travis County Medical Society and the Texas Medical Association (TMA). Drs. Chenault and Malone have served as presidents of the local medical society, Dr. Fox as the president of the Texas Orthopedic Society, Dr. Greenway as president of the Blood and Tissue Center of Central Texas, Dr. Malone as a TMA board member and a delegate to the American Medical Association, and Dr. Stephen Pearce as an examiner for the American Board of Orthopedic Surgery.

Left to right, Stephen Pearce, M.D., John Pearce, M.D., Earl Kilbride, M.D., Bruce Malone, M.D., Don Greenway, M.D., and Christopher Chenault, M.D.

AUSTIN COLON & RECTAL CLINIC ASSOCIATION

THE AUSTIN COLON & RECTAL CLINIC Association was the first clinic in the city to specialize in Colon and Rectal Surgery. The clinic grew out of the practice of Dr. Andrew Hibbert, Jr., who became Austin's first board-certified colon and rectal surgeon in 1973. It is now under the joint direction of David C. Fleeger, M.D., and

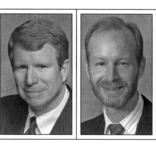

Ernest D. Graves, III, M.D., who are both board certified and fellows in their specialty. The clinic operates at two locations, which both feature amenities specific to colon and rectal surgery. The partners focus on the diagnosis and treatment of colon cancer, inflammatory bowel disease, anorectal disease, colonoscopy, and laparoscopic colon surgery.

Dr. Fleeger, who arrived in Austin in 1991, attended medical school at Texas A&M University, performed his General Surgery residency at the Mayo Clinic, and completed his fel-

lowship in Colon and Rectal Surgery at Louisiana State University at Shreveport. Dr. Graves, who joined the clinic in 2000, attended medical school at Louisiana State University in New Orleans, performed his general surgery residency at the Ochsner Clinic in New Orleans, and completed his fellowship in Colon and Rectal Surgery at the University of Texas Health Science Center in Houston.

The partners were both inspired to specialize in Colon and Rectal Surgery by the enthusiasm of their physician mentors, who impressed upon them that doctors who become expert in a finite specialty can provide more efficient, quality care to patients. As a result, Doctors Fleeger *(pictured left)* and Graves *(pictured right)*, who are committed to maintaining a high-level of patient care, continue to expand their practice with state-of-the-art colon and rectal techniques.

AUSTIN ENDOMETRIOSIS AND FEMALE INFERTILITY CENTER

AFTER BOUNDING ACROSS CONTINENTS TO DEVELOP his medical skills, Dr. Kavoussi brought his passion—treating infertility and pelvic pain in women—to Austin. Since 1983, he has led the Austin Endometriosis and Female Infertility Center with his wife, Homa, by his side, and has become the city's most experienced doctor in treating endometriosis.

Even before his schoolboy days in Yazd, Iran, Kavoussi—inspired by his pediatrician—wanted to be a doctor. His father, a hard-working entrepreneur responsible for bringing electricity to their town, encouraged him to pursue higher education. Young Kavoussi traveled to the United States, where he attended Columbia University, learned English, and accumulated pre-med prerequisites at Baylor University. He received a scholarship to attend medical school in Shiraz, Iran, and then returned to the United States for an Ob/Gyn residency at Bayview Hospital at Johns Hopkins University.

He then did a fellowship in Reproductive Endocrinology and Infertility at the University of Maryland Hospital.

After completing his education, Dr. Kavoussi taught in Iran and then at Brackenridge Hospital as an assistant professor from the University of Texas Health Science Center in Houston. He was designated as Director of Obstetrics/Gynecology at Brackenridge Hospital in Austin for a year. Thereafter, he opened his clinic, which now includes laparoscopic and hysteroscopic treatment for fibroid tumors, and infertility treatment. He mostly enjoys helping women through his gynecology and fertility practice, especially those who have previously encountered challenges.

Two of his three sons have adopted his zeal for medicine. His oldest son, Shahryar, completed a fellowship in Reproductive Endocrinology and Infertility and joined the clinic in 2007. His youngest son, Parviz, is completing his Urology residency.

AUSTIN GASTROENTEROLOGY, P.A.

AS A BOY GROWING UP IN JALANDHAR, in Punjab, India, Harish Gagneja received intramuscular injections from his family physician that were so unpleasant that he swore he would get back at him by becoming a doctor and giving those same shots to the physician. He never got back at the physician, but he did become the first doctor in his family. Dr. Gagneja now enjoys the relief and comfort he provides his patients with digestive disorders.

Dr. Gagneja completed his residency training at Cleveland Clinic

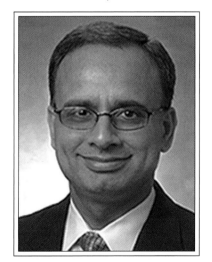

Health Care System in Cleveland, Ohio and did a gastroenterology fellowship at State University of New York in Buffalo, New York. He then served as Assistant Professor and Co-director of the GI fellowship program at University of Texas M.D. Anderson Cancer Center in Houston.

While in Houston, he sometimes ventured to nearby Austin. "I should practice here," thought Dr. Gagneja, impressed with the landscape, the quality of medical care, and the friendly people. Though he did not know a single person there, he moved his family and put his anchor down in Austin. He joined the staff at the Austin Medical Education Program and began his gastroenterology practice.

After only two years, he has attracted loyal clients who appreciate his willingness to patiently listen to their concerns. In August 2004, Dr. Gagneja joined Austin Gastroenterology, PA, the field's premier and largest group in central Texas, further establishing himself in the city and field he loves, and allowing him more time for family, hobbies, and community work.

AUSTIN ORTHOPAEDICS, SPINE, AND SPORTS MEDICINE ASSOCIATES

A BOARD-CERTIFIED ORTHOPAEDIC SURGEON, NEWT Hasson, M.D. is in private practice with Austin Ortho-paedics, Spine, and Sports Medicine Associates in South Austin. He has a general orthopaedic practice with a special interest in sports medicine, knee arthro-scopy and ligament reconstruc-tion, as well as total joint replace-ments of the hip and knee. A football and lacrosse player him-self for many years, Hasson treats athletes from all over Central Texas. On staff at South Austin Hospital since 1983, when it was but a small community hospital, Hasson is notorious for perform-ing surgeries "with his boots on" —literally. As a concession to his passion for football at the Uni-versity of Texas, the hospital ad-ministration agreed to paint his operating room burnt orange, the school's color.

A native of Baltimore, Dr. Hasson attended Duke Univer-sity on a football scholarship, majoring in physics. While at Duke, he was a two-year varsity letterman as an offensive line-man, and was the team's "Scholar-Athlete" in his senior year. As a midfielder on the Duke lacrosse team, Hasson was voted "Rookie of the Year," "Best Offensive Player," and "Captain." Hasson also was named to the Atlantic Coast Conference Honor Roll for "Outstanding Academic Achievement" and was president of the senior class at Duke.

Hasson returned to Duke University for his Doctor of Medicine degree, did his internship and residency in Or-thopaedic Surgery at Stanford University, and completed

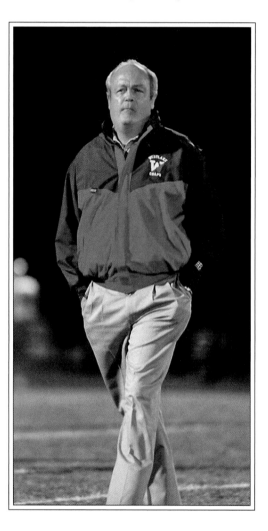

Dr. Newt Hasson of Austin Orthopaedics, Spine, and Sports Medicine Associates has been recognized by the Consumers' Research Council as one of "America's Top Physicians," most recently in 2007.

a fellowship in Sports Medicine at the renowned Hughston Orthopaedic Clinic in Columbus, Georgia.

Moving to Texas because he wanted to be where "football is king," Dr. Hasson has been on the sidelines as a team physician for more than 20 years with Westlake High School. In this role, he is able to combine his passion for the game with his gift for practic-ing medicine and the desire to be involved with the youth of the community. Previously, he has served as team physician for schools in California, Georgia, Alabama, and close to home at Del Valle High School and the Texas School for the Deaf. Hasson is active in Eanes ISD middle school athletics and has coached in numerous West Austin/West-lake youth sports programs.

Committed to giving back to the community, Dr. Hasson has invested his time with a select number of boards related to medi-cine, sports, or ministry. He cur-rently serves on the board of di-rectors of the Greater Austin Chapter of the National Football Foundation and College Hall of Fame. Previously, he has served both as medical director and on the board of directors for the Texas Special Olympics, and on the board of South Austin Chap-lain Ministries and the Greater Austin Chapter of the Fel-lowship of Christian Athletes. Hasson has received the "Champions of FCA" and "You Make a Difference in EISD" awards, and the "Contribution to Amateur Football" award.

Hasson and his wife, Pam, have three children, Lauren, Duke, and Meredith.

AUSTIN PEDIATRIC SURGERY

IN 1972, DR. ABRAHAM BESSERMAN FOUNDED THE Austin Pediatric Surgery Association and brought to this area a previously unrealized ability to care for children with complex congenital anomalies and with severe prematurity. He was joined by Dr. Robert Schlechter in 1984. In the midst of a rapidly expanding need for children's health services, Drs. Schlechter and Besserman were essential motivating forces in the 1988 construction of the Children's Hospital of Austin. Dr. Mark Smith, and subsequently Dr. Jeff Horwitz, came to Austin in the 1990s and grew a large practice of their own called Children's Surgical Associates. Similarly, in the first years of the new millennium, Dr. Schlechter was joined by Drs. Tory Meyer, Julie Sanchez, and Michael Josephs to meet the growing needs for pediatric surgical services. In 1995, the pediatric surgeons joined the pediatric community in calling for the transfer of management of Children's and Brackenridge Hospitals from the city to the Seton healthcare network. Only 10 years later, with urging from the medical community, Seton agreed to build a new children's hospital as an anchor to the new development at the old Mueller Airport site. In 2007, The Dell Children's Medical Center of Central Texas was opened with expanded capacity and capabilities and the pediatric surgeons had once more played instrumental roles in the design and programs of this new hospital. Dr. Smith and Dr. Schlechter played key positions in the building of the Strictly Pediatrics medical office building and outpatient surgery center adjacent to the new hospital. Also in 2007, the two previously separate pediatric surgery groups merged to form one group of six surgeons called Austin Pediatric Surgery (APS).

The most senior partner of present-day APS is Dr. Robert Schlechter who did his surgery residency at Tulane University and his fellowship in pediatric surgery at McGill University-The Montreal Children's Hospital before coming to Austin.

Dr. Mark Smith also completed his surgery residency at Tulane University and did a fellowship in pediatric surgery at LeBonheur Children's Medical Center. In addition, Dr. Smith did a pediatric surgical oncology fellowship at M.D. Anderson Cancer Center.

After his general surgery residency in Philadelphia at the Medical College of Pennsylvania, Dr. Jeff Horwitz did a surgical critical care and ECMO fellowship in Houston at the University of Texas. His pediatric surgery fellowship was done at Yale University.

Dr. Tory Meyer completed both his general surgery residency and pediatric surgery fellowship at the University of Cincinnati and the Cincinnati Children's Hospital Medi-

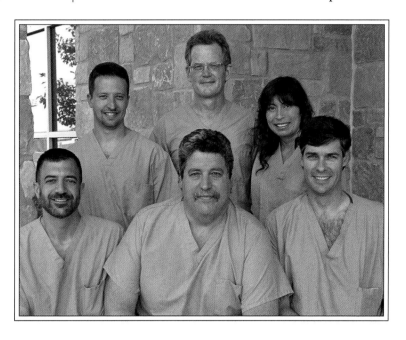

Austin Pediatric Surgery, clockwise from left, Jeffrey Horwitz, M.D., Michael Josephs, M.D., Robert Schlechter, M.D., Julie Sanchez, M.D., Tory Meyer, M.D., and Mark Smith, M.D.

cal Center. He also completed a two-year research and ECMO fellowship at the University of Cincinnati.

Although raised in Houston, Dr. Julie Sanchez completed both her general and pediatric surgical training in New York at the SUNY Health Sciences Center and finished a trauma and research fellowship at Johns Hopkins as well.

Dr. Michael Josephs came to Austin after completing his general surgery residency at the University of Florida in Gainesville. His pediatric surgery fellowship was served at the Cincinnati Children's Hospital Medical Center.

The surgeons of APS remain committed to providing state-of-the-art surgical care for the children of Central Texas and to being leaders in the advancement of pediatric services.

AUSTIN RADIOLOGICAL ASSOCIATION

THE ROOTS OF THE AUSTIN RADIOLOGICAL ASSOCIATION (ARA) can be traced back to 1954, when Dr. Robert Snider arrived in Austin and began work as the first full-time radiologist at the original Seton Hospital. His goal was to offer "excellent patient care and radiological services to the Austin community." He strove to make imaging services convenient for patients both in and out of the hospital and wanted Austin to have access to the best technology possible. Toward this end, he began offering outpatient radiology services in a remodeled house at 2410 Rio Grande in 1956. His equipment then consisted of a diagnostic x-ray unit with fluoroscopy and two state-of-the-art radiation treatment units. By that time, his practice had grown enough to hire another radiologist and became known as the Austin Radiological Group (ARG).

As Austin's population expanded over the next 30 years, the group kept pace, and in 1968 it was officially chartered as the Austin Radiological Association (ARA). In 1990, the association added nine new radiologists; six years later, they merged with Radiology Consultants and added ten more. Since then, more than 30 additional doctors have joined the practice.

Today, ARA is one the largest providers of outpatient imaging in central Texas. Their more than 70 radiologists include physicians with subspecialty training in interventional radiology, diagnostic and interventional neuroradiology, body imaging, mammography and women's imaging, musculoskeletal imaging, nuclear medicine, and pediatric radiology. With 14 outpatient imaging centers and 13 hospital locations in the area, every area resident has access to all modalities of outpatient imaging.

For over 50 years, ARA has committed itself to investing in the latest technology in order to provide the highest quality of care to referring physicians and patients in Central Texas. ARA is the only radiology practice in town with pediatric radiology and outpatient nuclear medicine studies. Two new imaging centers have opened, one dedicated to pediatric patients. ARA is also adding the first SPECT CT scanner in Austin to complement its two PET CT units.

Since 2001, ARA has led the nation in filmless outpatient imaging. ARA's Picture Archiving and Communication System (PACS) is one of the largest and most sophisticated digital communication systems in the world.

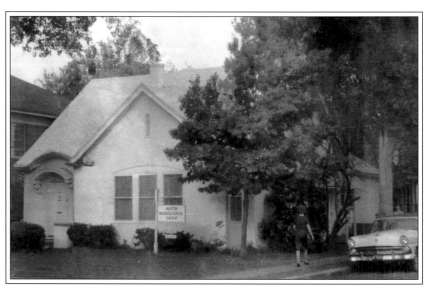

Austin Radiological Association started in this modest house.

Radiologists and other physicians have immediate, secure access to patients' images and image interpretations anywhere any time. ARA also provides PACS services and IT support to the seven hospitals of the Seton Healthcare Network, the largest hospital system in the region.

ARA is a leader in providing imaging services to the uninsured and underinsured both on an inpatient basis at all of the region's major hospitals and on an outpatient basis at its imaging centers and at Brackenridge Hospital clinics. ARA is the leading provider of outpatient imaging for the Project Access program of the Travis County Medical Society as well as all programs serving those in need of assistance with medical care. ARA supports medical research both financially (designated as a Visionary in Practice group by the Radiological Society of North America) and as a participating research site for ACRIN, the clinical research arm of the American College of Radiology. ARA is committed to keeping pace with the rapid growth of the Austin area as well as with rapid advances in technology. "Excellent in imaging" is the stated goal and continuing reality of ARA.

AUSTIN REGIONAL CLINIC

IN THE SPRING OF 1980, THE population of Austin was 345,496 and a trip to the country to see the blooming wild flowers meant driving to Cedar Park, Pflugerville, or Round Rock. Highway 183 was a two-lane country road and Whole Foods Market was about to open its very first store at 10th and Lamar.

At that time, Austin's health care community included mostly solo and small group practices and patients who paid for their care at the time of services with the expectation of reimbursement from their health insurance carriers. As frustration with the system grew, the health care field in the United States began to change and employers demanded relief from the spiraling cost of health care. New laws were passed in an attempt to contain costs, and health maintenance organizations (HMOs) began to spring up across the country with the hope of decreasing costs.

Austin Regional Clinic (ARC) opened its doors during this time of industry transformation. The medical group was founded by family practitioner Norman Chenven, M.D., who invited pediatricians Thomas Zavaleta, M.D. and Carol Faget, M.D. to join him in establishing what is now the largest, multispecialty group practice in Greater Austin. The small group took the unprecedented step of entering into a partnership with PruCare, which was Prudential Insurance Company's experiment in developing Austin's first health plan and health maintenance organization.

The trio envisioned a medical group that would be a part of every community in Austin, and they recruited physicians and opened new facilities throughout the city. ARC distinguished itself by offering services and conveniences that smaller practices could not afford and by establishing a system of quality assurance that ensured a high standard of care throughout the organization. Throughout the 1980s, ARC continued to grow and gain the loyalty of Austin residents.

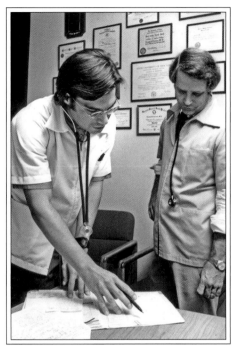

Norman Chenven, M.D. (left) with former associate James Sharp, M.D. (c. 1985).

"ARC's original mission—to provide access to quality, affordable medical care—remained the same even as it grew. In 2006, ARC served over 240,000 patients, or about 15 percent of residents in the Greater Austin area. It keeps its commitment to provide broad geographic access with clinics throughout Austin, Round Rock, Cedar Park, Pflugerville, and Hutto, with plans to add more to be able to grow with the community.

Contracting with a wide variety of insurers, approximately 50 health plans, and many government programs, including Medicaid, CHIP (Children's Health Insurance Program), and Medicare, ARC has initiated processes to foster responsiveness to patients' needs by providing same-day access, urgent care appointments, after-hours availability on weekends and holidays, and an all-night phone advice center. Patients enjoy the convenience of on-site lab and digital radiology at ARC locations and online services on the ARC website. The group continues to expand its areas of expertise, offering comprehensive medical care in pediatrics, family practice, internal medicine, obstetrics and gynecology, allergy and immunology, dermatology, ENT, endocrinology, podiatry, physical therapy, rheumatology, and nutritional counseling. ARC is especially known for its disease management programs and much emulated physician peer review program, designed to monitor and continuously improve the overall quality of care for the patients ARC serves.

ARC physicians contribute their time to hospital staff activities as departmental chairs and through service to various hospital committees. Their physicians have served on the executive board and many committees of the Travis County Medical Society, as delegates to and participants in the Texas Medical Association, and on committees of the American Medical Association. ARC physicians donate innumerable hours of professional time with direct service charity clinics in Austin and medical missions abroad.

AUSTIN PEDIATRIC OPHTHALMOLOGY

FOR F. KEITH BUSSE, JR., M.D., SETTING UP A PEDIATRIC ophthalmology practice in Austin was a chance to come home to the place he loved most. Having a father in the military afforded his family the opportunity to live all over the world as a youngster, settling in Austin by the time Busse was a teenager. A graduate of Anderson High School, Busse says "it's enjoyable when you treat children of former classmates."

The most common problem Busse sees is strabismus, or "wandering eye." If left untreated, not only will a child's sight suffer, but he may suffer ridicule when other children notice nonparallel eyes. At least once a month, Busse gives the gift of sight, restoring vision to a child who suffers from bilateral congenital cataracts. Busse calls these cases

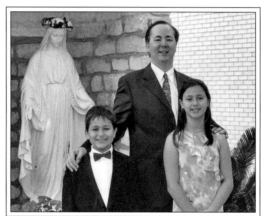

"enormously rewarding." One such case involved a mother who brought her baby from Mexico seeking Dr. Busse's help. Despite the fact that two Mexican doctors told the woman her child was fine and not in need of help, the woman knew deep in her heart that that was not the case. She decided to risk arrest by bringing her child to the United States in hopes of finding an answer. Dr. Busse was able to diagnose and treat the child for bilateral congenital cataracts, saving the child's sight. Also rewarding for Dr. Busse is diagnosing and treating cancers of the eye where he sees about two new cases a year. It is rewarding for him because he saves not only a child's sight, but their life as well.

F. Keith Busse, Jr. M.D. with son Philippe and daughter Christine.

AUSTIN RETINA ASSOCIATES

IN 1977. M. COLEMAN DRIVER, MD, AN Austin native, completed a retina fellowship in Portland, Oregon, and was board certified that same year. In those days, Austin residents felt that specialized medical care could only be obtained in the big cities, so he had to break out-of-town referral patterns. This required the purchase of specialized equipment and training specialized staff. He paid for this without the assurance of support from local hospitals, but he was determined to have a practice that was state-of-the-art in retina care. In the end, the hospitals and the medical community embraced the idea of sub specialization.

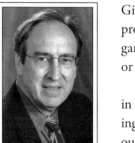

In 1980, Dr. Driver recruited the first of seven partners and founded Austin Retina Associates. With patients coming from all parts of Texas, a satellite office was opened in Waco, followed by branches in San Angelo, Brownwood, College Station, Lockhart, Marble Falls, Midland, Marshall, Odessa, San Marcos, Temple, Round Rock, Killeen, and

Giddings. The mission of the association is to provide excellent retina care to all patients regardless of their proximity to a medical center or their ability to pay.

Dr. Driver has blazed new paths for medicine in Central Texas and as a result of his pioneering efforts, Austin has become known throughout the country as an important center for retina research. He was elected president of both of the state professional organizations in the early 90s and his medical office, Austin Retina Associates, has become nationally known and respected by the ophthalmic community.

In 2006, Dr. Driver and his wife, Jody Driver, PA-C, turned over control of ARA to the remaining partners and established Angelo Retina Associates, 180 miles west of Austin. He plans to continue to practice at a reduced level for many more years, bringing to San Angelo the same quality of care and innovation that he brought to Austin 30 years ago.

BROOKSIDE WOMEN'S MEDICAL CENTER

DR. L. L. "TAD" DAVIS HAS ALWAYS BELIEVED IN A holistic approach to medicine. He opened his private medical practice, Brookside Women's Medical Center, in 1976. His philosophy has continuously set him apart, attracting patients who desire an obstetrician/gynecologist who will educate them, talk about the advantages and disadvantages of medical options, and allow them to fully participate in the decisions regarding their medical care. Meeting his patients' needs and respecting their choices led him to new and innovative practices, including some of the most sophisticated surgical procedures.

Dr. Davis was one of the first physicians in the nation, and the first physician in Austin, to allow fathers in the operating room during a C-section. He was also the first in Austin to perform an elective vaginal delivery after a C-section and to deliver a baby at a birthing center. Although sometimes controversial, he was one of the first doctors in the nation to provide artificial insemination for single women. He was also at the medical forefront using hypnosis during delivery and permitting the father to cut the umbilical cord.

Dr. Davis was also one of the first doctors to perform certain major gynecological surgeries, including laparoscopic-assisted vaginal hysterectomies and laparoscopic supracervical hysterectomies. In Austin, he performed the earliest Pfannenstiele (bikini) incision and ablations of the endometrium to avoid hysterectomies. He has always supported a woman's right to choose her own reproductive options and has provided abortion services throughout his career.

In addition to providing a path for other doctors to follow, he has served as chief of Ob/Gyn and as vice chief of staff at South Austin Medical Center, has held three clinical faculty positions at the University of Texas Medical Branch Galveston, at the University of Texas Medical School Houston, and at Texas A&M Medical School. He has also served as acting medical director of Planned Parenthood and as the medical director of People's Community Clinic.

THIEU BUI, M.D.

DR. THIEU BUI, A 1961 GRADUATE OF SAIGON UNIVERSITY Medical School, spent two years as an internal medicine resident at West Virginia University in the 60s, a break in his longtime service as a surgeon for the Vietnamese Airborne Division. After finishing his residency, he rejoined the division in Vietnam. In 1975, when Saigon fell, Dr Bui, his wife, Simone, and their children escaped to the United States and began their American life in Fort Chaffee, Arkansas, a temporary home for over 50,000 Vietnamese and Cambodian refugees.

Also in 1975, a wealthy Arkansas farmer was searching for a doctor to practice in the underserved town of Wilmot. After hearing of medical professionals at the refugee camp, he found Dr. Bui and convinced him to come to the rural town. He asked Dr Bui, "Do you want to be a small fish in a big pond, or a big fish in a small pond?" Dr Bui accepted the small pond. Newsmen, reporters from *Time* magazine, *People*, and

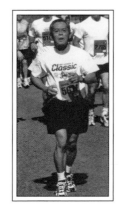

National Geographic rushed to the "small pond" and published articles about Dr. Bui and his family. His name was even mentioned in the second edition of *America, Past and Present*, a college history text.

For seven years in Arkansas, Dr Bui and his family enjoyed the hospitality of the appreciative residents until 1982, when, while visiting friends in Austin, they found a bigger pond and decided to make Austin their home. "We liked it because it was an intellectual, education-focused city, physically surrounded by nature—lots of hills, lakes, rivers, and shady trees," explains Dr Bui.

Dr Bui joined the Travis County Medical Society in 1982. At his office on North Lamar, where he has now practiced family medicine for 22 years, Dr Bui feels comfortable serving the nearby community. He inspires his patients with his lively optimism and healthful pursuits—from playing piano to running marathons at the age of seventy.

AUSTIN THYROID & ENDOCRINOLOGY CENTER

BEFORE DR. SIMONE SCUMPIA MOVED TO THIS COUNTRY and decided to pursue her interest in endocrinology or started her own clinic, she worked as a general practitioner in the Carpathian Mountains in Romania. She covered the medically underserved population of seven Romanian villages by making rounds with a horse and wagon. It was 1980, and medicine was more advanced in these parts than their transportation methods—or so it seemed. One of her duties included delivering babies. Her first delivery after medical school graduation was in a two-room cabin with the delivering mother in one room and her husband and their 11 children eating in the room next door. When she realized she did not have a tool to cut the umbilical cord, she called out to the father for help, trying to disguise her panic. The comparatively stoic father quickly arrived in the room with a pair of kitchen scissors. "'I can't use these,' I said, "they're just scissors, and they haven't been sterilized, and, and...," He looked at me and said, "They worked the first eleven times ... He was already eleven deliveries ahead of me,' laughed Dr. Scumpia.

Since then, she has gained the experience along with the training to continue advancing the quality of care for her patients. Although today's patients in Austin are often more educated and astute in their medical knowledge than those in her early days, they are just as grateful to have her expertise in Central Texas. The clinic she founded in 2002, the Austin Thyroid & Endocrinology Center, is the only specialized thyroid clinic of its kind between Dallas and San Antonio.

In 1983, she moved from Romania to Toronto, Canada for an internship in Internal Medicine, where she continued her European/French medical training, which stresses clinical diagnosis and bedside manner. Inspired by great Romanian endocrinologists that came before her, such as Dr. Constantin I. Parhon and Dr. Ana Aslan, who was one of her professors at the Medical School of Bucharest in Romania, Dr. Scumpia accepted an Endocrinology and Metabolism fellowship at San Antonio's University of Texas Health Science Center. She completed her formal subspecialty studies at the University of Pittsburgh School of Medicine in 1992. From Pittsburgh she moved to Austin

and began her clinical practice in Endocrinology at the Austin Diagnostic Clinic, where she stayed for ten years. She also became involved with the Central Texas Medical Foundation, serving as director of the Endocrinology division for eight years.

Dr. Scumpia's fascination with Endocrinology and its related fields prompted her ongoing research involvement. Her career research has included approximately 100 studies, which include studies in diabetes, osteoporosis, obesity, women's health, gastroenterology, neurology, and ophthalmology. From 1997 to 2000, she served as medical director of Obesity Treatment and Research at the Austin Diagnostic Clinic. In 2001, she combined her passion, her experience, and her expertise to form the Austin Thyroid & Endocrinology Center, where she specializes in non-diabetic endocrinology services. "The clinic is unique in its integrative approach to treating thyroid and hormone issues. After all, hormones affect every part of the body, so we look at it from all different angles."

Dr. Scumpia thrives on the detective work of diagnosis. Though her days at her clinic are impressively full, she says she is always smiling when she comes in and is still smiling when she leaves. With her own clinic, she feels that she has found a way to make the biggest difference for her clients by providing the most comprehensive thyroid practice she can, and in a manner that is more convenient, quicker, and less expensive for her patients. For example, her thyroid patients are guaranteed to get an appointment within 24 hours, if needed, and benefit from her state-of-the-art treatment equipment with modalities including ultrasound, radioactive iodine, and bone density scans. Dr. Scumpia is one of the few endocrinologists trained and licensed for radioactive iodine treatment.

As an accomplished expert in her field, Dr. Scumpia also serves as a consultant, advisor, and speaker for several pharmaceutical companies, and is invited to give medical lectures in the form of grand rounds and evening lectures on various topics in Thyroidology, Lipid Management, Metabolic Syndrome, and Osteoporosis. She is a fellow of the Royal College of Physicians and Surgeons of Canada and the American College of Endocrinology, and a member of the Texas Osteoporosis Board and the American

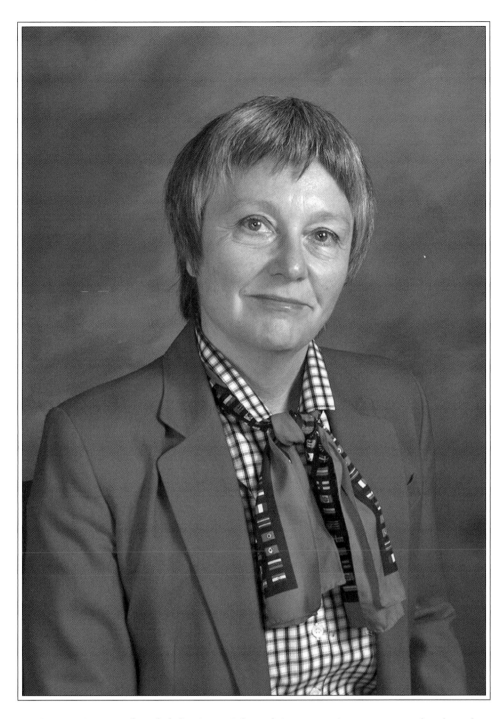

*Dr. Simone Scumpia founded the Austin Thyroid &
Endocrinology Center in 2002.*

faculty member at the Internal Medicine program at Brackenridge Hospital. From 1992 to 2000, she served as division chief of Endocrinology of the Central Texas Medical Foundation, and in 1996, as associate clinical professor of Medicine at the University of Texas Medical Branch in Galveston. Her target pupils also include the greater community. "It's known that 10 to 11 percent of the population has thyroid disease, most commonly hypo- or hyperthyroidism, and half of them don't know it," said Dr. Scumpia. Her public lectures also include information on Metabolic Syndrome (also called Syndrome X), which includes a cluster of medical conditions—abdominal obesity, high blood pressure, high blood sugar and triglycerides, low good cholesterol, polycystic ovaries, and hirsutism. One in three people has this syndrome, and it can lead to diabetes, heart attack, and stroke. Her quest to educate the population includes information on symptoms, preventative measures, and early and aggressive treatment.

In addition to educating the public on her area of medical specialty, she also enjoys the benefits of Austin's cosmopolitan growth, supporting the Austin classical music scene, the Austin Lyric Opera and the Western Civilization Program at the University of Texas. She says that Austin has been a great place to raise her family and practice medicine. "Unlike in other cities, there is healthy competition in Austin. The people here and the members of the medical community are very warm. I feel very fortunate that I've been able to learn so much from my colleagues."

Thyroid Association. Dr. Scumpia recently had the honor to become the first physician in Austin certified by the American College of Lipidology as a diplomat in Lipids, the science of cholesterol.

Like the endocrinologists she admired during her training, Dr. Scumpia feels that it is "important to impart expertise to younger doctors." She has taught at Brackenridge Hospital for ten years. From 1989 to 1991, she served as a

AUSTIN SURGICAL ARTS

IT WOULD BE DIFFICULT TO FIND A MEDICAL PRACTICE IN central Texas with doctors more educated than the physicians at Austin Surgical Arts (ASA). All three of the maxillofacial surgeons have advanced degrees in both medicine and dentistry which makes this practice unique in central Texas. Drs. William Buchanan, John Jones, and H. Paul Casmedes are able to provide patients with a wide range of oral and facial surgical services, from the removal of wisdom teeth to rhinoplasty to corrective jaw surgery to major facial reconstruction for accident and assault victims. The three joined forces when Dr. Buchanan left a larger practice to partner with Dr. Jones. Drs. Jones and Casmedes had previously worked together in San Antonio, so Dr. Jones knew Dr. Casmedes would be a perfect fit for the practice.

To provide patients with maximum care and privacy at a reasonable cost, the doctors even have their own operating room, making a hospital visit unnecessary. The operating room has passed the rigorous standards set forth by the Joint Commission on Accreditation of Healthcare Organizations (JCAHO) and is one of a very small number of private practices to receive JCAHO certification. Word of the excellent standards of this office has spread through the dental community and 60 percent of all patients are referred by area dentists, with the other 40 percent being patient-to-patient referrals. To that end, the surgeons all provide a great deal of consultation time to each patient, both before and after surgery, addressing individual concerns and making the patient as comfortable and relaxed as possible. "It's not like a big office," notes Dr. Buchanan. The doctors all agree that a "cozy, more intimate" atmosphere is something they're proud of achieving. Dr. Buchanan says the entire staff is "really laid back."

Because of their vast experience and education, the doctors are able to help patients make more informed choices in deciding upon a surgery. "Sometimes patients come asking for a smaller nose when in fact a larger chin might be

what they need," says Dr. Jones. Few patients are aware that jaw reconstructive surgery is even an option for them, so they don't know to ask for it. The satisfaction rate is extremely high. "We're expecting it to come out right and the patients are very grateful." As Dr. Jones explains, "we

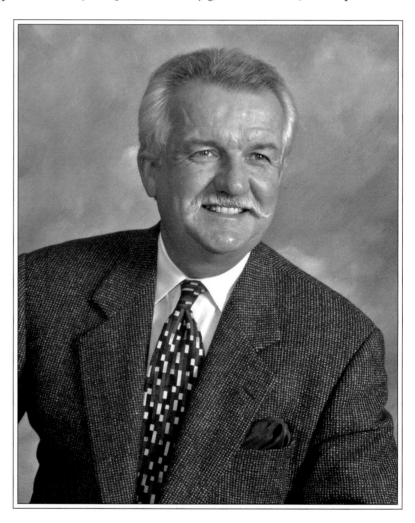

Dr. William Buchanan of Austin Surgical Arts.

live in a very visually critical society that emphasizes youth, fitness, and beauty. If the individual has aesthetic liabilities that are occupying their emotional health, they have the option of changing something to give them a better disposition." The range of the services provided at Austin Surgical Arts is both broad and unique, stretching across the medical and dental arenas. Dr. Jones best sums up the practice, "We're medicine's bridge to dentistry and dentistry's bridge to medicine."

CENTRAL TEXAS PEDIATRIC ORTHOPEDICS AND SCOLIOSIS SURGERY

DURING HIS SECOND YEAR OF RESIDENCY AT ST. LOUIS University, Dr. Jay Shapiro discovered Orthopedics to be an enjoyable sub-specialty in practicing Pediatric Medicine. After completing a fellowship at Texas Scottish Rite Hospital in Dallas, he returned to his hometown of Austin and "hung out a shingle." When he arrived in Austin, there were only a handful of pediatric specialists and surgery at Children's Hospital was considered "day surgery." "In the early '90s, there were some cases I would hesitate to do because we didn't have the pediatric sub-specialist support," remembers Dr. Shapiro. After over a decade of helping recruit pediatric specialists and sub-specialists to Austin and supporting the development of a top-notch pediatric hospital, his practice is now second to none in its level of treatment.

Now with four pediatric orthopedists, his group, Central Texas Pediatric Orthopedics & Scoliosis Surgery (CTPO), specializes in treating spinal disorders, club feet, leg length discrepancy, and other orthopedic congenital abnormalities. In

Dr. Jay Shapiro

1992, Dr. John Williams joined Dr. Shapiro and began specializing in complex congenital abnormalities and other spinal disorders. In 1997, Dr. Tony Kahn joined the group, specializing in limb lengthening and deformity reconstruction. Dr. Michelle Prince arrived in 2003, specializing in orthopedic spine disorders. In 2006, Dr. Robert Dehne, specializing in the treatment of foot and ankle injuries, joined CTPO. Other members of the group include physical therapist Kevin McHorse, pediatric nurse practitioners Tracy Kuper, Dana Madden, and Michelle Poole, and Physician Assistants Jennifer Calaway and Amy Hurst.

Today, nearly all pediatric specialties are represented in Austin, available to support the pediatric orthopedists. "It's an amazing achievement considering there is not a medical school here," says Dr. Shapiro. A full pediatric team allows CTPO to provide better ancillary care than many medical centers can provide, with pediatric sub-specialists attending to the nuances of medical care for children in every important detail, from the way they draw blood from their young patients to providing the best environment for post-surgery care. "We're fortunate that the vast majority of sub-specialists here are excellent physicians," says Dr. Shapiro, "maybe because the non-academic setting attracts doctors who are truly interested in the clinical aspect of practice. They also tend to have a maverick thought process, willing to try something outside of a big-city medical center." The group's doctors also appreciate the independence of not practicing in a medical school setting, allowing them to balance time between clinical, research, family, and outside activities. "Austin seems to attract those who are searching for that balance," states Dr. Shapiro.

Continuing on the cutting edge of medicine, the group will be one of only a dozen or so groups in the country—and, most likely, the only group who is not a part of a major academic institution—to treat chest wall deformities and congenital scoliosis with the recently approved VEPTR, or titanium rib. The new procedure requires a team approach and Austin now has the kind of top-notch team to handle it.

DONALD COUNTS, M.D.

DR. DONALD COUNTS MOVED TO AUSTIN IN 1975 TO establish his practice in family medicine after completing two years of service on the Flathead Indian Reservation in Hot Springs, Montana. He has established a solo practice structured to deliver a high level of personalized attention to his patients offering an objective approach to each complaint. Dr. Counts became one of the first physicians in Texas to offer medical acupuncture.

Dr. Counts received his M.D. degree from the University of Texas Medical Branch (UTMB) at Galveston. He is a Fellow of the American Academy of Family Practice as well as the American Academy of Medical Acupuncture, is board certified in Medical Acupuncture by the American Board of Medical Acupuncture and board certified in Holistic Medicine by the American Board of Holistic Medicine. Dr. Counts serves as a Clinical Assistant Professor in Family Medicine to medical students and residents in Austin for UTMB Galveston and he also serves as a preceptor to the University of Texas Health Science Center at Houston to foster interest regarding integrative medicine. In 2006, Dr. Counts was appointed by Governor Rick Perry to the Texas Acupuncture Board. Dr Counts has volunteered for Caritas and helped organize the initial HIV clinic in Austin as well as volunteering as a preceptor for the David Powell Clinic. In addition, he serves as medical advisor for SafePlace, is on the medical advisory committee for the Breast Cancer Resource Center of Austin, and is a volunteer clinician for Project Access, MusiCares and The SIMS Foundation. He was an early advocate and organizer of the Health Alliance of Austin Musicians (HAAM). As a member of the Performing Arts Medical Association, Dr. Counts has a special interest in caring for musicians and performing artists in the Austin area.

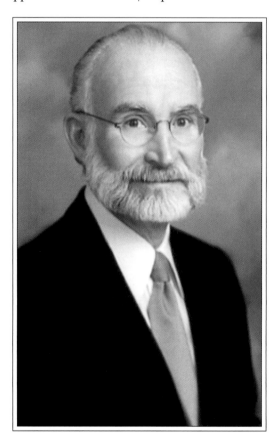

Dr. Donald Counts

Dr. Counts has been a member of the American Medical Association, the Texas Medical Association, and Travis County Medical Society for over 30 years. Recognized for his expertise in the field, Dr. Counts has consulted for multiple Texas Medical Association conferences on the topic of alternative and complementary therapies in health and wellness in medicine. He has consulted and lectured at universities, hospitals, and for various health care associations on the subject of integrative medicine and adding spirituality to the practice of medicine. As a delegate to the Texas Medical Association (TMA) in May 1998, Dr. Counts introduced a resolution to the House of Delegates of the TMA with the support and direction of the Travis County Medical Society delegation about the pros and cons of alternative therapies. The resolution provided the framework to begin formal training of medical doctors in Texas in various integrative medicine techniques.

Dr. Counts has contributed to the *Travis County Medical Society Journal* and *Texas Medicine*, the journal of the Texas Medical Association. In addition to his numerous medical writings, he also is co-author with his wife, Kathryn, of *A Texas Family's Cookbook*, a collection of recipes for healthy and satisfying Southwestern cuisine. Further, Dr. Counts was a consultant to the Continuing Medical Education joint project of Texas Medical Association and to the American Botanical Council's *Healthcare Professionals Guide to Commonly Used Herbs*. Dr. Counts served as an early consultant and supporter for the initiation of *Explore—The Journal of Science and Healing* and serves on the editorial board. Dr. Counts and Kathryn have been married for 29 years and have three children and eight grandchildren.

RONALD DEVERE, M.D.

WHEN THE SO-CALLED "SANDWICH" GENERATION, THE baby-boomers of today, find their parents are losing their ability to think and care for themselves, these adult children are faced with discovering whether Alzheimer's disease is to blame. That's when many seek the advice of neurologist, Dr. Ronald DeVere.

"The earlier we can diagnose this disease, the more likely we can improve the quality of this person's life," says Dr. DeVere. He finds baby boomers are bringing their parents to his office, often from other states, after a family visit in which the adult children see their parents are failing. "They (the Alzheimer's patients) may become paranoid, combative, and exhibit behavior disorders," says Dr. DeVere. With regard to Alzheimer's, he says "we can't stop it from progressing, but we can slow it down." That's just the sort of help many are seeking for their aging parents. Dr. DeVere does believe that in the near future "we'll be able to arrest the disease."

He says he likes helping people who suffer from memory loss in part because he has the opportunity to work with, and get to know, the patient's family. He had a close relationship with his own grandparents and feels a special bond with the older generation.

Symptoms of Alzheimer's typically occur in our mid to late 60s and older, though it can occur earlier. According to DeVere, each of us runs a 20 percent lifetime risk of developing Alzheimer's disease. Some run a higher risk than others. Risk factors include not only age, but also lower education, head injuries, family history, high cholesterol, diabetes, smoking, untreated depression, and excessive use of alcohol.

One of the curious things about Alzheimer's disease, and some other neurological disorders, is that patients frequently lose their sense of smell, thereby losing the ability to detect flavors. That is why Dr. DeVere is engaged in a pilot study that could help these patients compensate by stimulating other taste sensations with various types and intensity of spices and different textures, for example. He is currently developing a collection of recipes which he hopes will ultimately become a very useful "cookbook" for his patients.

Born in Winnipeg Manitoba Canada, Dr. DeVere completed medical school at the University of Manitoba. He became interested in neurology when he spent three months at the Mayo Clinic in Rochester, Minnesota as a senior medical student. He went on to do a neurology residency at the University of Minnesota in Minneapolis. Dr. DeVere worked in Houston for more than 25 years, but always had a deep attraction to central Texas, having a home here for most of that time. His love of the outdoors blossomed into hobbies which include sailing and bicycling. Finally, the appeal of Austin, and especially Lake Travis, lured him from Houston to set up practice in Lakeway. In addition to his interest in dementia and taste and smell disorders, he is a general adult neurologist, treating other common neurological disorders.

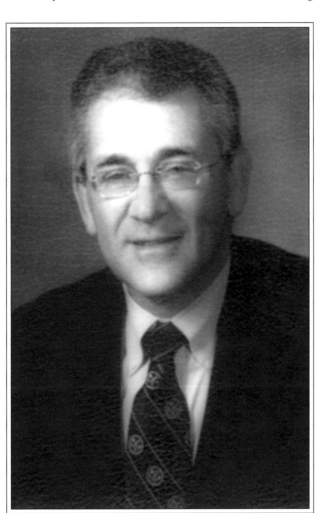

Ronald DeVere, M.D.

CENTRAL TEXAS OBSTETRICS AND GYNECOLOGY ASSOCIATES

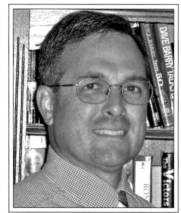

HOW CAN ONE MAN "IMPACT THE world?" That's a question asked by obstetrician/gynecologist Dr. Paul Locus. He is in constant search of ways to make a difference in people's lives, and one of the ways he's chosen is through the providing of health care to women. He provided this care for those less fortunate and in need through seven years of working within and directing the Obstetrics and Gynecology program at Bracken-ridge Hospital and its extensions in the Austin city clinics. He has also provided this care on a private level since 1992 through his private practice in Austin. "Women have been disregarded in medical history," he says, "so I think that feeling that I'm helping to correct that is my contribution."

His patients' needs are of chief concern, regardless of time of day. Fewer than seven percent of Dr. Locus's deliveries are primary cesarean sections, compared with a national average of around 26 percent. "It gets down to what's really important in medicine; it's that human to human interaction, the hands-on approach."

Dr. Locus stays active in charities, especially those involved with services to the deaf. He maintains a large patient base of deaf women, due to his fluency in sign language. He says he owes this skill to his deaf daughter, as he started learning sign language when she was a newborn.

While his practice is smaller than many obstetrics offices in Austin, he's proud to be able to deliver person-to-person care in a world that's gotten less and less personal.

EMMANUEL C. EDOKA, M.D.

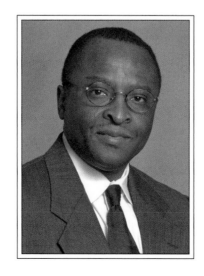

AS A YOUNG CHILD IN NIGERIA, EMMANUEL EDOKA accompanied his father on Sunday social visits to the family's physician. Impressed with the respect his father, an established businessman, had for the physician and the gift basket they brought, full of Irish potatoes, eggs, and a live turkey, Emmanuel decided at the age of six that he would become a doctor.

In 1965, at the age of 12, he accomplished the first step by passing the entrance exam to King's College, Nigeria's most elite secondary school. After civil unrest and a brutal war halted Nigeria's formal education system for two years, Emmanuel raced to complete his studies. He graduated from medical school in 1980, and although his father had died a year before, his inspiration lived on. After interning and serving in the National Youth Service Corps,

Emmanuel was a practicing physician, an accomplishment he knows his father would be very proud of.

Dr. Edoka migrated to the United States in 1984, and attended Meharry Medical College in Nashville, the first African-American medical school in the country. There he met his future wife, now a pediatrician and mother of their two children. They settled in Austin because "it seemed like a good place to start a family."

Since much of his internal medicine practice included geriatric care, Dr. Edoka educated himself on geriatric medicine and passed the board exams. Still excited by this emerging field, he enjoys "seeing how geriatrics is changing how we care for older adults and how more and more people are aging successfully."

EMERGENCY SERVICE PARTNERS

SINCE 1988, THE TEAM OF DOCTORS AT EMERGENCY Service Partners, L.P. (ESP) has provided emergency physician services to hospitals and health care systems in Central Texas, including Brackenridge Hospital, Seton Medical Center, Seton Northwest, Seton Southwest, and Seton Highland Lakes. Through the years, the group has responded to Austin's changing pulse. Although similar groups often survive for only five or six years, Emergency Service Partners has not only maintained its existence for three times as long, but has evolved into a team of established doctors, immersed in supporting the Austin community.

In 1983, there was only one hospital emergency department in Austin, located at Brackenridge Hospital. That year, following a nationwide trend, every hospital in Austin opened one. In 1983, Dr. Bruce Moskow began working in Seton's first emergency department and he was joined by Dr. Sam Roberts in 1985. In an effort to fill the void from the departure of a California company that had been staffing the hospital, the two doctors formed Third Coast Emergency Physicians, the predecessor of Emergency Service Partners, in 1988.

As Seton expanded to fill the emergency medical needs of Austin's growing population, Emergency Service Partners followed closely to match those needs. As strategies for attending to medical emergencies changed, they opened minor emergency centers at hospitals, working with hospitals to organize and staff them, and helped design and implement major hospital renovations. Soon ESP will be helping to open the first Children's Hospital, with an all children's emergency department, in Central Texas. With approximately 60 board certified doctors in their group, they now staff five area hospitals 24 hours a day, treating more than 230,000 patients in Austin a year. ESP eagerly anticipates further growth as the region grows.

In addition to responding to Austin's rapid growth, the group also continues to face one of the biggest challenges facing emergency facilities today—indigent care. Although Austin hospitals were never in the habit of "dumping" citizens who were without insurance or means of payment, the Emergency Medical Treatment and Active Labor Act of 1986 codified anti-dumping sentiment, entrusting emergency departments with the responsibility of serving any citizen who seeks emergency care, without regards for financial class. "Effectively sustaining this service will be one of the biggest challenges we'll face in the next ten to fifteen years," says Dr. Moskow.

Always strategizing to improve the system, Emergency Service Partners seeks to recruit the best trained doctors. "We look for doctors who are both competent and nice," says Cheryl Conner, RN, and CEO of the company. "And then we don't give them any excuse to leave." When these medical experts are not attending to the high-intensity demands of their careers, they are behind the scenes, working with hospital staff on the mundane details that affect patient safety in those critical hours of care. As hospital partners they provide more than a million dollars worth of charity care yearly, have initiated programs such as ACLS, and worked with state and local groups on liability legislation and emergency medical policies and protocols. As individuals, the physicians of ESP influence a vast array of organizations, serving as hospital chiefs of staff, on local peer review teams, residency teaching programs, and are actively involved in local and national professional and non-profit organizations.

We at ESP are proud of our first 20 years in Travis County and proud to be a part of the Travis County Medical Community. Our thanks to all who have helped us to help our patients.

The 2006-2007 Board of Directors at Emergency Service Partners are Patrick Crocker, D.O., Sam Roberts, M.D., Bruce Moskow, M.D., Robert Patton, M.D., Dennis Watts, M.D., and Christopher Ziebell, M.D.

ALBERT T. GROS, M.D.

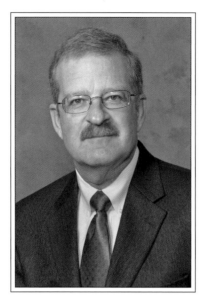

ALBERT GROS, M.D. HAS BEEN PRAC-ticing in the Austin area for more than 20 years. Originally a native of San Antonio, Gros attended St. Mary's University, graduating summa cum laude with a degree in Biology. After graduating from Baylor College of Medicine in Houston, Dr. Gros spent three years in the U. S. Navy on active duty. He returned to Baylor to finish his residency before moving to Austin and setting up private practice in 1983.

Today, Dr. Gros has an established medical practice specializing in Obstet-rics and Gynecology. Although he has hospital privileges all over town, he sees most of his patients at South Austin Hospital. He prides himself on providing one-on-one personalized care, taking the time to consult with patients before their exams, and

says, "We provide individualized atten-tion and we try not to make our pa-tients wait. My nurse, Teresa Miller, has been with me since the beginning, which provides continuity for the pa-tients. That is very important."

In addition to his nurse, many of Dr. Gros's patients have been with him the entire time he has been in practice. "I can't go anywhere in Austin without running into a patient. I find it very gratifying to meet a young person I have delivered. Over the past 21 years I have delivered several thousand young Austinites, and, in fact, I am starting to see patients that I delivered."

Dr. Gros is married with two children, son Jonathan and daughter Katha. His wife, Judy, also works in the medical profession as a nurse practitioner.

HENDRIX & SCHULZE

"I WENT INTO DERMATOLOGY TO PRACTICE medicine," says Thomas Schulze. That philosophy is what you will find at the dermatological practice of Hendrix & Schulze. Diag-nosis and treatment of diseases and tumors of the skin is the focus of these physicians.

Dr. Schulze grew up in Austin, graduating from Austin High School and the University of Texas. After graduation from the University of Texas Southwestern Medical School in Dallas, he served his country in Vietnam. He then pur-sued residency training in dermatology at the Mayo Gradu-ate School of Medicine in Rochester, Minnesota. Dr. Jay Hendrix grew up in Irving, Texas, and graduated from Rice University in Houston. He also attended the University of Texas Southwestern Medical School in Dallas. Following resi-dency training in internal medicine at Yale University, he stud-ied dermatology at Baylor College of Medicine in Houston.

Both men have seen major changes in the practice of dermatology over the years. They have incorporated many new treatments and techniques into their practice, but have

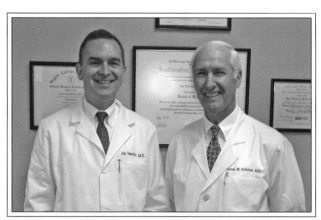

Jay Hendrix, M.D. (left) and Thomas W. Schultz, M.D.

steered clear of many others—mostly faddish cosmetic ser-vices—that seem to them to be of little value. Helping their patients with debilitating skin diseases to live productive lives has been the most gratifying challenge of their day-to-day practice.

KENNEDY DERMATOLOGY CENTER

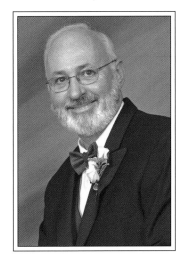

AFTER GRADUATING FROM THE University of Texas as a pharmacist and joining the Navy, the newly commissioned Ensign Bobby Joe Kennedy became Chief of Pharmacy Service at the Naval Hospital in Lemoore, California. During those early years of the Vietnam conflict, Ensign Kennedy, married with two children, decided to apply to medical school.

After graduating as a physician from the Texas College of Osteopathic Medicine in Fort Worth, Dr. Kennedy completed his rotating internship at Oaknoll Naval Hospital in Oakland, California, before being assigned as general medical officer aboard the *U.S.S. Samuel Gompers*. While serving aboard the U.S. Navy Destroyer *Tender* and completing a WESTPAC cruise to the Far East, he applied for and was accepted into the Dermatology residency program at Balboa Naval Hos-

pital in San Diego. Dr. Kennedy holds the distinction of being the first osteopathic physician accepted into the Navy residency at Balboa Naval Hospital, which was at that time the largest military hospital in the world. After completing his Dermatology residency and passing the board examination, Dr. Kennedy was certified by the American Board of Dermatology. His first assignment as a Navy dermatologist was as the Chief of Dermatology Service at the Naval Hospital in Millington, Tennessee, where he eventually became the Director of Medical Services at the Naval Hospital.

In 1984 upon completion of active duty, Dr. Kennedy returned home to Austin, used his extensive military medical experience as a basis for his reentry into civilian life, and established the Kennedy Dermatology Center.

LONE STAR PEDIATRICS

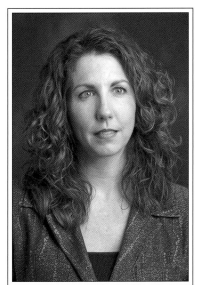

DR. KELLY THORSTAD RECEIVED HER medical degree from Baylor College of Medicine in Houston, Texas, in 1998. Originally from Austin, she graduated from the University of Texas with a bachelor's degree in Psychology in 1988. After completing her training at the Children's Hospital of Austin, Dr. Thorstad made the decision to establish herself in private practice.

Board certified by the American Academy of Pediatrics, Dr. Thorstad's specialty is pediatrics. She provides immunizations, primary care, and routine examinations for children of all ages, from birth to 18 years old. Her North Austin office, Lone Star Pediatriacs, reflects Dr. Thorstad's personalized approach to medical care. Her office has separate waiting rooms for sick and healthy children, as well as

a unique breastfeeding room reserved for nursing mothers.

Dr. Thorstad says, "My philosophy is to provide personalized service and high quality medical care in a more intimate setting. I truly feel it is a privilege to practice medicine. Every time parents walk in the door, they are trusting us with their children's health. I want all of our families to know we appreciate and are challenged by that responsibility."

On top of her growing medical practice, Dr. Thorstad stays involved in the community by giving talks at local PTAs, community centers, and churches. She is active in many hospital committees and a member of the Austin Physician Alliance. She is married with two children, son Cole and daughter Avery.

LONE STAR ONCOLOGY

WE AT LONE STAR ONCOLOGY (LSO) ARE DEDICATED TO the principle of compassionate medical care. We recognize that patients are whole persons with biological, economic, emotional, social, and spiritual needs. Meeting our patients' medical needs is our highest priority; because we never take for granted that our patients are individuals. We do our best to provide them with clear and comprehensive information so they can make informed decisions and participate in their own care. Like our relationships with our patients, our relationships with fellow employees and other members of the care team are based on concern, honesty, and trust. We believe compassion and mutual respect are essential to addressing successfully all human dimensions of cancer care.

As part of our commitment to our patients, Lone Star Oncology stays abreast of the most current cancer research. We are aggressive about finding treatments that are appropriate and beneficial for our patients' cancer care—from prevention, early detection, and diagnosis to treatment and long-term follow-up. Rest assured that our team will work together to give you and your family the best care possible.

Long Star Oncology's statement of patient care perhaps best conveys the heart of this practice. The people at Lone Star Oncology—a team of approximately 40 medical professionals—believe in caring for and treating a patient who has cancer, not in treating the cancer as a separate problem. The medical professionals work with patients not only on physical issues, but also to address psychological, emotional, and socioeconomic needs. This distinction provides the basis of compassionate care upon which this practice is founded. "If a doctor, nurse, or staff person doesn't think that way when they come on board, they get that way pretty quickly," says John J. Costanzi, M.D., president and chief executive officer. "Our nurses go the extra mile for our patients."

The only independent comprehensive treatment center in Central Texas, Lone Star Oncology offers its patients a very distinctive advantage in patient care. It is small enough to focus on compassionate individual care while providing state-of-the-art treatments arising from the tremendous progress the medical community is making annually in managing and treating cancer. In addition to traditional medical cancer treatments, patients may look to Lone Star Oncology for integrative or complementary medicine.

Dr. Costanzi is internationally known in the field of oncology. Before going into private practice in Austin, he was Professor of Medicine and Director of the Cancer Center at the University of Texas Medical Branch, in Galveston, Texas and then held a similar position at the Thompson Cancer Center in Knoxville, Tennessee. He is board certified in Medical Oncology and Internal Medicine and is an active participant in numerous scientific societies, which include the Southern Association for Oncology, the American College of Physicians, the American Society of Clinical Oncology, the American Association for Cancer Research, the American Society of Hematology, the American Federation for Clinical Research, the Central Society for Clinical Research, and the Southern Society for Clinical Investigations. Dr. Costanzi has received many honors which include being the Invited Lecturer by the German Cancer Society in Berlin, Munich, Frankfurt, Cologne, and Goettingen, and receiving the United States Air Force Surgeon General's Award for Scientific Achievement. He has published more than 150 peer-reviewed papers, numerous book chapters, and was editor of two volumes on Malignant Melanoma.

Uri M. Mintz, M.D., LSO Associate, attended medical school at Austria's Vienna University and the Hebrew University in Jerusalem, Israel, his birthplace. Mintz completed his residency at the Beilinson University Hospital in Israel, where he went on to serve as chief physician of its Medical Oncology department. He was a research fellow in the Genetics department at the Weizman Institute of Science in Tel Aviv and was a clinical fellow and instructor at the University of Chicago Cancer Research Center. Mintz was an attending physician in the Medical Oncology division of Mt. Sinai Medical Center in Cleveland, Ohio and was a partner and officer of Medical Oncology Associates in Beachwood, Ohio.

Brian J. Shimkus, M.D., partner of Lone Star Oncology, attended medical school at the Medical College of Georgia. Shimkus completed his internship and residency at the University of Virginia Hospital in Internal Medicine. During this time he conducted research in the areas of breast cancer and colon cancer. He is certified by the American Board of Internal Medicine and Medical Oncology and is an associate member of both the American Medical Association and the American Society of Clinical Oncology.

Glen R. Leupnitz, Ph.D., world-renowned biochemical nutritionist, consults with patients at Lone Star Oncology

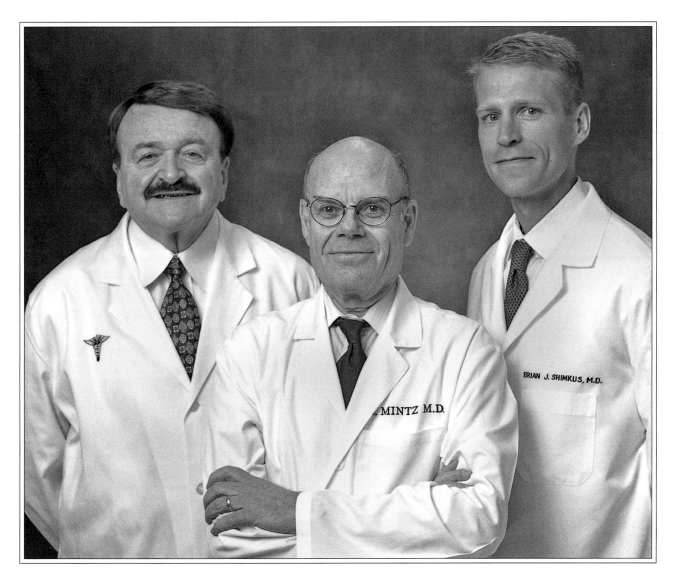

Long Star Oncology (left to right), John J. Costanzi, M.D., president and chief executive officer, Uri M. Mintz, M.D. and Brian J. Shimkus, M.D.

to customize the nutritional and immunological component of their treatment. He works with patients to coordinate all of their selected methods of treatment, helping to safeguard against any complications or neutralization of one treatment option by another. Dr. Leupnitz recommends cooperative, or adjuvant, therapies that boost effectiveness throughout the course of medical treatment. He is a member of numerous professional associations and works regularly with members of the U.S. Olympic men's and women's track team and women's swim team.

Many "non-medical" options are proven to be beneficial for the patient, particularly in the area of pain management. Rather than leaving the patient to seek out these options on his or her own, massage therapy, acupuncture, and lymphatic massage are among the complementary options that are available at Lone Star Oncology. This comprehensive approach is embraced by the patients, with approximately fifty percent at any given time utilizing complementary therapies that may help with direct cancer treatment, or achieve optimum pain management. "By having all elements under our control, we are best able to serve, and treat, the patient," Dr. Costanzi explains.

Lone Star Oncology regularly conducts investigative studies, or protocols, in the treatment of cancer. Highly selective in the trials in which it participates, Lone Star Oncology accepts roughly 20 percent of those with which it is presented. The medical team at Lone Star Oncology is dedicated to bringing patients the most advanced treatments and opportunities available. "The dedication of this team far exceeds what can be offered through in-house trials. We will work tirelessly to find the appropriate treatments for our patients," says Dr. Costanzi.

GABRIEL MILLAR, M.D.

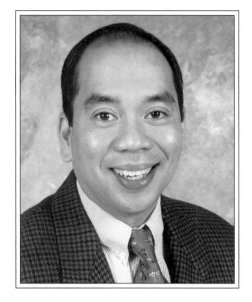

"MEDICINE IS BOTH ART AND science," says pediatrician Gabriel "Gabby" Millar. When you walk into his office, it is easy to see how Dr. Millar has both scientific and creative talents.

Nearly every painted piece, from pictures hanging on the walls to the beautifully detailed, custom children's furniture, is his handiwork.

But when Dr. Millar refers to medicine as both science and art, he isn't just talking about the accoutrements which adorn his office and waiting areas, he's talking about the "personal approach" he takes with each of his patients. "If the practice gets too large, you lose the art." Dr. Millar says he chose pediatrics because of the unassuming and honest nature that's inherent in chil-

dren. "Children will thank you profusely with sincerity and if they don't like you, they'll let you know that too!" Fortunately, the children who come to Dr. Millar like him a great deal, so honesty is never a problem.

A native of the Philippines, Dr. Millar says he's living out his dream practicing medicine in Round Rock. He's grateful to his entire family for their help, including his in-laws, his wife, a Harvard PMD graduate who runs the business end of his practice, and his parents. His father is a thoracic and cardiovascular surgeon practicing in the Philippines. He calls his office a "collaborative effort," saying he could never have achieved so much without the help of his family and staff.

BRIAN E. MONKS, M.D.

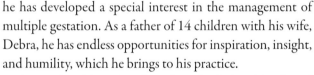

SINCE HIS ELABORATE MIDDLE SCHOOL PROJECT ON Embryology won the region's best-of-fair award, Brian Monks has been on the track to a rewarding career in Obstetrics and Gynecology. After completing his medical training at Texas Medical Center in Houston, Dr. Monks came to Austin to become an academic physician at Brackenridge Hospital, where he served as assistant director of the Ob/Gyn department from 1991 to 1994. In 1994, he began his private practice career which offers both low and high-risk obstetrics care, plus comprehensive office and state-of-the-art operative gynecological services.

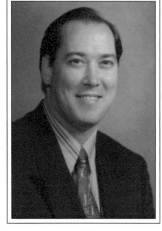

His personal life and professional life work as supporting components to each other. During his first son's 14-year battle with bone cancer, he experienced the medical field from a non-physician perspective. As a parent of two sets of fraternal twins,

he has developed a special interest in the management of multiple gestation. As a father of 14 children with his wife, Debra, he has endless opportunities for inspiration, insight, and humility, which he brings to his practice.

Attuned to his patients' needs—physical, spiritual, and emotional—his patients trust and confide in him the details of pivotal life periods and rely on his expertise during high-risk obstetric situations, while managing recurring miscarriages, or when performing advanced laparoscopic or conservative, minimally invasive gynecological surgeries. "I get a great deal of personal satisfaction from, and thank God for, the opportunities I have had to improve the quality of my patients' lives and share their experience of bringing new life into this world," confides Dr. Monks. "Hopefully, my efforts will consistently impact the lives of my patients in a positive way."

PAIN MANAGEMENT CONSULTANTS

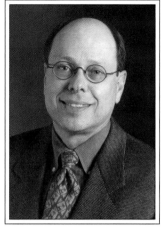

Pain Management is a field of medicine born from the discipline of Anesthesiology. The roots of pain are numerous, including disease, injury, and birth defects, but until the birth of pain management, there was little in the way of relief. The need for dealing with chronic pain was so strong that separate certification for this specialty became available in 1993. Austin doctor Julian Lowell "Sonny" Haro was among the first anesthesiologists to become board certified in pain management.

Haro's philosophy for alleviating his patients' pain involves treating "the whole patient." Whether that need requires injections, medicine, physical therapy, or psychological services, Haro uses a comprehensive plan to see to it that his patients receive the pain relief they need to lead productive lives. One method employed by Dr. Haro is radio frequency thermal coagulation. In this procedure, electric current in the tip of a needle is used to deaden pain. Liquid nitrogen is another pain defying procedure used by Haro to help his patients find relief.

An especially gratifying case of pain management was that of a cancer patient who had a leg amputated. The woman was on so much pain medicine that she was seldom awake. Her family could only watch her sleep away her life, until help came from Dr. Haro. He connected a pump of morphine to her spine with amazing results. "My sister's awake and not hurting. You gave me my sister back!" The gratitude of the woman's family made a lasting impression on Dr. Haro. He used just a small amount of the drug, but because he positioned the medication right at the woman's spine, she enjoyed the pain relief without sedation, something she had never experienced before.

THE PATIENT-PHYSICIAN PARTNERSHIP

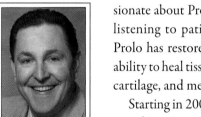

As a board-certified Physical Medicine and Rehabilitation (PM&R) specialist, Brad Fullerton, M.D. helps people be as functional as possible despite pain or disability. This focus has led Dr. Fullerton into a variety of leadership roles in Austin and Texas.

As Secretary and President-elect of the Texas PM&R Society, he has organized medical education meetings on degenerative musculoskeletal disease, ultrasound imaging of joints, and spasticity management for the Texas Medical Association (TMA). He serves as the Medical Director for the Spasticity Clinic at the Children's Hospital of Austin and has presented internationally on these topics. In 2000, he partnered with a local lung specialist to create a neuromuscular pulmonary clinic, the first of its kind in Austin.

In his private practice, The Patient-Physician Partnership, Dr. Fullerton focuses on patients with musculoskeletal pain related to sports injuries, arthritis, and accidents. Ask any of his patients and they will tell you that he is passionate about Prolotherapy or "Prolo." Years of listening to patients and treating them with Prolo has restored his faith in the body's own ability to heal tissues such as ligaments, tendons, cartilage, and meniscus.

Starting in 2000, he sought training in Ultrasound imaging to objectively evaluate tissue healing in response to Prolotherapy. He has presented this clinical research to physicians at the American Academy of PM&R, the American Association of Orthopedic Medicine, TMA, University of Pittsburgh, University of Wisconsin and the National Institute of Health. Dr. Fullerton now collaborates annually with the University of Pittsburgh/Pittsburgh VA to research ultrasound imaging in wheelchair athletes at the National Veteran Wheelchair Games.

Each patient is the only expert in their life history, values, symptoms, and intuition. Dr. Fullerton's goal is to partner with each individual patient and empower that patient to actively participate in their own healing.

KARIN MONTERO, M.D.

"PLASTIC SURGERY, THE MOST FUN SPECIALTY OF ALL," IS how Dr. Karin Montero describes her practice. We can treat children to seniors, from the toes to the head with conditions that are congenital or were acquired later, or which were created by trauma."

Dr. Montero is one of the plastic surgeons who participate in Austin Smiles, a not-for-profit group that donates services for people with congenital deformities who cannot afford surgery, from Austin to Central and South America and Asia. She has traveled with Austin Smiles to Ecuador and El Salvador many times. On some trips as many as 70 to 100 children have had cleft lips and palates repaired. "It's not the individual but the team," she states. "We all volunteer care for indigents at home. Going a step further has been possible thanks to many people before me and assuredly many more after."

Dr. Montero was the first female plastic surgeon in Austin. That was just one of her trailblazing efforts. Another was being the first-ever female graduate in Plastic Surgery from the University of Texas Medical Branch in Galveston. The decision to go into Plastic Surgery came after doing a General Surgery rotation at Children's Hospital in Philadelphia and a Pediatric Oncology rotation which Dr. Montero describes as "heartbreaking." Finally, a rotation in Plastic Surgery came along and this is where Dr. Montero found her niche and lifelong fulfillment.

Dr. Montero was sick a lot as a child, and because her family traveled to many countries due to her father's work, she felt she didn't fit in with other children. She, like most kids, felt the pressure of being different. "I was either too big or never thin enough, too athletic or hyperachieving, she says. This experience helped her be more empathetic to physical ailments and the emotional issues that accompany them.

Dr. Montero cares for a great variety of patients, performing reconstructions for cancer of the breasts, breast reductions, correction of asymmetries, and breast augmentations. "I am humbled by how much this means to them," she says of her grateful patients. "The majority have given it a lot of thought, they're well informed, and they do it for their own personal, intimate, self-esteem." Some of her pa-

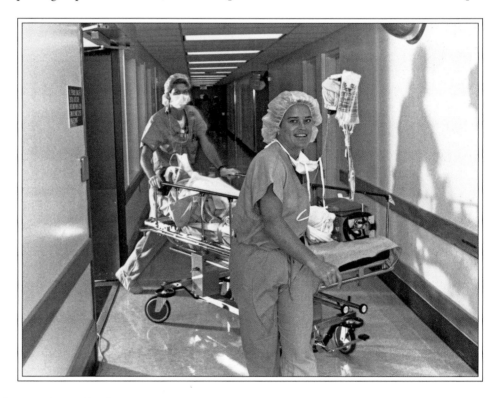

Dr. Karin Montero, the first female plastic surgeon in Austin.

tients are reluctant to wear a bathing suit or undress in front of another person prior to surgery. The change not only makes patients feel better about themselves physically, but their whole psychological outlook can change as well. They're doing it for themselves; you have to respect their choice, if they're realistic about their expectations.

In addition to breast work, Dr. Montero is skilled in body contouring and head and neck rejuvenation and keeps learning about new techniques and how to safely apply them.

Montero credits her 'wonderful staff' for making her office unique and welcoming, a place where people feel comfortable discussing their deepest feelings about changing something about their appearance which has been bothering them for many years.

PERSONIQUE

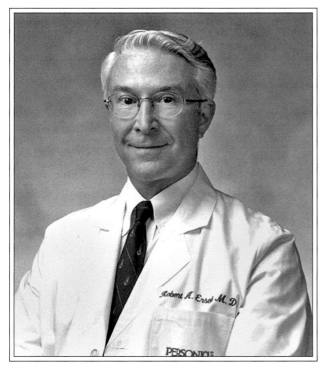

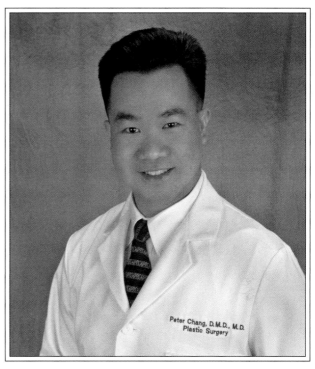

Dr. Robert Ersek (above left) and Dr. Peter Chang (above).

INTERNATIONALLY ACCLAIMED SURGEON, ROBERT ERSEK, M.D. established his Austin practice in 1978. Along with Peter Chang, M.D., Ersek performs only aesthetic, or cosmetic, surgery. Ersek has published more than 100 articles and delivered lectures around the world. His publications range from reconstructive surgical methods to skin grafting and technical reports on the suction-assisted lipectomy process. A pioneer in his field, Ersek has developed and invented numerous unique procedures for surgical techniques. He also invented the first intravascular stent (Patent No. 3,657,744), and is dedicated to the highest standards in the medical profession.

A highly sought after speaker and educator on plastic surgery, Ersek has been interviewed for national publications and television shows. He is a Clinical Assistant Professor of Plastic Surgery at Southwest Texas State University and an Instructor at the University of Texas. Certified by the American Board of Plastic and Reconstructive Surgery and a member of the American Medical Association and the Texas Medical Association, Ersek is affiliated with every major hospital in the Austin area. He is active in many civic organizations including the Austin Symphony and Ballet Austin, and is a member of Austin Smiles, a group of plastic surgeons and other volunteers who perform pro

bono cleft palate surgery for children from poor and undeveloped countries.

Dr. Chang is trained in all aspects of cosmetic surgery including liposuction, body contouring, and facial surgery. He is an active member of multiple national and regional medical societies. He has published many articles ranging from complex facial surgery to upper and lower extremity surgeries. He has also authored several books and articles on cosmetic surgeries.

Aesthetic surgery is often equated solely with facelifts and other age-related procedures. At Personique, cosmetic surgery is an elective procedure designed to alter a person's appearance in a positive way. All of Personique's employees are walking testimonials to the benefits of aesthetic surgery, as everyone has had at least one surgery. "If you want something special done, you go to a specialist. That's why our patients come here. We do 100 percent aesthetic surgeries, and we have more than 30,000 cases worth of experience, all done with sedation and local anesthesia," says Ersek. He adds, "Patient confidentiality is carefully respected here. We have complete facilities on-site, with a private recovery area right next door to the operating room."

PHYSICAL MEDICINE & REHABILITATION

TAKING PATIENTS FROM THE DEPTHS OF DESPAIR into the sunshine of hope through an intensive rehabilitationprogram by helping injured and disabled patients reach higher levels of independence has been the major emphasis of the professional life of Rodney J. Simonsen, M.D., board certified in Physical Medicine and Rehabilitation.

Simonsen was the first physiatrist to practice in Austin in 1974 at the invitation of neurologists Douglas Hudson, M.D. and Peter Werner, M.D. With them he established the first rehabilitation center at Shoal Creek Hospital, known as TRI, the Texas Rehabilitation Institute. He played a major leadership role in the development of both St. David's Rehabilitation Center and Brackenridge Hospital, which is now known as HealthSouth. In 1981, he was recognized for his work in rehabilitation both by the City of Austin and the State of Texas as Physician of the Year.

The concept of total inpatient rehabilitation could not happen without the many other additional staff members from the disciplines of rehabilitation nurses, especially Kit Goth, R.N., physical and occupational therapists, speech pathologists and therapists, social workers, cognitive therapists and psychologists, and the ever-present rehabilitation technicians. In addition, the orthopedic and neurosurgical specialists have been extremely supportive as they have turned their patients over to the rehabilitation team. There are countless patients and families who have benefited from the growth of rehabilitation in Central Texas.

In the 1980s, Dr. Simonsen introduced STAART (Sports Therapy and Advanced Rehabilitation Training) to the Austin community, a new concept of aggressive conditioning for work-related injuries similar to those used for athletes and now known as stabilization exercises worldwide.

Joe Powell, M.D. was the second physiatrist to practice in Austin and he has developed the concept of outpatient office-based physiatry. Currently there are several additional physiatrists practicing in the Austin metropolitan area. Everett Heinze, M.D., a neurologist, has sought additional training in rehabilitation and he, together with Dr. Simonsen, formed the first pain clinic in Central Texas in

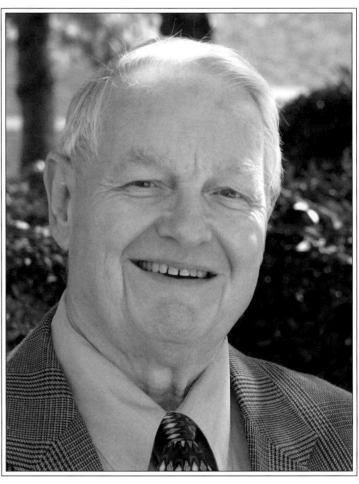

Rodney J. Simonsen, M.D. was Austin's first physiatrist.

1978, where they became a strong team in combining the skills of physiatry and neurology.

In the 1990s, Dr. Simonsen became fully credentialed, and then became a Diplomat of the McKenzie method of treating spinal pain which he introduced to Central Texas. He brought two McKenzie Institute International faculty members, Scott Herbowy and Mark Miller, to Austin where they are now established and have one of the premier nonsurgical spine clinics and teaching institutes in the world.

Dr. Simonsen and his wife Helga have raised their seven children in Austin and they will soon have 22 grandchildren. They will spend a great part of their retirement years providing healthcare to missionaries overseas, continuing to make life better for those in need. Much heartfelt appreciation is expressed to the many that have played a vital role in rehabilitation in Travis County.

RENAISSANCE WOMEN'S GROUP

THE RENAISSANCE WOMEN'S GROUP (RWG) WAS FORMED in the mid-1990s with the goal of quality, caring women's health care, attempting to retain the advantages of a solo or small group practice, but achieving the efficiencies and benefits that a larger group of physicians has to offer to their patients. The group is comprised of eight physicians: Linda Litzinger, Laura Meritt, Byron Darby, Melanie Collins, Sherry Neyman, Laurette Smith, Michele Gilbert, and Tara Mills who practice primary Obstetrics and Gynecology and share call to provide quality obstetric and gynecologic care to their patients around the clock. Byron Darby's practice is dedicated to prenatal diagnosis and Ob/Gyn ultrasound and he sees patients on a referral basis from both inside and outside the group. Donna Hurley recently retired from the group but remains a strong influence on the group's dedication to quality patient care.

Dr. Litzinger, Dr. Meritt, Dr. Hurley, and Dr. Darby were already practicing in Austin for a number of years before joining forces under the RWG umbrella. Dr. Neyman and Dr. Collins also arrived early in the group's formative years after completing their residency programs in 1996. Other members joining the group immediately after completing their residency include Dr. Smith in 1999, Dr. Gilbert in 2000, and Dr. Mills in 2004. The practice is one of the busiest in Austin, delivering an average of 150 babies a month. The group utilizes North Austin Medical Center, part of the St. David's network, and one of the newest facilities in Austin.

While Obstetrics is a major focus, RWG treats women of all ages, from the teens into the menopause years. Other focuses of the group include well woman care, contraception, hormone therapy, basic infertility, endometriosis, and urinary incontinence. The members of the group strive to provide state-of-the-art care, staying on the cutting edge of Ob/Gyn practice. Dr. Darby is recognized as one of the pioneers of prenatal diagnosis and ultrasound in central Texas, and his ultrasound practice is one of the few in Austin accredited by the American Institute of Ultrasound in Medicine.

In addition, the physicians of the Renaissance Women's Group work closely with a number of experienced and highly qualified advanced nurse practitioners and physicians assistants who provide excellent patient care for uncomplicated problems and achieve immense patient loyalty from the patients they care for. The group also pro-

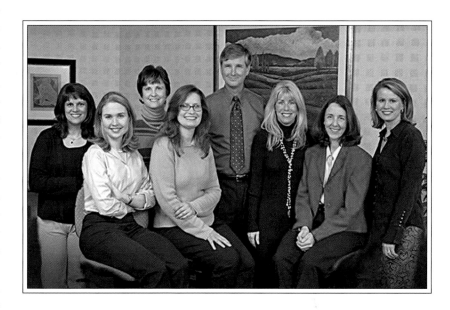

Renaissance Women's Group, left to right, Laurette Smith, M.D., Tara Mills, M.D., Sherry Neyman, M.D., Michele Gilbert, M.D., Byron Darby, M.D., Linda Litzinger, M.D., Laura Meritt, M.D., and Melanie Collins, M.D.

vides a number of ancillary services to its patients. RWG offers childbirth preparation classes, given by nurses who all have a wealth of experience caring for pregnant women. It also offers a class to teach new parents how to care for newborns and a class to help siblings prepare for the arrival of their new baby brother or sister. Another service RWG provides is on-site bone density testing and treatment of bone loss.

Since its inception, the Renaissance Women's Group has grown tremendously, in spite of moving from a southwest Austin location to north Austin in 2001. The group is grateful to its loyal patients, which is the reason RWG continues to grow. Regardless of where a woman is in her life cycle, she can trust the knowledgeable physicians and staff of the Renaissance Women's Group to provide excellent Ob/Gyn care and to offer a variety of valuable services.

DEIRDRE M. RHOAD, M.D.

WITH A FAMILY BACKGROUND THAT INCLUDES TEXAS roots and success in the sciences, it seems appropriate that Dr. Rhoad became a part of local history by assuming the practice of Dr. Frank Morris, the first plastic surgeon in Austin. Even as a child, Dr. Rhoad was attracted to biology. She raised tadpoles, was fascinated with her mother's volunteer work at a leprosy colony, and dreamed of the chance to see open-heart surgery. She was excited to learn that her grandfather was a noted geneticist who received an honorary degree for developing the Santa Gertrudis breed of cattle for the King Ranch in Texas. It also inspired her to follow her dreams.

As she pursued medicine, her sisters Sharon and Melissa provided both financial support and a ready

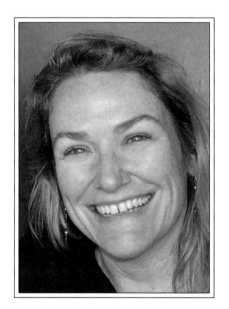

cheering team, and, in 1987, Dr. Rhoad graduated from medical school. Although she encountered some who were suspicious of her motives and questioned her resolve to continue on a path less traveled by women, she continued to claim her rightful place. At her residency program in General Surgery at New York Medical College, she was pleased to discover she had a natural aptitude for plastic surgery and patients often appreciated that she was a woman. She completed programs in Burn Surgery and Plastic Surgery in Detroit and Cosmetic Surgery in New York. Now many know how perfectly suited Dr. Rhoad is for her profession and she is grateful to be making people happy by blending her artistic abilities and technical talents.

ROXANA A. RHODES, M.D.

A VISIT TO THE OFFICE OF DR. ROXANA RHODES IS A VISIT to a third-generation Texas physician. She is the daughter of two Corpus Christi doctors and the granddaughter of the first Hispanic physician in Fort Worth. Dr. Rhodes's family has been healing Texans for over 100 years!

A large number of Dr. Rhodes's patients are from the University of Texas (U.T.) community. Students, faculty, and other U.T. staff seek her council when it comes to their health, because of her strong emphasis on keeping them well. "I think the big difference is that I'm into prevention. I try to make sure they're up to date on all their mammograms, cholesterol screenings, and inoculations," says Dr. Rhodes. Another area of consideration for U.T. and other patients is that

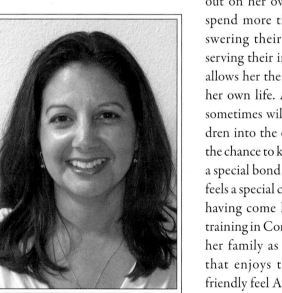

they can plan their schedule around an appointment with Dr. Rhodes. "I run on time. Patients' time is valuable."

Dr. Rhodes left a large group practice in 1996 to branch out on her own. This allows her to spend more time with patients, answering their questions and better serving their individual needs. It also allows her the flexibility she needs in her own life. A mother of three, she sometimes will bring one of her children into the office. Her patients get the chance to know her family, and feel a special bond with them. Dr. Rhodes feels a special connection with Austin, having come here directly from her training in Connecticut. She describes her family as an "outdoorsy" group that enjoys the casual and family friendly feel Austin offers.

GIL ROEBUCK, M.D.

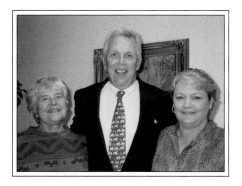

DR. GIL ROEBUCK OPENED HIS private practice in internal medicine in Austin in 1987. Over the past 20 years, this practice has become an extended family of friends. Shown in the photo are two of Dr. Roebuck's best friends: Karen Baker (on the right), who ran the practice for nine years until 1995; and Enge Meier (on the left) who became office manager and took over the duty of keeping Dr. Gil in line. Kind, good people like Karen and Enge make a practice work. The doctors who they supervise appreciate them and so do the patients, who are the extended family they try to help.

At Dr. Roebuck's office, most patients' voices are recognized when they call in, even before they identify themselves. Most have stayed with him through thick and thin over the past 20 years. It is an extended family of friends trying to work together in an increasingly stressful world.

This extended family—our patients—are very much appreciated and valued.

Also much valued are colleagues of all stripes. Austin has a wonderful blend of generalists and specialists. Two colleagues who have supported and sustained Dr. Roebuck are known to Austinites as Austin Allergy Associates; first, Dr. Lob Exline, and now Dr. Thurman Ray Vaughan. Dr. Roebuck is indebted to them and could never repay this extended family of Austin Allergy Associates in full or in kind.

Finally, all doctors' families know that patience on their part is the ultimate keystone to any medical practice. Dr. Roebuck's bride, Lisa Marie Weinheimer, is his touchstone.

We should all be thankful every day. Dr. Gil Roebuck is most thankful for all of you, his close and extended family, here in Austin, Texas.

RITA SCHINDELER-TRACHTA, D.O.

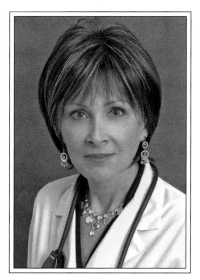

A UNITED STATES AIR FORCE VETERAN, Dr. Rita Schindeler-Trachta was working directly with the astronauts as a contractor for Johnson Space Center NASA when she recognized that she had not yet discovered her life's work. She experienced her "aha" moment when dissecting a cat for a natural science course and there was no looking back. After 22 years in aerospace, she entered medical school at age 43. Schindeler-Trachta says that, to her knowledge, she held the honor of being Brackenridge Hospital's oldest graduating resident at age 49. Those who know Schindeler-Trachta know that she probably ran circles around her younger counterparts.

Within one week of her entering medical school, Schindeler-Trachta's son, now a United States Navy F/A-18 pilot, started college. They graduated virtually simultaneously and now live their dreams. A teenage runaway, Schindeler-Trachta is no stranger to hard work, perseverance, and standing on her own two feet. Her intense passion and dedication was evident at her former practice, the Austin Family Medical Clinic, which she founded and operated for four years.

Schindeler-Trachta is now the Medical Quality Director for the State of Texas in the Department of Aging and Disability Services where she helps thousands of people in Texas nursing homes and the developmentally and physically impaired. She continues to practice clinical medicine part-time on the weekends, and serves as a volunteer physician in a tattoo removal clinic, helping primarily teens with gang-related tattoos.

SENSORY VIEW

Though it may seem unorthodox for a highly trained surgeon to go into the business of finding medical therapeutics to alter the course of nervous system disorders, Dr. Kendal Stewart has spent years making his previous surgical expertise less of a necessity for his and other doctors' patients. Even during high school, Dr. Stewart was eager to become a doctor. He had the benefit of having a father, Landon Stewart, M.D., and an uncle, Sidney Stewart, M.D., to peak his interest during his childhood years. When he was only 20 years old, he began medical school at the University of Texas Medical School at Houston. He completed his formal medical education in Ear, Nose, and Throat/Head and Neck Surgery at the University of Texas at Houston/MD Anderson Hospital System and continued his training with a fellowship in Neurotology/Skull Base Surgery from Baylor University Medical Center in Dallas.

In 1994, he arrived in Austin and began focusing on the treatment of complicated inner ear and nervous system syndromes using surgical procedures. In rapidly increasing numbers, patients suffering from severe neurological syndromes such as vertigo, imbalance, progressive hearing loss, and memory disorders, such as dementia and Alzheimer's, began arriving at his doorstep. These patients had previously met countless obstacles in their search for a cure, or even a diagnosis, and, at best, had found treatment only for their symptoms. By necessity, Dr. Stewart gradually became an expert in these areas. At the same time, he became attracted to a new field of medicine called "neurotrophism," which focuses on new methods for altering or reversing the progression of degenerative syndromes of the nervous system. As a surgeon focusing on the skull base, he was already an expert at testing nerves in the skull region. He started recognizing that the patients who are unable to process information normally were not being fed accurate information from their sensory system. He also noticed correlations between the severity of symptoms and the degree of misinformation being sent to the brain. "If a patient has chronic dizziness, they are probably also experiencing other symptoms including clumsiness, difficulty sleeping, thinking, concentrating, formulating words and sentences, more emotionality, and just not feeling good. These are all complaints that doctors can't see and the patient is easily misdiagnosed, and may be eventually labeled as a hypochondriac" admitted Dr. Stewart.

In an attempt to better understand these patients' needs, Dr. Stewart acquired a large array of FDA-approved diagnostic equipment from many different manufacturers in his office setting. Some of these systems were developed 20 years ago, others more recently. Some of the systems were developed in the NASA program. Using these diagnostic methods, he noticed many correlations between the different tests and, in a sense, he began to 'see' the symptoms. Despite some raised eyebrows from the medical community, he began using medical therapies aimed at reducing inflammation of the nervous system and returning the body's hormonal and nutritional status to a better state. His non-conventional approach worked well and today is accepted and utilized by many physicians throughout the country. In 2002, Dr. Stewart was granted a U.S. patent for the network integration of these specific diagnostic testing devices.

In 2003, Dr. Stewart assembled a team of Austin business experts and software engineers to develop and distribute a software product designed to incorporate the diagnostic systems he had used. This software, Sensory View,™ incorporates all testing data from the individual tests and stores it in a central database. Instead of using the overwhelming human resources of large academic centers to gather data and write publications, the team created a query system to access diagnostic outcomes and make correlations between diagnostic data. The doctor support was so overwhelming after creating Sensory View that an idea of creating a nationwide network of specialty facilities utilizing this software was proposed. To that end, a new company, NeuroSensory Centers of America, Inc., was born.

Although it took the hi-tech community and entrepreneurial spirit of Austin to launch his product, it seems that it is attracting attention from sophisticated professionals, as well as some rural doctors, enabling them to provide diagnostic services equivalent to that of a major medical center in any location. By testing the brain and the information it is receiving and how it is responding to that information, a doctor has an objective picture of symptom-based diseases. "If you compare a human body to a computer, the sensory system of the body—vision, three-dimensional processing, touch, feel, etc.—is like the software program for a computer. Even if the computer is perfect, if the program is bad, the computer will not work

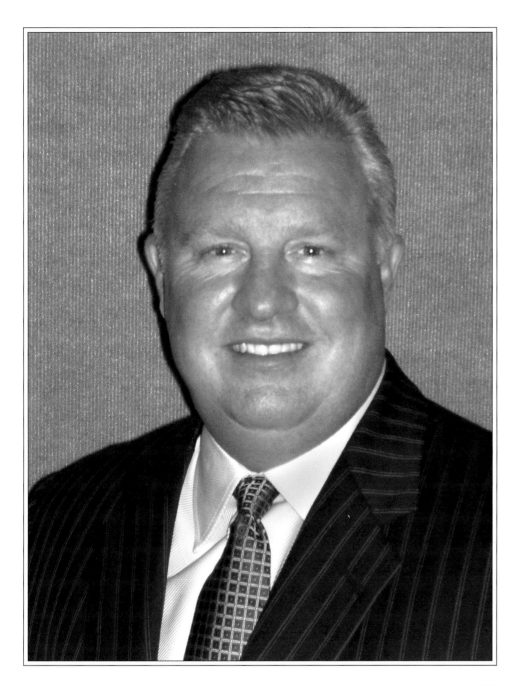

Dr. Kendal Stewart, developer of the diagnostic systems incorporated into Sensory View™ software.

munity. He followed the advice of a now famous "dizzy doctor," John Epley, who suggested trying a less political path than the usual one of publications and conferences. "After all," comments Dr. Stewart, "the products we utilize are all FDA-approved and widely accepted. Putting them together just creates a better picture of the patient's abnormality. I'm just eager for other doctors to use the same objective systems and utilize their own individual medical protocols; then we can compare data utilizing the same diagnostics and judge each protocol's effects." Together, doctors can then determine the best patient protocol. With ongoing use, Dr. Stewart foresees the database of diagnostic information growing with each patient's use, perhaps setting the stage for many other important discoveries. Sensory View™ software is currently being utilized in 13 different facilities in places like Dallas, Houston, Austin, Kansas City, Abilene, Midland/Odessa, Lincoln, Nebraska, Indiana, and New Mexico.

Patients throughout the nation seek out Dr. Stewart's clinic and its services. The Sensory View™ can show concerned patients who have spent years of searching and studying, as well as thousands of dollars on previous attempts at diagnosis, that they indeed have a problem. It can display the abnormalities objectively to fellow doctors and patients. Even better, it can objectively reveal when a specific treatment has reversed the condition. "I originally got into medicine to take care of people, and now I really feel like I am. I'm no longer merely a technician. It's so exciting to be out here on the cutting edge of medicine."

properly," explains Dr. Stewart. "We created a diagnostic model using up to 15 variables that results in a highly accurate statistical model of how the body is utilizing its senses. If all the variables match, theoretically, it can only be wrong once in a billion times."

After working with colleagues at The University of Texas and the University of Southern California Medical School, as well as other academic centers, and after years of clinical research and development, Dr. Stewart followed a surprisingly quiet path of presenting his model to the medical com-

SETON FAMILY OF HOSPITALS

THE SETON FAMILY OF HOSPITALS WAS founded in Austin by the Daughters of Charity more than a hundred years ago. Today, it bears little resemblance to the original Seton Infirmary, which brought Central Texans their first professional nurses in 1902. Since then, Seton has become the leading provider of healthcare services in Central Texas with more than 23 hospitals and healthcare facilities across the region, including five urban acute care hospitals, two rural hospitals, a mental health hospital, several outpatient service facilities, and three primary care clinics. Seton, a member of Ascension Health,

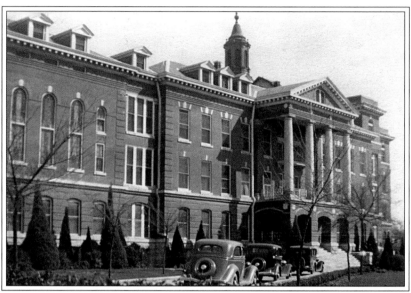

the nation's largest non-profit Catholic healthcare system, is Central Texas's largest community service organization and second largest private employer. While many things have changed over the years, Seton's mission has never wavered: to provide health care to the greater Central Texas area with special regard for the sick and the poor.

For more than a century, Seton has faced challenges and risks, from smallpox to flu epidemics. In 1930, during the Great Depression, Sister Philomena Feltz, a member of the Daughters of Charity and supervisor of the Diet Kitchen, opened a soup kitchen and, after feeding patients, provided food to long lines of hungry Austinites waiting outside the back door of the Infirmary.

Over time, the Infirmary changed its name to Seton Hospital and expanded its services to include intensive care, heart surgery, imaging, maternity, and skilled nursing care. As the community continued to grow, it became apparent that Seton needed to grow as well. In 1975, Seton Hospital closed its doors on 26th Street and reopened at its present location as Seton Medical Center. Seton Medical Center Austin has continued to expand over the years, becoming a referral center for complex patients requiring highly skilled care for cardiac, cancer, surgery, and maternity services and home to the region's only neonatal center. Seton also added new facilities, opening a community health center, Seton McCarthy, to provide primary medical care and social services for the working poor. Two additional primary care clinics have been added since then: Seton Topfer and Seton Kozmetsky. Simi-

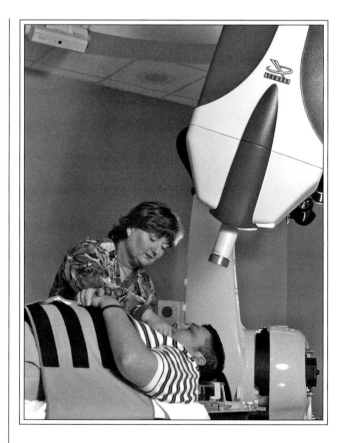

larly, Seton Northwest Hospital opened in 1991 in response to the need for convenient care for those living in the rapidly expanding area north of Austin.

In 1995, Seton and the City of Austin entered into an historic lease agreement that sought the network's expertise in operating the region's only dedicated pediatric hospital, the only Level II Trauma Center, Brackenridge Hospital, and the only children's hospital, Children's Hospital of Austin. In addition, at the request of leadership in each community, Seton acquired Highland Lakes Hospital in Burnet and Seton Edgar B. Davis Hospital in Luling, bring-

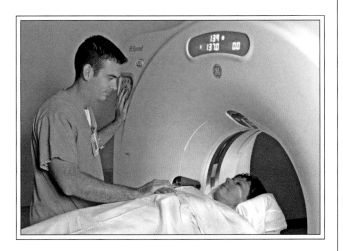

The Seton Family of Hospitals has grown from the original Seton Infirmary (opposite page, above) to more than 23 hospitals and healthcare facilities across Central Texas. Modern technology at Seton includes CT scans (above) and Cyberknife (opposite page below), a painless, non-invasive treatment for previously inoperable tumors.

ing them into the Seton family. When Seton opened additional medical service centers in Cedar Park, Pflugerville, and near Oak Hill—the largest being Seton Southwest Hospital—the Seton Family of Hospitals was born.

As Seton entered the twenty-first century, it faced new challenges, including an aging population and continued dynamic growth. It continues to address the healthcare needs of Central Texans by expanding its hospitals, creating new services, adding state-of-the-art technology and planning new hospitals to meet demand. The new Dell Children's Medical Center, which is located at the former Robert Mueller Municipal Airport, opened in June 2007. It is approximately three times larger than the former children's hospital and will help address overcrowding challenges in patient beds, surgery, emergency care, and parking that existed. The 170-bed hospital includes a 33-room emergency department and a 12-suite surgery center, along with associated patient prep, recovery, diagnostic, and outpatient capacity.

To meet the healthcare needs of Williamson County, Seton Medical Center Williamson is scheduled to open in Feb-

ruary 2008 on 74 acres in Northeast Round Rock. The 365,000-square-foot medical center will include more than 180 beds, with the ability to expand to 350 beds by 2020. It will offer the most advanced care and the latest available technology and will be the lynchpin of major new growth and economic development in the area. In order to meet the needs of the exploding population south of Travis County, representatives with the Seton Family of Hospitals have approved the purchase of property in Hays County. Seton is developing a major medical center at the site to add to its growing family of hospitals across Central Texas.

Seton's efforts over the years have brought not only much-needed and often unique services to Central Texas, but have also garnered national recognition. In 2002, four of Seton's acute care hospitals were awarded the coveted Magnet status, the highest level of recognition given by the American Nurses Credentialing Center for excellence in nursing. Two years later, Seton Medical Center Austin and Brackenridge Hospital became the first hospitals in Texas to be recognized as Primary Stroke Centers by the Joint Commission on Accreditation of Healthcare Organizations for offering comprehensive stroke prevention and treatment programs. Also a first for Central Texas, the Brain and Spine Center at Brackenridge Hospital offers the CyberKnife, a painless, non-invasive treatment approach to irradiating cancers of the head, neck, and spine, which can be used to treat tumors or lesions, once considered inoperable, anywhere within the body. Responding to the urgent need for more physicians, nurses, and other health care staff in central Texas as well as the nation, Seton has joined forces with The University of Texas at Austin, Austin Community College, and the University of Texas Medical Branch-Austin Programs to collaborate on a unique interdisciplinary education center. The Clinical Education Center at Brackenridge (CEC), includes flexible classroom spaces equipped with built-in multimedia technology, a state-of-the-art medical and surgical simulation center, facilities for teaching patient-provider communication, clinical areas set up as skills labs for health professionals, a computer lab, and a learning resources area.

The Seton Family of Hospitals continues to build on a century of service, committed to providing access to comprehensive, leading edge, compassionate health care to all patients, regardless of their ability to pay. In the future, Seton wants to further that proud tradition, successfully addressing the ever-growing demand of our changing community. Through leadership, collaborative efforts, and good stewardship, Seton can meet those demands and truly make an impact on those it serves.

SMART CARE OF TEXAS

ALTHOUGH NOT ENTIRELY SATISFIED WITH A TERM THAT accurately depicts his practice model, Sidney Robin, M.D. knows what his patients get out of it—more of his time. And that's exactly the way he likes it. In family practice since June 1976, Robin changed his practice mode in January 2001 to what is often called "concierge medicine." Eschewing that term, which he says sounds a bit "uppity," Robin explains that the "retainer medicine" approach allows him to limit his practice to about 1,000 patients. Each patient pays a predetermined fee in exchange for an unlimited number of office visits and routine lab work. "This allows me to spend my time on what's important—my patients," says Robin, one of the earliest pioneers of this approach. "I can spend an hour performing a physical exam. The patients are more relaxed and I can help guide them to where they need to be, if they need to be somewhere else. And we don't have nearly the paperwork hassle."

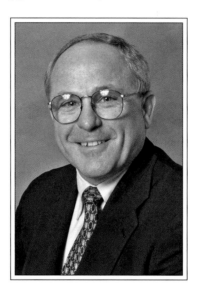

In addition to the rewards of a practice that allows him to establish the doctor-patient relationship he values, Robin derives great pleasure from mission work that has taken him as far as Africa. A medical team of 120 Americans and 80 Zambians saw 19,000 people in a period of seven days during his 2003 trip. Robin's wife and two adult children accompanied him.

Dr. Robin and his wife Susan have two children. Brett, previously a running back for the University of Texas football team, now attends the University of Texas Medical School at San Antonio and Berkeley attends Texas Christian University.

SOUTH AUSTIN ORTHOPEDIC CLINIC

IN 1978, WHEN THERE WERE FEW specialists and no hospitals south of the Colorado River in Austin, Drs. Michael Elliott and Gary Phipps opened their own orthopedic clinic on South Lamar Street, and became Austin's first orthopedic group south of the river. In 1982, a hospital opened in South Austin. The area's population swelled, another medical center formed, and the demand for orthopedic services increased.

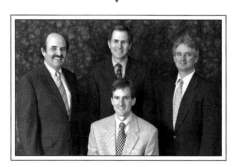

Clockwise from left, Doctors Race, Savage, Blais, and Westmoreland.

To help meet those demands, the group recruited Dr. Clark Race, who completed his orthopedic training at Southwestern Medical School, in 1983; Dr. David Savage, who trained at Emory University, in 1995; and Dr. Robert Blais, who trained at UTMB Galveston, in 1997. The team relocated to their current Westgate location in 2000, and two years later recruited their latest orthopedist, Dr. Greg Westmoreland, following his sports medicine fellowship in Knoxville, Tennessee. In June 2003, the group further expanded. They opened the South Austin Rehab and Wound Clinic on Ben White Boulevard to provide comprehensive wound care and full-scale rehabilitation services, including aquatic, occupational, physical, and speech therapy.

Despite the broad spectrum of services, the doctors manage to maintain reasonable schedules, allowing time for personable doctor/patient relationships to develop and for patients to become part of the care team. Employees of the clinic, three of whom have been with the clinic for twenty years, are also entrusted to be a part of that team. The result is quality treatment that is top choice for even medical professionals who are seeking care.

SOUTHWESTERN COLON & RECTAL SURGERY

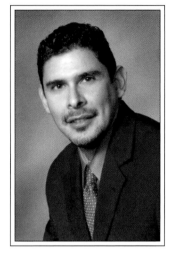

IT MAY BE DIFFICULT TO FIND A COLO-rectal surgeon in Austin, as there are but a small handful. Among the select few is Dr. Ricardo Solis. Dr. Solis says the other colorectal surgeons in Austin are very supportive and encouraging of one another, often working together to find the best treatment for patients.

Although neither of his parents finished high school, Dr. Solis says "ever since I was a kid, a little boy, I wanted to be a doctor." Solis turned that dream into a reality and married his longtime sweetheart along the way. His wife, Julie is also a physician. Solis's mother was just 50 years old when she died of a stroke, another factor that helped fuel Dr. Solis's desire to become a doctor. He credits the Texas Medical Associa-tion (TMA) with getting his office up and running. He says the TMA's physician services department helped him arrange everything from the office space itself to the equipment he uses to treat patients.

One patient he recalls had severe abdominal pain. She was the wife of a friend and had been evaluated by several other doctors. She credits Solis with being the first in a long line of physicians willing to take the necessary time to properly explain her disease and treatment options. The time following surgery was the first time she had relief from the terrible symptoms she had been suffering from for years. Dr. Solis says it gives him great pleasure to be able to give people the gift of good health and the ability to lead productive lives.

BENJAMIN SUPNET, M.D.

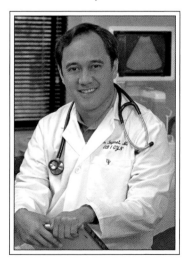

WOMEN LOOKING FOR A GYNECOLO-gist/obstetrician they can count on for years to come have been able to rely on the South Austin Ob/Gyn practice of Dr. Benjamin Supnet. "Sometimes your patients become your friends," he says. Without a doubt, an obstetrician has the opportunity to develop a lifelong friendship with patients and their families, and that's something Dr. Supnet looks forward to in his growing practice.

The son of two physicians, medicine seemed a natural fit for Dr. Supnet. And as the only boy in a family of four children, attending to women's health was an extension of that fit. "I like delivering babies; it's rewarding and gratifying, and you establish strong relationships with patients."

At his former practice, South Austin Ob/Gyn*, Dr. Supnet had more than his share of unusual cases. He once stayed up all night with a woman who had a ruptured uterus. She continued to hemorrhage even though she received a blood transfusion. Dr. Supnet did an emergency hysterectomy which stopped the hemorrhaging, saving the woman's life.

Patient education is a passion for Dr. Supnet. It is important to him to answer all of his patients' questions, no matter how many there are, or how long it takes. He feels strongly that his patients should have all the information and knowledge they need to lead healthy lives. Whether it is routine care or a life-saving emergency, Dr. Benjamin Supnet wishes to care for the gynecological and obstetric needs of his patients for many, many years to come.

*As of November 5, 2007, Dr. Supnet relocated his practice to his home town of Corpus Christi.

'SPECIALLY FOR CHILDREN

A SERIOUS ILLNESS CAN BE A DIFFICULT AND CHALLENGING step in a child's development. Such a diagnosis also can be especially trying for families. For these children and adolescents, a dedicated team of physicians, nurses, and other care givers offers hope for a healthier future—and a positive, healing atmosphere close to home and family.

The only practice of its kind in Central Texas, 'Specially for Children (SFC) is a group of pediatric subspecialists who provide expert treatment and a family-focused healing environment to meet the special medical needs of patients with a wide range of complex medical problems. The physician specialists of SFC are experts in many different areas of pediatric medicine and provide comprehensive diagnostic care and treatment of most childhood illnesses and diseases. They offer specialty services in the areas of: Allergy/Asthma/Immunology, Clinical Genetics, Endocrinology, Gastroenterology and Nutrition, Hematology/Oncology, Infectious Disease, Nephrology, Neurology, Palliative Care, and Rheumatology.

Physicians and staff provide inclusive, high-quality clinical care for children and adolescents from birth through eighteen years of age. Patients are accepted by physician referral when the child or adolescent is newly diagnosed or suspected of having a disease or illness requiring treatment from a pediatric subspecialist.

The Seed of Pediatric Subspecialty Care in Central Texas

SFC is one of the few pediatric medical subspecialty practices of its size and breadth in the country that has developed outside of the typical, large urban area medical school environment model. As the Austin and Central Texas community grew, it reached the point where the region needed and would support comprehensive and multidisciplinary, subspecialty care for children and adolescents. In 1996, SFC

BELOW: *James Sharp, M.D. (left) and Donald Wells, M.D.*
OPPOSITE PAGE, TOP TO BOTTOM: *Linda Shaffer, M.D., Jeff Kerr, M.D., and Sharon Lockhart, M.D.*

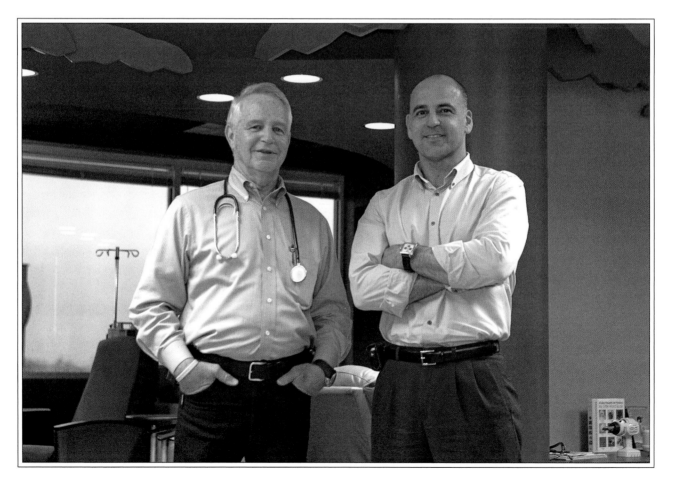

was formed as a joint venture between the founding group of pediatric subspecialists (James Sharp, M.D., Sharon Lockhart, M.D., and Donald Wells, M.D. in Pediatric Hematology/Oncology, and David Anglin, M.D., Kenneth Maslonka, M.D., and Nancy Felsing, M.D. in Pediatric Intensive Care) and the Seton Family of Hospitals. The primary goal of the joint venture was to develop and expand a pediatric subspecialty program to service a 46-county region specifically associated with Children's Hospital of Austin, a member hospital of Seton. As part of Seton's mission, care is provided to pa-

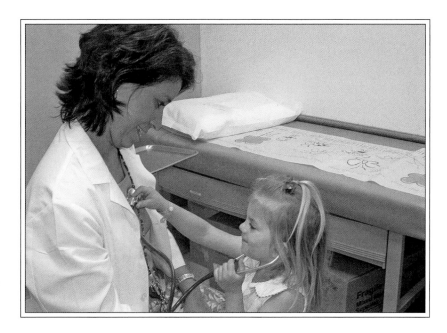

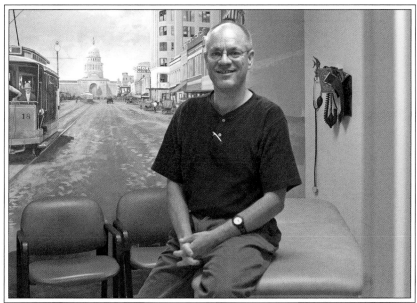

tients regardless of their ability to pay. Today, pediatric patients with the most chronic or complex illnesses no longer have to travel to larger Texas metropolitan areas to receive the multidisciplinary specialty care they require. More than 15,000 patients are seen by the 26 pediatric subspecialists of SFC each year. Most are treated on a continuing outpatient basis with utilization of hospitalization and outpatient programs at Children's Hospital as necessary.

Having most of the pediatric subspecialists included in one group makes

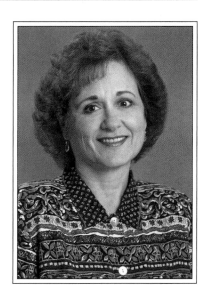

for easy communication and enables physicians to have easy access to each other's expertise informally, and for consultation. Financial backing by the Seton Family of Hospitals has allowed the practice to grow and serve the needs of its patients by attracting and recruiting more specialists to the area.

Growing with the Community

Central Texas is one of the fastest growing regions in the country, and the need for quality health care for the pediatric population is keeping pace. SFC is ready for growth.

In late June 2007, Children's Hospital closed and moved to a brand new facility, Dell Children's Medical Center of Central Texas. Full of innovative design elements that optimize the healing and family environment as well as state-of-the-art technology, Dell Children's is three times the size of the current hospital. In March 2007, SFC moved to the Dell Children's campus and opened its new offices at the Strictly Pediatrics medical office building. Once again, with Dell Children's, SFC is poised at the forefront of future children's health care in Central Texas and to meet the needs of a rapidly growing community.

SOUTHWEST SKIN & CANCER CLINIC, P.A.

SINCE OPENING HIS SOUTH Austin dermatology office in 1977, Dr. Houston has seen the area expand in population and available medical services. "I enjoyed growing up in South Austin," he says. "The people here are so friendly and appreciative!"

After graduating from the University of Texas in Austin and the UT Medical School in San Antonio, Dr. Houston studied Dermatology at Baylor College of Medicine in Houston. During his early career as a general dermatologist in Austin, Dr. Houston received invaluable support from fellow physicians, including Allen Sonstein, Henry Dittert, Glenn Graves, Joe Malleske, Eric Weidmann, Dennis Berger, Robert Stroud, Richard Helmer, Lee Arnold, V. C. Smart, and Charles Ferrin.

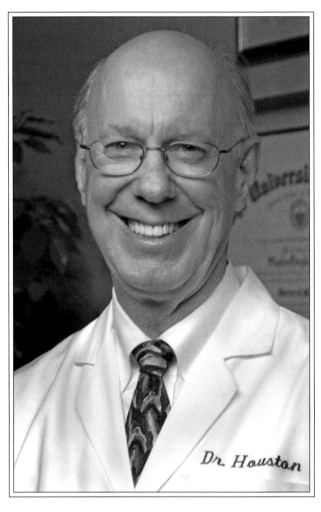

Dr. Stephen D. Houston

our clinic is that we have a dedicated, highly competent, and above all, compassionate staff," reflects Dr. Houston. "When a patient walks through the door and feels warmly greeted, valued, and cared for, it makes everyone's job easier, especially the patient's! It is gratifying to have seen dermatology in Austin steadily improve because of the high quality of medical professionals that have moved into the community," continues Dr. Houston. "We now have an excellent group of general dermatologists, surgical dermatologists, and dermato-pathologists." He gives a special note of appreciation to fellow dermatologists with whom he often works very closely: William Ramsdell, Anne Epstein, Mary Ann Martinez, Robert Jackson, John Fox, Janet Dubois, Michael Coverman, John Ghidoni, and Brian Townsend.

Later, during the 1990s, Dr. Houston's dermatology practice evolved into a surgical one, leading him to found the Southwest Skin & Cancer Clinic, P.A. Currently, most of his time is spent caring for patients with skin cancer, frequently using Mohs Micrographic Surgery. This technique helps to assure the complete removal of difficult skin cancers through careful microscopic examination of excised tissue. Having earned his degree in Microbiology from the University of Texas, Dr. Houston says, "It feels very natural to move back and forth between removing skin cancer from the patient in the surgical suite and examining their tissue under the microscope."

Since 1998, Dr. Houston's clinic has been enhanced by the help of Austin's first dermatology physician assistant, Connie Sterritt, M.P.A., PA-C. "The key to the success of

Dr. Houston appreciates the fact that his dermatology practice allows him to care for persons of all ages over an extended period of time. "It's much like family practice in that way, seeing patients through the years," explains Dr. Houston. He realizes how important connecting to his patients has been to his success as a doctor and to his patients' progress. "I see myself as my patients' coach. I want them to feel empowered as participants on a team, the same way I would want to feel as a patient."

"My patients are much like my extended family, and I owe so much in my professional life to them." He emphasizes, however, that "I am most grateful to my wife Dixie, and my children Chris, Emily, and Kate, who have been so inspiring and supportive of me all these years."

KAREN TEEL, M.D.

ALTHOUGH SOME OF HER COLLEAGUES AND CO-WORKERS refer to Dr. Karen Teel as Austin's matriarch of pediatrics, Dr. Teel likes to think of herself as an "active facilitator" for a very worthy cause. Without her integral role in developing Austin's pediatrics residency program, the Children's Hospital of Austin, and the Pediatric Physician Alliance of Central Texas (PediPact), none of the programs would likely have emerged as successfully and perhaps not at all. In 1963, Dr. Teel received her M.D. degree from Baylor University College of Medicine. After an internship in Cincinnati, a pediatric residency at Baylor, and a two-year fellowship in Pediatric Infectious Disease at Baylor, she practiced general pediatrics at Bergstrom Air Force Base. During the early 1970s, Austin's handful of pediatricians taught rotating interns at Brackenridge Hospital, and Dr. Teel was asked by them to help start a residency program to raise the quality of teaching and attract conferences to the area. After settling in Austin with her husband, Carl Teel, she worked with the Central Texas Medical Foundation, University of Texas Medical Branch Galveston and Dr. Bill Daeschner for one to two years to get the residency program approved and operational. The program now has fully merged with the UTMB Galveston pediatric residency training program. The Austin Pediatric residents now number 42 physicians in training. Their annual outstanding pediatric resident award is named in her honor.

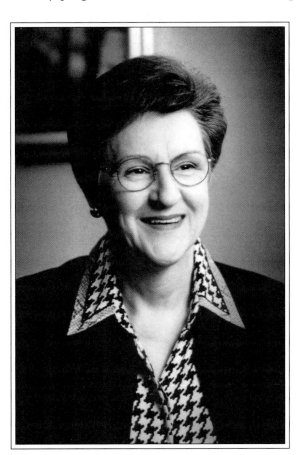

Dr. Karen Teel

After serving as Director of Pediatric Education at Brackenridge Hospital from 1972 to 1977, Dr. Teel traded in her role as an administrative physician for that of a pediatrician in private solo practice. From 1976 to 1986, she also served as an official oral examiner for the American Board of Pediatrics. In 1982, Brackenridge Hospital honored her with the Physician of the Year Award. A year later, the hospital administrator met with Dr. Milton Talbot and Dr. Teel to discuss the prospects of a children's hospital to accommodate the city's growth and the large increase in the number of children to be served. "Great. How can we help?" they replied. Soon, she and Dr. Talbot were co-chairing a steering committee, establishing working groups to include members of each of Austin's growing pediatric practices, and meeting with architects and others until the Children's Hospital of Austin was ready to open on February 14, 1988. "Everyone had an opportunity for input and all of the pediatric physicians were on the same page," said Dr. Teel.

To further assist the growing number of pediatric physicians in the Austin area to speak with a unified and effective voice, she helped create the Pediatric Physician Alliance of Central Texas. Dr. Teel served as its president for the first five years beginning in 1995. The Alliance, which now has over 200 pediatric physician members, supported the hospital's transition to professional hospital management by the Seton Health Network.

Prior to her retirement in November 2005, Dr. Teel focused on leading the medical team at her private practice, providing an environment where they could take the time to give the kind of quality care that her patients had come to expect and appreciate even years after their children had grown. "I don't think there is really any substitute for the opportunity that we as physicians are given to serve people in such valuable and important ways," says Dr. Teel.

TEXAS CARDIOVASCULAR CONSULTANTS, P.A.

JOHN A. DIECK, JR., M.D. AND THOMAS N. Tracey, M.D. co-founded Texas Cardiovascular Consultants, P.A. in 1990. From an initial group of three physicians, the practice has grown to 39 doctors who are dedicated to the detection and treatment of cardiovascular diseases and heart rhythm disturbances.

Texas Cardiovascular Consultants has built a reputation for maintaining an exemplary standard of care. Dieck explains that by maintaining six offices throughout Austin, the doctors can best provide patients with continuity of care. "From a business standpoint, it makes more sense to gather all the physicians in one building. It's far more efficient to dedicate some physicians to making rounds and others to the office on any given day. But it's not the best way."

Providing quality patient care demands the best that technology has to offer. For this reason, Texas Cardiovascular Consultants was the first in Texas to acquire the GE Medical Systems Lightspeed° angiography CT scanner. "Our practice is young and forward-thinking and we understand the value of state-of-the-art technology when it comes to patient care," says Dieck. Clearly, at the core of quality patient care stands the physician. Doctors enjoy being part of Texas Cardiovascular Consultants. By operating several separate offices, each feels more personable. "Our doctors like to take care of the patient and they're well trained. Their contracts are fair; when physicians are happy here, they stay. The patients appreciate the opportunity to develop an ongoing relationship with their doctor," says Dieck.

Patients from around the state have put their trust in Texas Cardiovascular Consultants which, following a merger with a physician group of electrophysiologists, offers a full spectrum of cardiovascular care.

Practice members are: Nima Amjadi, M.D., Shane M. Bailey, M.D., David G. Burger, M.D., Robert C. Canby, M.D., Edward R. Chafizadeh, M.D., Fotini Chalkias, M.D., Manish S. Chauhan, M.D., Mary Beth Cishek, M.D., John A. Dieck, M.D.**, Kara A. Dlabal, M.D., Elizabeth A. Ebert, M.D., Paul W. Dlabal, M.D., Gary L. Foster, M.D., J. Todd Gage, M.D., G. Joseph Gallinghouse, M.D., Michael

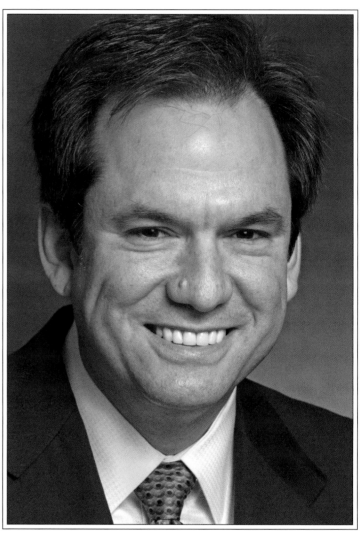

John A. Dieck, M.D., F.A.C.P., F.A.C.C, President/CEO, Texas Cardiovascular Consultants, P.A.

S. Grad, M.D., Rodney P. Horton, M.D., Gerald V. Levy, M.D., Jeffrey B. Michel, M.D., Tuan D. Nguyen, M.D., Vinh D. Nguyen, D.O., Vu D. Nguyen, M.D., F. Javier Otero, M.D., Erol H. Ozdil, M.D.*, Larry D. Price, D.O., Paul J. Roach, M.D.*, Matthew T. Rogers, M.D., Javier E. Sanchez, M.D., Jonathan I. Sheinberg, M.D., Matthew B. Stahlman, M.D., David W. Terreson, M.D., Thomas N. Tracey, M.D.**, Paul A. Tucker, II, M.D.*, Paolo V. Venengoni, M.D., Michael G. Watkins, M.D., Robert J. Wozniak, M.D., Jason D. Zagrodzky, M.D., and Mo Zeineddin, M.D.

* Senior physician   ** Co-founder

TEXAS OCULOPLASTIC CONSULTANTS

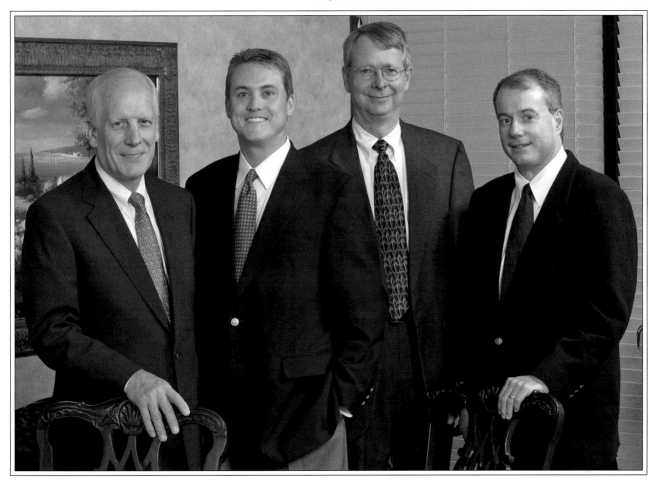

TEXAS OCULOPLASTIC CONSULTANTS (TOC) IS A PRIVATE practice partnership devoted to providing high quality oculoplastic care including surgical and medical management of eyelid, lacrimal, orbital, and aesthetic facial issues. TOC is the first and only practice in Austin to specialize in oculoplastic surgery.

The roots of Texas Oculoplastic Consultants can be traced to the founding partner, Russell W. Neuhaus, M.D., who, in 1982, assumed the practice of Otto Lippmann, M.D., Austin's first board-certified ophthalmologist. In 1997, Dr. Neuhaus partnered with John W. Shore, M.D., F.A.C.S., to launch Texas Oculoplastic Consultants. Today, TOC numbers four partners including Sean M. Blaydon, M.D., F.A.C.S. and Todd R. Shepler, M.D., ophthalmologists with equally extensive training in oculoplastic surgery and diseases.

Teaching and research play a significant role at TOC. The four partners are on the voluntary clinical faculty in

Left to right, John W. Shore, M.D., Todd R. Shepler, M.D., Russell W. Neuhaus, M.D., and Sean M. Blaydon, M.D.

the Department of Ophthalmology and provide faculty supervision at the University of Texas Medical School in San Antonio in Oculoplastic Surgery. They also supervise and instruct a fellow-in-training from the M.D. Anderson Medical Center in Houston, Texas.

TOC provides pre- and post-surgical and aesthetic facial care in an adjoining aesthetic center, staffed by the TOC doctors and registered nurses with special training in skin management including Botox, Juvederm, Restylane, and other laser light therapies. Texas Oculoplastic Consultants have established a state-of-the-art, laser-equipped, ambulatory surgical center (ASC) that is dedicated to eyelid and orbital surgery and is state licensed and federally approved. The partners perform approximately 90% of their operations in their ASC and the remainder at various Austin hospitals.

TEXAS ASTHMA & ALLERGY CENTER

DR. JAMES HAS BEEN TREATING Austinites, especially the younger ones, for asthma and allergies since 1977, and from his North Austin office on Jollyville Road for the past 20 years. When he would visit the family pediatrician at the age of three, Dr. James became interested in becoming a pediatrician. During medical school at Louisiana State University, he worked with renowned allergist Dr. John Salvaggio, who whetted his appetite for the challenge of diagnosing allergies and related conditions.

His subsequent training at Charity Hospital in New Orleans provided an excellent clinical education and a sturdy foundation to further develop the essential patient history-taking skills and bedside manner. In 1977, after two years in the army

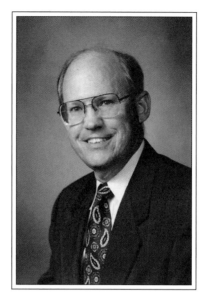

at Fort Bragg, North Carolina, where he worked in the busiest of environments as chief allergist, he moved to Austin, where he could enjoy living in a progressive city that was close to his home state of Louisiana.

Over the past 30 years, Dr. James has seen the emergence of three different paradigms and various technological advances in his field. To his dismay, he has also witnessed the role of insurance companies change the way he and other doctors practice medicine. One constant over the years has been the pleasure he receives from working with his patients, solving their problems, and watching them get well. You can still find him in his office, on the floor with a young patient, lowering his voice to a calming whisper to better connect with and care for the young patient.

TEXAS PAIN REHABILITATION INSTITUTE, P.A.

WHEN ANESTHESIOLOGIST DR. GRAVES OWEN'S OWN chronic back pain did not respond to available medical procedures, he began to explore other methods and disciplines. After finding reprieve from a combination of sources, the Texas doctor wanted to learn more and completed a pain fellowship at Pain Evaluation and Treatment Institute in Pittsburgh, Pennsylvania.

The native Austinite returned to the Hill Country and opened the Texas Pain Rehabilitation Institute, P.A., in Round Rock, Texas, where he and an interdisciplinary team of psychologists, nurses, physical therapists, and other providers take an intradisciplinary approach to pain management. The Texas Pain Rehabilitation Institute utilizes a variety of interventional, rehabilitative, and pharmaceutical strategies for individualized treatment of chronic pain. The best outcome occurs when the patient takes an active role in his or her treatment.

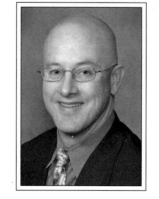

"Our goal is to improve the patient's daily functioning, reduce pain and suffering, and then empower the patient to manage any remaining pain. We want to teach patients to help themselves," says Dr. Owen. "By implementing tools taught in our clinic, they become less concerned about reinjury and painful flare-ups." One of the biggest challenges the clinic faces is patients' conceptions about pain and treatment. "They want a quick fix, but the reality is that only a minority of patients respond to only medical procedures, without utilizing other strategies. There is no known 'cure' for chronic pain," explains Dr. Owen. Patients' perceptions, however, usually change when they see positive and lasting outcomes from the clinic's comprehensive approach, especially when patients can remove the suffering from the pain and begin to take control of their lives again.

BRYAN TOWNSEND, M.D.

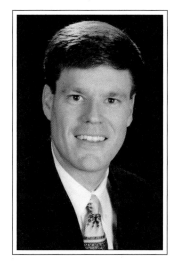

DURING AUSTIN'S GROWTH SPURT, DR. Bryan Townsend, a board certified dermatologist specializing in Mohs micrographic surgery for skin cancer, joined the ranks of the medical profession, providing an important service for the growing Central Texas population. Dr. Townsend first came to Austin from southeast Texas to attend the University of Texas. He began his Austin dermatology practice in September 1998, after receiving medical training in Houston and New Orleans.

Especially for those who have previously battled skin cancer, the specialized micrographic surgery he provides in his office is a welcome referral. Mohs micrographic surgery is an advanced surgical technique for the complete removal of skin cancer, performed by highly trained surgeons who are specialists in Dermatology, Pathology, and Reconstructive Surgery. With this unique combination of training, Dr. Townsend is able to remove only diseased tissue, preserving healthy tissue and minimizing the cosmetic impact of the surgery.

Skin cancer now represents half of all new cancers. More than one million new cases of skin cancer will be diagnosed in the United States this year, of which 80 percent are basal cell, 16 percent are squamous cell, and 4 percent are melanoma. By 2010, approximately one in 50 Americans will have a lifetime risk of developing melanoma, the most dangerous type of skin cancer.

Since his arrival in Austin in 1998, Dr. Townsend continues to teach his staff that the patient is always—and always should be—their number one priority. *The patient comes first. The patient comes second. The patient comes third. That's what medicine is—it's about the patient.*

VICTORY MEDICAL AND FAMILY CARE

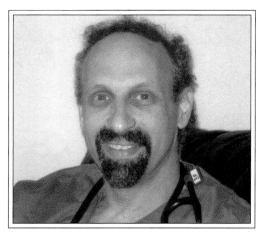

WILLIAM G. FRANKLIN, M.D. IS in private practice at Victory Medical and Family Care, which he founded in 1996 in Austin, Texas.

Dr. Franklin was born in Detroit, Michigan and raised in Houston, Texas where he graduated magna cum laude from Bellaire High School. His undergraduate work was done at the University of Texas at Austin where he received a Bachelor of Arts in Philosophy and graduated summa cum laude. He received his Doctorate of Medicine from the University of Texas Medical Branch at Galveston.

Dr. Franklin has been a health care provider since 1983 and some of his postgraduate activities include being a member of the Associate Teaching Faculty at UTMB Galveston; serving as Medical Director at Victory Medical and Family Care; being a member of the American Academy of Anti-Aging Medicine; being a member of the Caritas (Charity Clinic) staff; being a member of the Baylor Medical Center Family Practice Review, and being on the Committee for Physician's Health and Rehabilitation. Dr. Franklin is a Certified Medical Review Officer for the Texas Department of Transportation and is an active teacher in Family Practice.

Board certified in Family Practice, Dr. William Franklin also has special training in Natural Hormone Replacement Therapy, Age-Management, Workers' Compensation, Sports Medicine, Addiction Medicine, Depression, and Weight Loss.

GORDON L. WHITE, M.D.

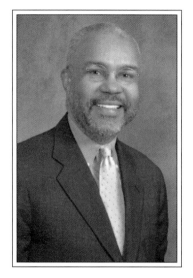

IN PRIVATE PRACTICE IN AUSTIN SINCE 1987, Gordon L. White, M.D. specializes in neurological surgery. As a general neurosurgeon, Dr. White's practice includes adult as well as pediatric/neonatal patients. He is affiliated with St. David's Medical Center in Austin and performs spinal, cranial, and peripheral nerve procedures. Dr. White and his surgical team performed the first successful separation of Siamese twins (craniopagus) in Austin in 1995.

White holds his medical degree from M.S. Hershey College of Medicine at Pennsylvania State University. He served his general surgery and medical internship, neurological residency and fellowship (Leo M. Davidoff Department of Neurological Surgery) at Albert Einstein Affiliated Hospitals in New York City. Dr. White currently maintains memberships with the American Medical Association, the Texas Medical Association, the Travis County Medical Society and the Texas Neurological Society.

When Dr. White is not with patients or running his practice, he enjoys investing his time pursuing various activities that fulfill his personal commitment to serve the community. While quite active in this realm, he typically prefers to do so anonymously. In addition, he spends time nurturing his garden, which has been featured in a number of national publications. He is involved with Girl Scouts-USA, and with the School of Architecture at the University of Texas, sharing and further developing his interest in garden design/architecture. An avid reader of non-fiction books, Dr. White also is an accomplished gourmet cook.

DAVID WOERNER, M.D.

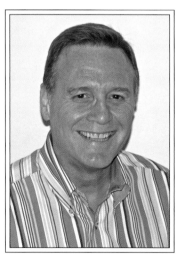

WHEN DAVID WOERNER FIRST BEGAN practicing medicine it was at a small clinic in a village outside Guadalajara, Mexico where he was enrolled as a medical student. He and some classmates set up a small office to see patients who most of the time could not pay, and when they could the currency was often chickens!

A lot has transpired since those early years, and now Dr. Woerner has a thriving family practice in Austin. But in between, he has had his share of medical adventures including setting up an office in an old house built in the 1880s in Salina, Kansas, a house which had to be retrofitted with plumbing and electricity. "In Salina, I rode my bike to work everyday, except when we had ice, then I rode my tractor!"

Woerner longed to return to Texas and made that move in 1984. Although he grew up in Houston, Austin was smaller and not too far removed from the quaintness of Salina. The philosophy of his family practice took shape. He made care a collaborative effort between doctor and patient. "I actively consider each person's religious, economical, cultural, spiritual, and psychological make-up." The idea is to treat the whole person, not just symptomatic ailments. "Being a good listener is foremost" says Dr. Woerner.

The atmosphere in the office is relaxed and casual. Dr. Woerner wears jeans and casual shirts rather than the more traditional attire. Artwork by his children, and pictures of his and the staff's children adorn the walls. He is very proud of all six of his children, some of whom are pursuing careers in medicine. The next generation of Dr. Woerners may join dad in treating patients, but it is unlikely any of them will be paid with chickens.

HARVEY WORCHEL, M.D.

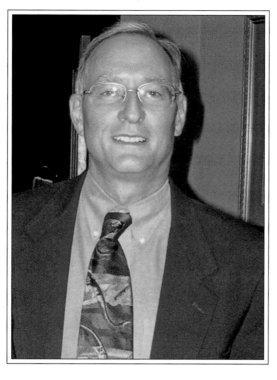

A BOOK HE READ IN SIXTH grade changed the course of Harvey Worchel's life. He knew he wanted to be a surgeon and a summer working with surgeons at an Army hospital in Bangkok, Thailand during college reinforced his career choice. "I like interacting with people and every day is different. I cannot imagine a more interesting and challenging profession than general surgery."

Born and raised in Austin, Dr. Worchel came to Bastrop, a town with a population of 3,000, in 1979 to begin his practice. He was the only general surgeon in the county at that time. He helped Bastrop Hospital become updated, ordering ventilators, blood gas machines, central venous catheters and other advanced devices, all of which were firsts for Bastrop.

Dr. Worchel moved back to Austin with his family in 1983. He has tried to keep his practice personal, maintaining a solo practice from the same office and the same one-person office for 24 years. His practice centers around hernia repairs, gallbladder and bowel surgery, and breast cancer surgery. "I feel blessed to have the life and practiced the profession I have always dreamed of."

DR. GRACE YEH

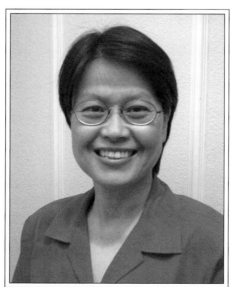

"BEING A FAMILY PHYSICIAN IS a privilege," says Dr. Grace Yeh. "Patients come to you not only with their physical problems, but they also share their personal stories." Dr. Yeh feels very fortunate to be in a position of helping people to achieve good health. She strongly believes in the importance of a proactive holistic approach to health by taking physical, mental, and spiritual factors into consideration when treating patients. Dr. Yeh encourages her patients to live a healthy lifestyle as a preventive approach to achieving overall good health. "Blend exercise into your everyday routine and make eating fun and healthy! Also, take time to nurture your spiritual needs."

Dr. Yeh was born in Taiwan and was trained at the University of Minnesota and the University of California at Los Angeles in Family Medicine and Public Health, respectively. She is fluent in English, Taiwanese, and Mandarin. This cultural diversity has made her more receptive to alternative treatments such as acupuncture and herbal medicine as complementary approaches to western medicine. "Both of these practices have been used in Asia for thousands of years with good results," says Dr. Yeh. As a Christian, Dr. Yeh shares that she has used her medical practice in any way possible "to heal others with broken hearts, minds, and bodies."

PAST PRESIDENTS OF THE TRAVIS COUNTY MEDICAL SOCIETY

1930 AND 1946 DR. C. P. HARDWICKE	1941 DR. G. F. THORNHILL	1956 DR. C. HAL McCUISTION
1931 DR. L. E. EDENS	1943 DR. J. C. THOMAS	1957 DR. FRED LOWRY
1932 DR. BEN R. EPPRIGHT	1945 DR. WILLIAM M. GAMBRELL	1958 DR. RALEIGH R. ROSS
1933 AND 1944 DR. H. A. SCOTT	1947 DR. O. W. SUEHS	1959 DR. GEORGE W. TIPTON
1934 AND 1942 DR. TRUMAN MORRIS	1949 DR. J. EDWARD JOHNSON	1960 DR. C. B. DILDY
1935 DR. HENRY HILGARTNER, JR.	1950 DR. SAM KEY, SR.	1961 DR. M. D. McCAULEY
1936 AND 1948 DR. JOE T. GILBERT	1951 DR. M. F. KREISLE	1962 DR. RUTH M. BAIN
1937 DR. C. M. DARNALL	1952 DR. R. G. CARTER	1963 DR. GEORGE CLARK
1938 DR. J. T. (PAUL) ROBISON	1953 DR. JOHN F. THOMAS	1964 DR. DOUGLAS F. BARKLEY
1939 AND 1940 DR. W. R. HOUSTON	1954 AND 1955 DR. J. M. COLEMAN	1965 DR. WALTER S. MOORE

1966
DR. P. CLIFT PRICE

1967
DR. CHARLES F. PELPHREY

1968
DR. DANIEL B. POWELL

1968
DR. ALBERT F. VICKERS

1969
DR. SAM N. KEY, JR.

1970
DR. ROBERT F. ELLZEY

1971
DR. DARRELL FAUBION

1972
DR. HARDY E. THOMPSON

1973
DR. GROVER L. BYNUM

1974
DR. ROBERT A. DENNISON

1975
DR. H. S. ARNOLD

1976
DR. JAMES M. GRAHAM

1977
DR. HOMER R. GOEHRS

1978
DR. EARL L. GRANT

1979
DR. V. C. SMART

1980
DR. G. WOOTTEN BROWN

1981
DR. WILLIAM G. GAMEL

1982
DR. MAC BRANNEN

1983
DR. STUART S. NEMIR

1984
DR. THOMAS D. KIRKSEY

1985
DR. MILTON W. TALBOT

1986
DR. DONALD C. SPENCER

1987
DR. JAMES F. REEVES

1988
DR. WILLIAM A. WALKER

1989
DR. JOSEPH M. ABELL, JR.

1990
DR. BRUNO YBARRA

1991
DR. ROBERT E. ASKEW, SR.

1992
DR. C. BRUCE MALONE

1993
DR. CHARLES E. FELGER

1994
DR. WILLIAM J. DEATON

1995
DR. THOMAS B. COOPWOOD, SR.

1996
DR. JAMES A. PRENTICE

1997
DR. PHILLIP J. CHURCH

1998
DR. HECTOR E. MORALES

1999
DR. HAROLD SKAGGS, JR.

2000
DR. STEPHEN S. CLARK

2001
DR. TOM S. MCHORSE

2002
DR. CATHERINE L. SCHOLL

2003
DR. JAMES R. ESKEW

2004
DR. CHRISTOPHER S. CHENAULT

2005
DR. GUADALUPE "PETE" ZAMORA

2006
DR. PEGGY M. RUSSELL

2007
DR. DAVID C. FLEEGER

2008
DR. PHILLIP C. COLLINS

SELECT BIBLIOGRAPHY

BESIDES SPECIFIC CITATIONS, NUMEROUS ADDITIONAL sources were used for verifications, especially those from Texas Medical Ass ociation and Travis County Medical Society archives, and many official government, institutional, organizational, physician, topical, and geographic Web sites. [Most Web site addresses have been condensed to the main address and some may no longer be available.]

Abell, Joseph M., Jr. "The President's Message. The Kemp Years." *TCMS Journal* 35, (November) 1989: 4-6. Also, other papers and archives on Whitman provided to Texas Medical Association

Alexander, Richard J. "People's free clinic." *Texas Medicine* 68 (February 1972): 94-100.

American Medical Association. "Ethics Timeline: 1847 to 1940." www.ama-assn.org; AMA's Principles of Medical Ethics; and the *American Medical Directory*.

"Annis (Joseph P.), MD, elected to the AMA Board of Trustees." American Medical Association. Press release. June 13, 2006.

"Arc Celebrates 25 Years." Austin Regional Clinic. www.austinregionalclinic.com (Cached).

"A Short History of Magnetic Resonance Imaging (MRI). " Tesla Memorial Society of New York. www.teslasociety.com.

Association of American Medical Colleges. www.aamc.org.

The Austin American. "Council Takes Fluoride Bid Under Advisement." July 21, 1967:1.

Austin American-Statesman. (Numerous news items, features, and obituaries.)

The Austin Diagnostic Clinic. www.adclinic.com.

Austin Fire Department, Historical Highlights 1841-1975; 1976-2002. www.ci.austin.tx.us.

Austin History Center/Austin Public Library vertical files. "Austin: Hospital; No. 8-Historical Highlights of the Capital City of Texas." City of Austin Public Information Department. Also other AHC vertical files, census information, telephone books, Austin city directories, and other sources.

Austin-Travis County Emergency Medical Services. ATCEMS System Synopsis. Area hospitals. www.atcems.org.

"Austin Treasures: Just Outside Austin, Rural Travis County Communities." "Austin Beginnings. An Exhibit of Memorable Austin Firsts." City of Austin. www.ci.austin.tx.us.

Bain, Ruth M., with Baker, Marilyn Miller. *Doors Will Open for You: Memorable Experiences in My Life as a Doctor*. Ruth M. Bain, M.D. 1997.

Baker, Marilyn Miller. *The History of Pathology in Texas*. Texas Society of Pathologists. 1996.

Baker, Marilyn Miller. *Caring for the Children: The History of Pediatrics in Texas*. Texas Pediatric Society, A Chapter of the American Academy of Pediatrics. 1996.

Barker, Eugene C. *The Life of Stephen F. Austin, Founder of Texas 1793-1836, A Chapter in the Westward Movement of the Anglo-American People*. Austin, Texas: The Texas State Historical Association, 1949.

Barkley, Mary Starr. *History of Travis County and Austin 1839-1899*. Waco: Texian Press, 1963.

Bastrop County Historical Markers. www.forttours.com

Bastrop County, Texas. Copyright T. Owen. www.rootsweb.com.

Bellis, Mary. "Vitamins-Production Methods. History of the Vitamins." www.inventors.about.com.

Bellis, Mary. "The History of Penicillin." www.inventors.about.com.

Bennett, J. D. C.: Medical Advances Consequent to the Great War 1914-1918. *Journal of the Royal Society of Medicine* 83 (November) 1990: 738. www.pubmedcentral.nih.gov.

Black, Hulon W. "Remarks at the Laying of the Cornerstone of St. David's Hospital." December 19, 1954. Vertical files, Austin History Center.

Blair, Lyman C. "Anson Jones, MD, Physician-Statesman." *Texas State Journal of Medicine* 58 (December) 1962: 1045-1046.

Boggy Creek Farm, History of the Farm. www.boggycreek farm.com.

Brown, Frank. *Annals of Travis County and the City of Austin (from the Earliest Times to the close of 1875),* Chapters IV-V. Austin History Center.

Brown, Paul. "Best Kept Secrets: Stories behind UT buildings." October 17, 2005, 5 a.m. News8Austin. www.news8austin.com.

Burns, Chester R., M.D., Ph.D., via Oertling, Sarita B, of The University of Texas Medical Branch Truman G. Blocker, Jr., History of Medicine Collection, Moody Medical Library. E-mails February 2006.

Cantrell, Gregg. *Stephen F. Austin: Empresario of Texas.* New Haven and London: Yale University Press, 1999.

Carrier, John P.: "Medicine in Texas: The Struggle with Yellow Fever, 1839-1903." *Texas Medicine* 82 (November) 1986: 62-68.

Census Records (federal) via TexShare Databases. Heritage Quest Online (various years) and other census records online and at Austin History Center.

Chatman, J. A. *The Lone Star State Medical, Dental, and Pharmaceutical History.* Printed as a Myers Yearbook, 1959.

Chemsoc Timeline, 1928. Fleming-Penicillin. Royal Society of Chemistry. London. www.chemsoc.org.

CHG Cornerstone Healthcare Group. www.cornerstone healthcaregroup.com.

Children's Hospital of Austin. www.childrenshospital.com.

"Children's medical center gets $2 million grant." *Austin Business Journal.* February 2, 2006. www.bizjournals.com.

"Chronic Disease Overview." Centers for Disease Control and Prevention, Department of Health and Human Services. www.cdc.gov.

Civil War Home. "Biography of William Joseph Hardee." www.civilwarhome.com.

Coleman, James M. *Aesculapius on the Colorado, The Story of Medical Practice in Travis County to 1899.* Austin, Texas: A Waterloo Book, The Encino Press for The Friends of the Austin Public Library, 1971.

Coleman, James M. "Medical Journalism in Texas." *Texas State Journal of Medicine* 51 (July) 1955: 486-488.

Cox, Geo. W. *History of Public Health in Texas.* Austin: Texas State Department of Health, 1950.

"Death Rates by Cause of Death, 1900-2002 (per 100,000 population)." United States. Infoplease. www.infoplease.com.

DeShields, James T. *Border Wars of Texas.* Matt Bradley, revising editor. Austin, Texas: State House Press, 1993.

Directory of Medical Specialists, American Board of Medical Specialties (published under various titles). Also, current information online at www.ABMS.org.

"Disease and mortality." Various articles. Pearson Education, publishing as Infoplease. www.infoplease.com.

"Dr. John Genung." Texas Longhorns, The Official Site of University of Texas Athletics. www.texassports.com.

"Drugs and Drug Substitutes in the South, Articles from Civil War Newspapers." Compiled by Vicki Betts, Robert R. Muntz Library, The University of Texas at Tyler. www.uttyler.edu.

Eckels, Jet Graham, and Graham, James M. *Oh, To Be a Doctor! A Biography of James M. Graham, M.D.* 2006. Privately published.

Ellzey, Robert F., M.D. "The Birth of Mammography." *TCMS Journal* 47 (November/December) 2001:12. Various other papers, including correspondence with Robert L. Egan, M.D.

Esquivel, Irene Louise, October 4, 2004. *The Dallas Morning News* (family-placed obituary). www.nl.newsbank.com.

Esquivel, Sandy (Also Esquivel, Sandi). "Sandi Esquivel, Cross Country (1923-25) Track (1925-26) Basketball (192426, Forward)." Texas Longhorns, Men's Athletic Hall of Honor. www.texassports.com.

Fahrenthold, Lisa, and Rider, Sara. *Admissions: The Extraordinary History of Brackenridge Hospital.* Austin, Texas. Brackenridge Hospital, City of Austin, 1984.

Fehrenbach, T. R. *Lone Star, A History of Texas and the Texans.* New York: Collier Books, a Division of Mac-millan Publishing Co., Inc., 1980.

Flexner, Abraham. *Medical Education in the United States and Canada*, A Report to The Carnegie Foundation for the Advancement of Teaching. The Carnegie Foundation for the Advancement of Teaching, Bulletin Number Four, New York City. Boston: D. B. Updike, The Merrymount Press, 1910.

Ford, Joseph H., Colonel. Prepared under the direction of Ireland, M. W., Major General, The Surgeon General. The Medical Department of the United States Army in the World War: Volume II. Administration American Expeditionary Forces. Washington, DC, United States Government Printing Office, 1927. www.history.amedd.army.mil.

Fox, Kermit W. *A Son of La Bahia Remembers, 1991,* privately published.

Future Directions for Medical Education. A Report of the Council on Medical Education. Adopted June 16, 1982, by the House of Delegates of the American Medical Association, Chicago, Illinois, 1982.

Gambrell, Herbert. *Anson Jones, The Last President of Texas.* Austin: University of Texas Press, 1947. Second edition, 1964. (Copyright 1947, 1948. Second copyright 1964.)

Gammel's The Laws of Texas, Nineteenth-Century Texas Law Online, University of North Texas Libraries (various entries). www.texinfo.library.unt.edu.

Gilbert, Joe Thorne, M.D. Presidential Address (1966). Texas Surgical Society. Typewritten copy.

Goehrs, Homer, R. Taped oral histories with Austin physicians Eugene P. Schoch, Jr., M.D., R. Vincent Murray, Jr., M.D. (10/27/87). Also, W. Burford "Dutch" Hahn, M.D., and George W. Tipton, M.D.

Gonzales, Texas June 30, 1909, Burton, J. W., Editor. "Extracted from tablets made by Kathleen Spring, 1991. Tablets are in Gonzales County Archives." www.roots web.com.

Graduate Medical Education. Seton Family of Hospitals. www.seton.net.

Greater Kansas City Community Foundation. Shields, Heloise. www.gkccf.org.

"Guide to the Records of the U.S. House of Representatives at the National Archives, 1789-1989 (Record Group 233); Chapter 22. Records of the Select Committees of the House of Representatives." Legislative Branch, The Center for Legislative Archives, The National Archives. www.archives.gov.

Gulf Coast Regional Blood Center. "Our History." www.giveblood.org.

"Haig, Douglas, 1st Earl Haig, Viscount Dawick, Baron Haig of Bemersyde." Encyclopedia Britannica Online. www.britannica.com.

Handbook of Texas Online, The, s.v. "Anderson, Washington," "Austin, Catholic Diocese of," "Austin, Texas," "Borden, Gail, Jr.," "Catholic Health Care," "Garcia, Alberto Gonzalo," "Gilbert, Joseph," "Gotier's Trace," "Health and Medicine," "Hilgartner, Henry Louis (1868-1937)" "Holy Cross Fathers and Brothers," "Hornsby, Reuben," "Medical Journals In Early Texas," "Medical Societies," "Public Health," "Shriners Hospitals For Crippled Children, Galveston Burns Unit," "Stagecoach Lines," "Texana, TX," "Travis County," "Webberville, Texas," "Wilbarger Creek." A Joint Project of The General Libraries of the University of Texas at Austin and the Texas Historical Association. www.tsha.utexas.edu.

Hardwicke, C. P., M.D., with introduction by Yeakel, Earl L., M.D. "A Personal Account of the Move of the Texas Medical Association from Fort Worth to Austin 1948-1951." Texas Medical Association archives.

"Health, Medicine, and American Culture, 1930-1960." University of Pennsylvania History of Sociology and Science. www.ccat.sas.upenn.edu.

"Historical Milestones. Methodist DeBakey Heart Center." The Methodist Hospital System. www.methodist health.com.

History of the 1964 Surgeon General's Report on Smoking and Health, CDC. www.cdc.gov.

"History of the Department of Veterans Affairs—Part 4. GI Bill." U.S. Department of Veterans Affairs. www1.va.gov.

"History of Minimally Invasive Surgery." Minimally Invasive Surgery Center, Mount Sinai School of Medicine. www.mssm.edu.

"The History of Pharmacy" cited by The Lindsay Drug Company. www.lindsaydrug.com.

Hood, R. Maurice. "John Salmon (RIP) Ford, MD, 1815-1897." pp. 130-149. Chapter in *Early Texas Physicians, 1830-1915.* R. Maurice Hood, M.D., ed. Austin, Texas: State House Press for The Texas Surgical Society, San Antonio, Texas, 1999.

Hood, R. Maurice. *The Collected Published Papers and Presentations on Surgery, History, Sermons and Medical Evangelism of R. Maurice Hood, M.D.,* Volumes I and II. 2000. Private papers.

Hornsby Bend. Website owned by Hornsby Bend families. www.hornsbybend.com.

"Hospital for Negroes Opens." *Austin American-Statesman,* August 4, 1940.

Houston Academy of Medicine-Texas Medical Center Library. John P. McGovern Historical Collections and Research Center. www.mcgovern.library.tmc.edu.

"Historical Medical Tour of Galveston." The Virtual Tour of Galveston Island. University of Texas Medical Branch, Galveston. www.utmb.edu.

"Illinois Trails Presents Chicago Institutions in 1901 from the Historical Encyclopedia of Illinois ©1901." www.iltrails.org.

"Impact of Vaccines Universally Recommended for Children-United States, 1990-1999. April 2, 1999." CDC, Division of Media Relations, MMWR, Morbidity and Mortality Weekly Report, April 2, 1999, Centers for Disease Control, Office of Enterprise Communications, Media Relations. www.cdc.gov.

Interviews, personal, telephone, and/or e-mail: Joseph M. Abell, Jr., M.D.; Gerald A. Baugh, M.D; Belinda Clare; Thomas B. Coopwood, M.D; Marshall Cothran; Marvin R. Cressman, M.D; Robert F. Ellzey, M.D; Kermit W. Fox, M.D; Howard Gatewood; Homer R.

Goehrs, M.D; R. Maurice Hood, M.D; Glen E. Journeay, M.D, PhD; Albert A. La Londe, M.D; Marjorie G. Lawlis, M.D; Virgil B. Lawlis, M.D; Carey Legett, Jr., M.D; Georgia F. Legett, M.D; Mary Micka; Jack W. Moncrief, M.D; Hector E. Morales, M.D; James A. Prentice, M.D; Linda Gilbert Prentice, M.D; P. Clift Price, M.D; Margie Pohl; Donald E. Pohl, M.D; Arthuree Quander; Joseph P. Quander, Jr., M.D; J. Nelson Sanders, M.D; Leonard J. Sayers, M.D; Eugenia Schoch; Eugene P. Schoch, Jr., M.D; V. C. Smart, MD; Robert N. Snider, MD; Lansing S. Thorne, MD; John P. "Jack" Schneider, MD; George W. Tipton, Sr., M.D; Judy Talbot; Milton W. Talbot, Jr., M.D; Albert F. Vickers, M.D; John P. "Pete" Vineyard, Jr., M.D; William A. Walker, M.D. Also, prior interviews by Betsy Tyson of the following: Drs. Abell, Coopwood, Ellzey, Hood, Georgia Legett, Schneider, Tipton, Robert E. Askew, Sr., Mathis W. Blackstock; Grover L. Bynum, Jr.; Albert L. Exline; Charles E. Felger; Earl L. Grant; Sam. N. Key, Jr., James E. Kreisle, Sr.; John D. "Chip" Oswalt; Karen Teel; Jeffrey T. Youngkin, and others.

In The Matter Of Karen Quinlan, An Alleged Incompetent [no number in original]. Supreme Court of New Jersey 70 N.J. 10; 355 A.2d 647; 1976 N.J. LEXIS 181; 79 A.L.R.3d 205 January 26, 1976, Argued March 31, 1976, Decided. www.philosophy.wisc.edu.

"Isolation of the Iodine Compound Which Occurs in the Thyroid." (Kendall, E. C. (1919) *J. Biol. Chem.* 39, 125–147) in "The Isolation of Thyroxine and Cortisone: the Work of Edward C. Kendall." Robert D. Simoni, Robert L. Hill, and Martha Vaughan. *J. Biol. Chem.*: 277, Issue 21, 10 (May 24) 2002. www.jbc.org.

"Jackson County Historic Interest," Jackson County Chamber of Commerce and Agriculture. www.ykc.com.

Jones, Ralph W. "The First Roots of the University of Texas Medical Branch at Galveston," in *The Southwestern Historical Quarterly* LXV (April) 1962: 465.

Jones, Ronald Coy. "Second Chief of Surgery (1900) in "History of the Department of Surgery at Baylor University Medical Center." From the Department of Surgery, Baylor University Medical Center, Dallas, Texas. *Proc Bayl Univ Med Cent.* 2004 April; 17(2): 130–167. © 2004, Baylor University Medical Center. www.pubmedcentral.nih.gov.

Kemp, John. "From the Executive Vice President, A Report on the Progress of the Central Texas Health Plan." *TCMS Journal* 32 (June) 1986:5. Also, "From the Executive Director." *TCMS Journal* 27 (September) 1981:3.

"Kenney Fort" in "History of Williamson County and Round Rock, Texas." Williamson County Historical Museum. www.wchm-tx.org.

Key, Sam N., M.D. "The Etiology of Winter Hay-Fever in Texas." *Texas State Journal of Medicine* 13 (January 1918): 308-309.

King, William Harvey. "History of Homoeopathy and Its Institutions in America." www.homeoint.org.

"Knee Arthroscopy." American Academy of Orthopaedic Surgeons. www.orthoinfo.aaos.org.

"Kodak X-Omat processor, first roller transport processor for x-ray film, reduced processing time to six minutes. A History of Pioneering Innovations. 1956." Kodak Research and Development. www.kodak.com.

Koepsel, Loretto. Texas Medical Association Alliance. E-mail communication, March 10, 2006.

La Londe, A.A, and Gardner, W. J. "Chronic Subdural Hematoma; Expansion of Compressed Cerebral Hemisphere and Relief of Hypotension by Spinal Injection of Physiologic Saline Solution, *New England Journal of Medicine*, 239:493-496 (1948).

Leach, Karen Branz. "Thomas M. Runge, MD Leads Research in External Cardiac Assist." *TCMS Journal* 41 (July-August) 1995.

Lester, Paul. *The Great Galveston Disaster*. Pelican Publishing Company, Gretna 2000.

Liaison Committee on Medical Education. Directory of Accredited Medical Education Programs. www.lcme.org.

McCarrick, Pat Milmoe: "Ethics Committees in Hospitals," National Reference Center for Bioethics Literature. Citation of Teel, Karen: The Physician's Dilemma; A Doctor's View: What the Law Should Be, Baylor Law Review. 27:6-9, 1975. www.georgetown.edu.

McGovern (John P.) Historical Collections and Research Center. Texas Healthcare Postcards: Austin. www.mcgovern.library.tmc.edu.

McVey, Kate: "A Doctor with Heart." *Austin Business Journal*, April 20-26, 2001, republished in "In the Media." Cardiovascular and Thoracic Surgeons. www.ctvstexas.com.

"Medical Convention" in *Texas State Gazette*. Austin. December 11, 1852. Microfilm, Austin History Center.

"Medicine and Madison Avenue." The National Humanities Center. John W. Hartman Center for Sales, Advertising and Marketing History, and the Digital Scriptorium, Rare Book, Manuscript and Special Collections Library, Duke University. www.scriptorium. lib.duke.edu.

"Michael & Susan Dell Foundation Grants $50 Million to University of Texas to Bring Excellence in Children's Health and Education to Austin." News Release. The

University of Texas System. May 15, 2006. www.ut system.edu.

Micka, Mary. Files on the history of the Brackenridge Hospital (Austin) internship and residency programs.

Micka, Mary. "Memories of a Living Legend." *Travis County Medical Society Journal* 37 (September) 1991:14.

Miller, E. T.: "The State Finances of Texas during the Civil War." In *Southwestern Historical Quarterly*. Vol. XIV, No. 1, July, 1910 (SHQ Online, 014, No. 1) www.tsha.utexas.edu.

Morbidity and Mortality Weekly Reports (MMWR), Centers for Disease Control and Prevention (CDC), Department of Health and Human Services. Various reports. www.cdc.gov.

Morrison and Fourmy's *Austin City Directory* 1937. Morrison and Fourmy's Directory Company.

Moursund, Walter H., Sr. *A History of Baylor University College of Medicine 1900-1953.* Houston: Gulf Printing Company, 1956.

National Board of Health, Records of, 1879-84, 90.11, in Records of the Public Health Service, (PHS), 1912-1968, Record Group 90, 1794-1990; 1879-84. www.archives.gov.

National Center for Biotechnology Information, National Institutes of Health, National Library of Medicine, PubMed, Medline. Various searches.

National Defense University, Institute for National Strategic Studies. www.ndu.edu.

National Institutes of Health, Department of Health and Human Services. "The NIH Almanac-Historical Data." "Chronology of Events." "Legislative Chronology." www.nih.gov.

National Oceanic and Atmospheric Administration (NOAA), Central Library. "World War II: Mapping the World." www.lib.noaa.gov.

Neel, Spurgeon. Medical Support of the U.S. Army in Vietnam, 1965-1970 (Vietnam Studies). Washington, DC: Department of the Army, 1973.

Newsbank.com (including Obitsarchive.com and Newslibrary.com). www.newsbank.com. Various obituaries and archived news items.

The New York Eye and Ear Infirmary. "About the Infirmary, History & Mission." www.nyee.edu.

Nixon, Pat Ireland. *A History of the Texas Medical Association, 1853-1953.* Austin: University of Texas Press, 1953.

Nixon, Pat Ireland. *The Medical Story of Early Texas, 1528-1853.* Mollie Bennett Lupe Memorial Fund. Lancaster, Pennsylvania: Lancaster Press, Inc., 1946.

The Nobel Foundation, www.nobelprize.org. The Nobel Prize in Physiology or Medicine.

Osler, William. *Aequanimitas, With other Addresses to Medical Students, Nurses and Practitioners of Medicine.* 3rd edition. Philadelphia: The Blakiston Company, 1947.

Pakor, Inc. "History." www.pakor.com.

Patrick S. Pevoto, M.D., P.A., Curriculum Vitae. Medem, Inc. www.austinobdoc.yourmd.com.

Paul, Lee. "The Legend of Josiah Wilbarger." Old West Legends, People Legends. www.theoutlaws.com.

Pelphrey, Charles F., MD. *Reflections, The Pulse of an Era.* 2005. Austin. Private publication.

Perri, Anthony J., III, and Hsu, Sylvia. A Review of Thalidomide's history and current dermatological applications. Department of Dermatology, Baylor College of Medicine, Houston, TX. *Dermatology Online Journal,* Volume 9, No. 3. *Dermatology Online Journal* 9 (3): 5 www.dermatology.cdlib.org.

Pevoto, Patrick Scott, M.D. Travis OB/GYN Associates. www.travisobgyn.com.

"Pioneers in Kidney Dialysis: From the Scribner Shunt and the Mini-II to the "One-Button Machine." November 1996. University of Washington, Office of Research. www.washington.edu.

Polk, R. L. (Multiple directories published by R. L. Polk under different titles, comprising physicians, hospitals and sanitaria, medical laws, and medical schools for selected years.).

"Polio Report." *TIME* Magazine, Monday, July 30, 1945.

"Preserving the Charitable Trust: Nonprofit Hospital Conversion in Texas." July 1998. Consumers Union www.consumersunion.org.

"Privatization of Public Hospitals: Summary of Findings." The Henry J. Kaiser Family Foundation. January 1999. www.esresearch.org.

Race, George J., Tillery, G. Weldon, and Dysert, Peter A., II. "A history of pathology and laboratory medicine at Baylor University Medical Center." Department of Pathology, Baylor University Medical Center, Dallas, Texas. www.pubmedcentral.nih.gov.

Rajkumar, S. Vincent. "Thalidomide: Tragic Past and Promising Future," *Mayo Clin Proc.* 2004; 79:899-903 © 2004 Mayo Foundation For Medical Education And Research.www.mayoclinicproceedings.com.

Red, George Plunkett (Mrs. S. C. Red). *The Medicine Man in Texas.* Houston: Standard Printing & Lithographing Co., 1930.

"Ross, Alonzo Alverly Centennial Chair." Meeting No. 869.

The Minutes of the Board of Regents, The University of Texas System. April 1, 1993. San Antonio, Texas. Pp. 5 and 71. www.utsystem.edu.

Rude, Joe C. "TMA's 100 Annual Sessions. *Texas Medicine* 63 (March) 1967: 48.

Sage, Robert: Evergreen Cemetery. Austin Genealogical Society. www.austintxgensoc.org.

Schuhardt, Vernon T. *Pathogenic Microbiology*, Philadelphia, New York, San Jose, and Toronto: J. B. Lippincott Company, 1978.

ScienceWatch. "Making Penicillin Possible: Norman Heatley Remembers." The Thomson Corporation. www.science watch.com.

Seton Family of Hospitals. www.seton.net.

Shivers Cancer Center. 1993 pamphlet. Austin History Center.

Silverthorne, Elizabeth. *Ashbel Smith of Texas, Pioneer, Patriot, Statesman, 1805-1886*. College Station, Texas: Texas A&M University Press, 1982. (Especially pp. 209-210.)

"Sister Celine is Honored." *Austin American-Statesman*, April 30, 1964. Vertical Files, Austin History Center.

Smithwick, Noah. The Evolution of a State, or Recollections of Old Texas Days. www.oldcardboard.com.

Snider, Robert N. "ARA (Austin Radiological Association) 50th Anniversary." Address to ARA physicians, September 11, 2004.

Snider, Robert N. Oral history for Seton Hospital. (Revised November 2003).

Snider, Robert N. "Remembrances about Brackenridge Hospital X-Ray Training. A Brief History of the Seton School of X-Ray Technology," Typewritten notes, September 2006.

"Some Images and Histories of Old New Orleans Hospitals," www.geocities.com.

Spaner, S. J., and Warnock, G. L. "A brief history of endoscopy, laparoscopy, and laparoscopic surgery." *J Laparoendosc Adv Surg Tech A*. 1997 Dec. 7(6):369-73. www.ncbi. nlm.nih.gov.

Sparkman, Robert S., et al. *The Texas Surgical Society, The First Fifty Years.* Robert S. Sparkman, M.D., ed. Dallas: The Texas Surgical Society, 1965.

"Stalnaker, Dr. P. R." (Obituary). *Texas State Journal of Medicine.* Vol. 60 No. 7 (July 1964), p. 619.

"State-of-the-Art Facility." St. David's Bailey Square Surgery Center. www.baileysquare.com.

St. David's Community Hospital, Pamphlet, p. 14, Vertical files, Austin History Center.

St. David's Health Care. www.stdavids.com.

"St. David's Hospital: Historical Chronological Summary." Provided to Betsy Tyson by Patricia Rodriguez, St. David's Hospital.

"St. David's Replaces Cobalt Unit," *The Austin American*, January 21, 1971.

St. David's South Austin Hospital. http://stdavids.com

"Stents." www.inventors.about.com.

Terrell, Alex W. "The City Of Austin From 1839 To 1865." In *The Southwestern Historical Quarterly* XIV (October) 1910, No. 2 (SHQ Online, 014, No. 2.) www.tsha. utexas. edu.

Texas Almanac. The Dallas Morning News. Various entries, including "Searchable Town Database." www.texas almanac.com.

Texas Courier-Record of Medicine. Daniel, F. E., and Brooks, W. B., eds. "Travis County Medical Association." 2, No. 6 (February) 1885: 341-342.

"Texas Declaration of Independence." Texas State Library & Archives Commission. www.tsl.state.tx.us.

Texas General Land Office: Archives & Records: Texas History, Texas Maps. www.glo.state.tx.us.

"Texas Healthcare Facility Postcards-Austin." John P. McGovern Historical Collections and Research Center. Houston Academy of Medicine.Texas Medical Center Library. www.mcgovern.library.tmc.edu.

Texas Infant Mortality Rates. Infant Mortality Rate Analyzer. Texas Department of State Health Services. www. dshs.state.tx.us.

Texas Medical Association. Transactions (Minutes) of the Twenty-First Session. 1889. (TMA library stored in hall of Travis County Medical Society and in office of F. E. Daniel, M.D., TMA secretary.)

Texas Medical Association. Various Proceedings and Transactions of the association and the House of Delegates; membership directories; taped oral histories; archival files; and online information. www.texmed.org.

Texas Medical Board. "Physician Demographic Information (M.D.s & D.O.s)." www.tmb.state.tx.us.

Texas Medical Journal. "A Noble Work." 23, (September) 1907: 95-97.

Texas Medical Journal, various issues.

Texas Medical News. multiple issues.

Texas Medicine. "Efficient Care of Sniper Victims Shows Worth of Disaster Plans." 62 (August) 1966: 84-86; and "Governor's Committee Recommends Health, Safety Measures for UT Campus." 62 (October) 1966:120,122.

Texas Medicine. "Free-standing surgical center—a first for Texas." 70 (March) 1974: 106.

Texas Osteopathic Medical Association. www.txosteo.org.

Texas State Cemetery. www.cemetery.state.tx.us.

Texas State Journal of Medicine. "Three Patients at Parkland." 60 (January) 1964:60-74.

Texas State Journal of Medicine (Texas Medicine). Texas Medical Association. (Numerous issues, 1905-2006.)

Texas State Library & Archives Commission. "Texas Treasures." www.tsl.state.tx.us.

"The Constitution of the Republic of Texas, 1836." www.republic-of-texas.net.

"The Road to the Biotech Revolution: Highlights of 100 Years of Biologics Regulation." U.S. Food and Drug Administration. FDA Consumer magazine, www.fda.gov.

Tiggelin, R. Van. "Since 1895, Orthopaedic Surgery Needs X-Ray Imaging: A Historical Overview. From Discovery To Computed Tomography." JBR–BTR, 2001, 84: 204-213. www.radiology-museum.be.

Tipton, George W. "Profiles in Surgery. Surgery under stress: World War II, Anzio Beachhead." *Bulletin, American College of Surgeons* 91 No. 6 (June) 2006: p. 44.

Tipton, George W. "The Tissue Audit Committee in an Open Staff Hospital; Three Years' Results from Brackenridge Hospital." *Bulletin, American College of Surgeons.* 39, No. 4 (July-August) 1954:159-161; 191, 192.

Tisdale, Marie C., and Albert A. *Texas Cousins: Correll, Tisdale, and Related Families.* Austin, Texas: 1986.

Torok, Simon. "Howard Florey: The Story; Maker of the Miracle Mould." www.abc.net.au.

Travis County Healthcare District. www.traviscountyhd.org.

Travis County Medical Society. *TCMS Journal*; membership directories; assorted files and papers. Also, www.tcms.com.

Travis County, Texas. Hornsby Bend Cemetery. RootsWeb. ftp.rootsweb.com.

"Treatments of Tuberculosis, Phrenic Nerve Crush (Phrenicotomy)." www.lung.ca.

"Tuberculosis (Clinical Overview)." Texas Department of Health (later Texas Department of State Health Services). www.tdh.state.tx.us.

United States National Library of Medicine, National Institutes of Health. www.nlm.nih.gov.

University of Texas at Austin, The. School of Biological Sciences. Vernon T. Schuhardt Centennial Memorial Scholarship. www.biosci.utexas.edu.

"University of Texas Building Collection, An Inventory of Drawings and Papers, 1882-ongoing. Part 2 of 3, Alexander Architectural Archive." The General Libraries, The University of Texas at Austin. www.lib.utexas. edu.

University of Texas Medical Branch at Galveston, The. *A Seventy-Five-Year History by the Faculty and Staff.* Austin & London: University of Texas Press, 1967.

University of Texas Southwestern Medical Center Library. Texas Physicians Historical Biographical Database. www4.utsouthwestern.edu.

UT System News Release. "Michael & Susan Dell Foundation Grants $50 Million to University of Texas to Bring Excellence in Children's Health and Education to Austin." The University of Texas System. May 15, 2006. www.utsystem.edu.

U.S. Civil War from 1861-1865, The. The History Place. www.historyplace.com.

Vernon, Walter N., Sledge, Robert W., Monk, Robert C., and Spellman, Norman W. *The Methodist Excitement in Texas, A History,* The Texas United Methodist Historical Society. Dallas: c/o Birdwell Library, SMU, 1984.

VintagePostCards.Com. "Buy Christmas Seals. Advertising Christmas Seals Texas Tuberculosis Association, Austin, Texas, 1932." www.vintagepostcards.com.

Watkins, Pruett, M.D. "Heroism at Parkland." *Texas State Journal of Medicine* 59 (December) 1963: 1129-1130.

"Webberville History." Webberville Village Commission. www.webberville.org.

Weller, Burford; Graham, G. M. "Relapsing Fever in Texas in Clinical Notes, Suggestions and New Instruments." *JAMA* 95, No. 24 (December 13) 1930:1834-1835.

White, E. B. "Patterns of development in Texas hospitals, 1836-1935: preliminary survey." *Texas Medicine* 82 (December), 1986: 55-60.

"Wilbarger's Indian Depredations in Texas." Fort Tour Systems, Inc. www.forttours.com.

Winkler, E. W. "Check List of Texas Imprints, 1846-1876. *Southwestern Historical Quarterly Online*, 47. No. 4. www.tsha.utexas.edu.

Yerwood, R.C.R., Physician & Surgeon, Advertisement, Cons. Coun., Gonz., TX 30 June 1909. The Conservative Counselor. RootsWeb. Extracted from Tablets made by Kathleen Spring, 1991. RootsWeb.Com.

Yerwood, Joyce. Letter to her Sister. Yerwood Center. www.yerwoodcenter.org.

INDEX

A PREEMINENTLY HEALTHY PLACE

INDEX TO PROFILES

PICTURE CREDITS

THE FOLLOWING ABBREVIATIONS are used for sources from which several images are used:

TCMS   Travis County Medical Association
TMA   Texas Medical Association
TSA   Texas State Library and Archives Commission

FRONT MATTER: ii-iii (both) Collection of the Texas Medical Association, photographs by Jim Lincoln. iv-v Austin History Center. iv-vii Collection of the Texas Medical Association, photograph by Jim Lincoln. viii-ix Library of Congress. x-xi Austin History Center, Austin Public Library. **CHAPTER ONE:** 3 TSA. 4 TSA. 5 (above) TSA; (below) The Center for American History, The University of Texas at Austin. **CHAPTER TWO:** 7 Austin History Center, Austin Public Library. 8 (both) TSA. 9 Austin History Center, Austin Public Library. 10 TSA. 11 (both) TSA. **CHAPTER THREE:** 12 TMA. 13 TMA. 14 Austin History Center, Austin Public Library. 15 Austin History Center, Austin Public Library. 16 TSA. 17 (both) TMA. 18 TSA. 19 TSA. **CHAPTER FOUR:** 20 Austin History Center, Austin Public Library. 21 Austin History Center, Austin Public Library. 22 Austin History Center, Austin Public Library. 23 Lawrence T. Jones, III Collection. 24 Austin History Center, Austin Public Library. 25 (both) Austin History Center, Austin Public Library. **CHAPTER FIVE:** 26 Lawrence T. Jones, III Collection. 27 TMA. 28 (above) Lawrence T. Jones, III Collection; (below) Austin History Center, Austin Public Library. 29 Austin History Center, Austin Public Library. 30 TCMS. 31 TMA. 32 Lawrence T. Jones, III Collection. **CHAPTER SIX:** 34 TMA. 35 Austin History Center, Austin Public Library. 36 Austin History Center, Austin Public Library. 37 TMA. 38 (above) Library of Congress; (below) TCMS. 39 Austin History Center, Austin Public

Library. **CHAPTER SEVEN:** 40 Library of Congress. 41 The Center for American History, The University of Texas at Austin. 42 Austin History Center, Austin Public Library. 43 Austin History Center, Austin Public Library. 44 Austin History Center, Austin Public Library. 45 TCMS. 46 TCMS. 47 (both) Private Collection. 48 TCMS. 49 TCMS. 51 TMA. 52 Lawrence T. Jones, III Collection. 53 TMA. **CHAPTER EIGHT:** 55 Austin History Center, Austin Public Library. 56 TSA. 57 TCMS. 58 Austin History Center, Austin Public Library. 59 Austin History Center, Austin Public Library. 60 Austin History Center, Austin Public Library. 61 TCMS. 63 Austin History Center, Austin Public Library. **CHAPTER NINE:** 64 Austin History Center, Austin Public Library. 66 TCMS. 69 TCMS. 71 Austin History Center, Austin Public Library. 72 TCMS. **CHAPTER TEN:** 75 TCMS. 76 (both) TMA, Kurt Lekisch Collection. 77 TCMS. 78 Austin History Center, Austin Public Library. 80 TCMS. 81 TCMS. 82 Austin History Center, Austin Public Library. **CHAPTER ELEVEN:** 85 TCMS. 86 TCMS. 87 Alexander Architectural Archive, University of Texas Libraries, The University of Texas. 89 TCMS. 90 TCMS. 91 TMA. **CHAPTER TWELVE:** 92 TMA. 93 TCMS. 95 TCMS. 97 TCMS. 98 TCMS. 101 TCMS. 102 (both) TCMS. **CHAPTER THIRTEEN:** 105 TCMS. 107 TCMS. 108 TCMS. 110 Lyndon Baines Johnson Library. 112 TCMS. 113 TCMS. 114 TCMS. 115 TCMS. 117 TCMS. **CHAPTER FOURTEEN:** 118 TCMS. 121 TMA. 123 Courtesy Dr. Karen Teel. 124 TCMS. 127 TCMS. **CHAPTER FIFTEEN:** 129 TCMS. 131 TCMS. **CHAPTER SIXTEEN:** 133 TMA. 134 TCMS. 135 TCMS. 136 TCMS. 137 TCMS. 138 (both) TCMS. 139 TCMS. **CHAPTER SEVENTEEN:** 140 TCMS. 141 TCMS. 142 TCMS. 143 TCMS. 144 TCMS. 145 TCMS. 146 TCMS. **PROFILES IN TRAVIS COUNTY MEDICINE:** 148 Library of Congress.